# THE MESOTHELIAL CELL
# AND MESOTHELIOMA

# LUNG BIOLOGY IN HEALTH AND DISEASE

*Executive Editor*

**Claude Lenfant**
*Director, National Heart, Lung and Blood Institute*
*National Institutes of Health*
*Bethesda, Maryland*

### ADDITIONAL VOLUMES IN PREPARATION

The opinions expressed in these volumes do not necessarily represent the views of the National Institutes of Health.

# THE MESOTHELIAL CELL AND MESOTHELIOMA

*Edited by*

## Marie-Claude Jaurand

*Institut National de la Santé et de la Recherche Médicale*
*Créteil, France*

## Jean Bignon

*University of Paris Val de Marne*
*Créteil, France*
*and*
*Institut National de la Santé*
*et de la Recherche Médicale*

**Marcel Dekker, Inc.**          **New York • Basel • Hong Kong**

**Library of Congress Cataloging-in-Publication Data**

The mesothelial cell and mesothelioma / edited by Marie-Claude Jaurand,
Jean Bignon.
    p. — cm. — (lung biology in health and disease : v. 78)
    Includes bibliographical references and index.
    ISBN 0-8247-9232-7 (alk. paper)
    1. Mesothelioma.  I. Jaurand, Marie-Claude.  II. Bignon, Jean.
III. Series.
    [DNLM: 1. Mesothelioma — physiopathology. W1 LU62 v. 78 1994 / QZ
340 M58005 1994]
    RC280.L8M46   1994
    616.99′2 — dc20
    DNLM/DLC
for Library of Congress                                    94-16595
                                               CIP

The publisher offers discounts on this book when ordered in bulk quantities. For more information, write to Special Sales/Professional Marketing
at the address below.

This book is printed on acid-free paper.

Marcel Dekker, Inc.
270 Madison Avenue, New York, New York 10016

Current printing (last digit):
10  9  8  7  6  5  4  3  2  1

PRINTED IN THE UNITED STATES OF AMERICA

# INTRODUCTION

C.S. Minot is credited with proposing the name mesothelium. As he wrote in Buck's *Handbook of Medical Sciences* in 1886:

> The whole of the mesoderm . . . does not go through this metamorphosis, but . . . a part remains closely compacted; but ultimately it is only the single layer of the cells immediately bounding the coelom . . . which remains thus close together. These cells, therefore, have all the characteristics of an epithelium so that the coelom is limited by an epithelium of cuboidal cells, for which I have proposed the name mesothelium.

In the pleural cavity, the mesothelial cells cover the lungs and the inner side of the chest walls.

This volume is not the first in the series of monographs "Lung Biology in Health and Disease" to address mesothelial cells and mesothelioma. In 1985, the series published *The Pleura in Health and Disease*, which contained several chapters on various aspects of the mesothelium. The inclusion of this new volume reflects the importance of this area of investigation and also the abundance of work that is being done. In addition, this book links the biology of the mesothelium to environmental factors.

The editors, Marie-Claude Jaurand and Jean Bignon, have assembled an international roster of distinguished contributors — an achievement that illustrates the worldwide interest in the biology of the mesothelium in health and disease. It has often been remarked that the many names given to the tumors of the mesothelium attest to the many controversies that surround them. This volume is a major step toward the resolution of these controversies.

It was only in 1909 that mesothelioma was first described (J. G. Abami). Many advances have occurred since, but much more remains to be done, as evidenced by some of the questions posed in this book. Both clinicians and researchers should be not only aided, but also provoked by this volume. If they are, and if progress results, it will be a tribute to the editors and authors.

**Claude Lenfant, M.D.**
Bethesda, Maryland

# PREFACE

Mesothelial cell biology is often studied in a toxicological context wherein the physiological responses of mesothelial cells to mineral fibers are determined. These investigations emphasize the enormous capacity of mesothelial cells to produce different sorts of molecules, called mediators, and their role in the development of important physiological processes such as inflammation. When the mesothelial cell's defense mechanisms against carcinogenic agents fail, however, it may undergo cytopathological processes that result in neoplastic transformation. How does such evolution take place? How can the harmonious arrangement of mesothelial cells at the pleural surface be impaired and changed to a diffuse malignancy?

A review of the literature made it apparent that a great amount of work has been done on mesothelial cells and mesothelioma that sheds light on some aspects of the biology of normal and neoplastic mesothelial cells, the mechanisms of cell transformation, and the elements essential for further progress in mesothelioma therapy. However, a new approach seems necessary to stimulate the development of further research on the physiology and biology of mesothelial cells and mesothelioma. Hopefully, such research efforts will satisfy the ultimate goals of biologists and physicians, which are the acquisition of knowledge about cell characteristics in a normal and a pathological state and the development of methods to cure malignant diseases.

This book takes a multidisciplinary approach, focusing on the historical and epidemiological aspects of malignant mesothelioma as well as on the most sophisticated molecular biological techniques. The volume provides readers with an up-to-date understanding of mesothelial cell transformation and the ways in which these cells respond to some toxicological agents.

This book also describes new in vitro pharmacological data on immune imbalance in malignant mesothelioma, particularly geared toward an understanding of the mechanism of cytokine response.

Several chapters deal with the diagnosis (thoracoscopy and tomodensitometry) and management (the development of new therapeutic approaches, particularly immunotherapy) in human mesothelioma.

We wish to thank all the outstanding contributors who so kindly agreed to participate.

*Marie-Claude Jaurand*
*Jean Bignon*

# CONTRIBUTORS

**Hoda Anton-Culver, Ph.D.** Director, Epidemiology Program, Department of Medicine, University of California, Irvine, California

**Philippe Astoul, M.D.** Hôpital de la Conception, Marseille, France

**J. Carl Barrett, Ph.D.** Director, Environmental Carcinogenesis Program and Chief, Laboratory of Molecular Carcinogenesis, National Institute of Environmental Health Sciences, National Institutes of Health, Research Triangle Park, North Carolina

**Jean Bignon, M.D.** Professor, University of Paris Val de Marne and Head, Unité 139, Institut National de la Santé et de la Recherche Médicale, Créteil, France

**Christian Boutin, M.D., A.C.C.P.** Head, Department of Pneumology, Hôpital de la Conception, Marseille, France

**A. Philippe Chahinian, M.D.** Mount Sinai School of Medicine, New York, New York

**John E. Craighead, M.D.** Professor, Department of Pathology, University of Vermont, Burlington, Vermont

**John M. G. Davis, M.A., Sc.D., F.R.C.Path.** Institute of Occupational Medicine, Edinburgh, Scotland

**Nicholas de Klerk, B.Sc., M.Sc., Ph.D.** Senior Research Officer, Department of Public Health, University of Western Australia, Perth, Western Australia, Australia

**M. Delahaye, C.T.** Department of Pathology, Cytology Section, Academic Hospital Rotterdam, Rotterdam, The Netherlands

**Jocelyne Fleury, M.D., Ph.D.** Histologist, Department of Pathology, Hôpital Henri-Mondor, Créteil, France

**Brenda I. Gerwin, Ph.D.** Senior Research Chemist, Laboratory of Human Carcinogenesis, National Cancer Institute, National Institutes of Health, Bethesda, Maryland

**Heddi Haddada, Sc.D.** CNRS, UA 1301, Institut Gustave Roussy, Villejuif, France

**Anne Hagemeijer, M.D.** Professor, Department of Cell Biology and Genetics, Erasmus University Rotterdam, Rotterdam, The Netherlands

**Henk C. Hoogsteden, M.D.** Pulmonary Physician, Department of Pulmonary Medicine, University Hospital Dijkzigt, Rotterdam, The Netherlands

**Marie-Claude Jaurand, Sc.D.** Directeur de Recherche, Laboratoire de Pathologie Cellulaire et Moléculaire de l'Environment, Unité 139, Institut National de la Santé et de la Recherche Médicale, Créteil, France

**Agnes B. Kane, M.D., Ph.D.** Associate Professor, Department of Pathology and Laboratory Medicine, Brown University, Providence, Rhode Island

**Sakari Knuutila, Ph.D.** Department of Medical Genetics, University of Helsinki, Helsinki, Finland

**Tom Kurosaki, M.S.** Principal Statistician, Epidemiology Program, Department of Medicine, University of California, Irvine, California

**Jacques F. Legier, M.D.** Department of Pathology, Riverside Regional Medical Center, Newport News, and Pathologist, Associate Clinical Professor, Eastern Virginia Medical School, Norfolk, Virginia

**Henry T. Lynch, M.D.** Professor and Chairman, Department of Preventive Medicine and Public Health, Creighton University School of Medicine, Omaha, Nebraska

**John C. Maddox, M.D.** Pathologist, Riverside Regional Medical Center, Newport News, Virginia

**K. Mattson, M.D.** Department of Pulmonary Medicine, Helsinki University Central Hospital, Helsinki, Finland

**Alison D. McDonald, M.D., F.F.P.H.M.** Professor, Department of Occupational Health, McGill University, Montreal, Quebec, Canada

**J. Corbett McDonald, M.D., F.R.C.P.** Professor, Department of Occupational and Environmental Medicine, Royal Brompton National Heart and Lung Institute, London, England

**Isabelle Monnet, M.D.** Centre Hospitalier Intercommunal de Créteil, Créteil, France

**Françoise Rey, M.D.** Hôpital de la Conception, Marseille, France

**Bruce W. S. Robinson, M.D., F.R.A.C.P., M.R.C.P.** Associate Professor, Department of Medicine, University of Western Australia and Sir Charles Gairdner Hospital, Perth, Western Australia, Australia

**Pierre Ruffié, M.D.** Institut Gustave-Roussy, Villejuif, France

**L. Tammilehto, M.D.** The Finnish Institute of Occupational Health, Helsinki, Finland

**Theodorus H. van der Kwast, M.D., Ph.D.** Associate Professor, Department of Pathology, Erasmus University Rotterdam, Rotterdam, The Netherlands

**Marjan A. Versnel, Ph.D.**   Senior Research Biologist, Department of Immunology, Erasmus University Rotterdam, Rotterdam, The Netherlands

**J.-R. Viallat, M.D.**   Hôpital de la Conception, Marseille, France

**J. Christopher Wagner, M.D., F.R.C.P.A.T.H., F.F.O.M.**   Consultant, Weymouth, Dorset, England

# CONTENTS

# 1

# Historical Background and Perspectives of Mesothelioma

**J. CHRISTOPHER WAGNER**

Weymouth, Dorset, England

## I. Introduction

Mesothelioma must be seen in the perspective of the overall biological effects of asbestos, and so I have considered the problems under the following headings with a reference to the review papers I have published on these different subjects (1–5).

## II. Biological Effects of Asbestos Dust Exposure

Asbestos may produce pleural thickening and plaques, asbestos pleurisy with effusion, interstitial lung disease, carcinoma of the lung, and mesothelioma of the pleura and peritoneum. The severity of the disease may reflect the degree of exposure (6–10).

### A. Pleural Plaques and Pleural Thickening

Pleural plaques (PPs) may occur in groups of subjects with moderate exposure to any type of asbestos. These plaques may have different radiographic patterns, or may not be seen at all on a plain x-ray film, even if at postmortem they are extensive. Pleural thickening can be more irregular and is even more difficult to see. Oblique films can be helpful, but a thoracic computed tomography (CT) scan is more reliable. Advanced cases may have a "crows feet" configuration running across the chest radiograph.

Clinical presentation is varied. Usually, PPs are found by chance on radiographs, being useful markers of exposure. Plaques are less likely to be associated with underlying interstitial disease than is diffuse pleural thickening. On their own, plaques cause virtually no disturbance of lung function, nor are they thought to be direct precursors of pleural mesotheliomas. The pathology of PP reveals areas of scarring that are found on the pleural surface lining the wall. They are usually bilateral and symmetric; large areas of scarring are also found on the diaphragm. Plaques vary in size from very small discrete disks to large thick layers that completely envelop the lungs. As the fibrous tissue becomes older, it is gradually infiltrated by $Ca^{2+}$ salts. It generally takes up to 20 years for sufficient $Ca^{2+}$ to accumulate to make the plaque sufficiently opaque for radiological visualization in a living patient. Plaques are thus seen by pathologists far more frequently than by radiologists.

### B.  Asbestos Pleurisy

Asbestos pleurisy was described by Harries, in 1970 (7), but is not recognized often because an adequate occupational history is not obtained. Clinical presentation may simulate pleurisy of infective origin, with pain, fever, and leukocytosis, which resolve, leaving widespread pleural thickening. Or it may be benign, self-limiting, and not recognized by either physician or patient. The relation to mesothelioma and lung cancer is not fully understood because, as yet, few cases have been properly identified. There is speculation that diffuse pleural thickening, which is often associated with underlying interstitial disease, may be a result of unrecognized asbestos pleurisy and is a quite different entity from discrete pleural plaques with no underlying disease, but occasional asbestos fibers will be present in the lung parenchyma (9).

### C.  Asbestosis

All forms of asbestos may cause pulmonary fibrosis, although it appears that the amphiboles are more potent than chrysotile in causing asbestosis. A certain amount of asbestos exposure is necessary; hence, the reasoning that there may be a "safe threshold" (varying with the type of fibers), below which fibrosis will not occur. Clinical presentation is usually with shortness of breath, initially on exertion, but progressing to breathlessness at rest, possibly accompanied by a productive cough, even in nonsmokers. On examination, late, crisp inspiratory crackles may be heard, particularly posteriorly at the bases, which do not clear with coughing and may be missed if the patient does not take in a really deep breath. Clubbing sometimes occurs, but is not a helpful sign, since it does not relate to the degree of fibrosis. Gross clubbing, present early on in the disease process, is unusual, and may make one reconsider the diagnosis.

The radiological appearance of asbestosis is rather like that of other forms of pulmonary fibrosis, with irregular opacities, preponderantly in the lower lobes. The clue relating this interstitial change to asbestosis is the finding of pleural thickening or plaques. Careful search for calcification on the diaphragm can be rewarding. The textbook description of shaggy heart border and indistinct diaphragm is rarely seen and, then, only in advanced cases. A helpful practical point is that the chest radiograph in asbestosis generally looks more untidy, with more aggregation than that of, for example, idiopathic pulmonary fibrosis.

Lung function tests classically reveal a restrictive pattern, with decreased lung volumes and decreased gas transfer. Those who have airway obstruction will show a mixed picture.

Asbestos bodies, now more correctly called ferruginous bodies, may be found in the sputum. They indicate exposure to asbestos, but are not a mark of disease.

The diagnostic criteria established by Parkes (8) are as follows:

1.  History of exposure (including presence of asbestos bodies)
2.  Dyspnea on exertion
3.  Persistent basal crackles, with or without clubbing
4.  Radiological evidence of diffuse interstitial fibrosis or pleural plaques, or both
5.  Restricted lung function and impairment

It is rarely necessary to obtain tissue to make the diagnosis, but if this is required, then an open-lung biopsy should be considered. Lung function changes may precede radiological and clinical evidence and, particularly, in the early stages, it is not uncommon to hear crackles, whereas the chest radiograph is still normal, although it is usually abnormal. Management should first revolve around persuading those who smoke to cease. This is imperative in all those exposed to asbestos, but particularly in those who show overt evidence of considerable exposure. Nonsmokers exposed to asbestos have a fivefold greater risk of lung cancer. The risk of developing lung cancer in smokers exposed to asbestos is about 50 times greater than in nonsmokers with no asbestos exposure.

The pathological appearance shows that inhaled asbestos fibers become trapped in the lung tissue, in the alveoli arising directly from the respiratory bronchioles. The fibers of more than 10 $\mu$m in length lodge in these air spaces, either within the macrophages or lying loose; some of the fibers are coated and appear as asbestos bodies. At this stage, some of the macrophages disintegrate and release enzymes, attracting fibroblasts that start secreting thin strands of collagen that eventually form a fine net of scar tissue. Unable to escape, more macrophages die and release yet more enzymes; the process progresses until the alveoli all along the respiratory bronchioles are replaced with a layer of scar tissue. Initially, only occasional respiratory bronchioles are involved, but gradually more and more of these airways become scarred. The fibrous tissue then spreads farther down the walls of the air sacs, at first as a thin layer, but gradually thickening; the extensions of the scarring between the individual units link up so that increasingly more lung becomes involved. The scarred walls of the respiratory bronchioles then become stretched because of respiratory movement and appear as small, thick-walled cystic spaces. The amount of scar tissue thus increases, but eventually, if the patient lives long enough, the scarring which starts at the base of the lower lobe of the lungs may continue, resulting in a shrunken lung that is a mass of scar tissue surrounding collapsed and useless air spaces.

Asbestos bodies are golden-brown rods found in the sputum and lung tissue (11,12). They consist of asbestos fibers, usually of amphibole type, and coated with an iron–mucoprotein complex. These bodies were thought to be evidence of occupational exposure to asbestos dust. However, as techniques became more sophisticated, it was realized that these bodies can be found in the lungs of most people living in urban communities (13–16). Electron microscopy has shown that only a small proportion of the inhaled fibers become coated and that most, which are uncoated, are rarely observed under the light microscope (17–20). In the study of the general population, up to a million fibers can be recovered from 1 g of dried lung tissue, without any evidence of disease being discovered in the individual.

### D.  Lung Cancer

The incidence of carcinoma of the lung is far more common than diffuse mesothelioma in populations of asbestos workers. Over the past 30 years, there have been numerous epidemiological studies confirming the association between asbestos and lung cancer, even in nonsmokers. This association is believed to be causal, although the rates quoted vary, depending on the method of the study. The latency period is about 20 years, with the risks being greater for those with higher asbestos exposure. It has been suggested that adenocarcinoma is the most common type of tumor in asbestos workers, in contrast with the general population.

### E. Mesothelioma of the Pleura and Peritoneum

Unlike other asbestos-related diseases, this tumor can develop after apparently minimal exposure, although there is evidence that the risk increases with greater exposure. There is ample evidence to implicate crocidolite, but this also suggests that other types of amphibole asbestos, tremolite and amosite, may also be responsible, to a lesser degree. The latent period between exposure and onset of disease may be 30 or 40 years. This long latent period, coupled with the fact that only a limited exposure is necessary, understandably contributes to public fears. Although these cases do arise, most patients have had occupational exposure. Interestingly, there appears to be no connection between smoking and mesothelioma. It is most important to recognize that spontaneous (or cryptogenic) mesotheliomas do occur.

Among the clinical features, the first symptom of pleural mesothelioma is often dull chest pain and, typically, shoulder pain. However, when the patients present, it is quite common to find pleural effusion, with weight loss, cough, and shortness of breath. The signs will depend on the stage of the disease. Clubbing is common, and acute arthropathy has been described. The diagnosis is best made by obtaining an accurate history of exposure and finding, if the facilities are available, malignant mesothelial cells in the pleural fluid. A biopsy should be avoided if possible. There is evidence that a CT scan is now necessary for early diagnosis and staging.

Peritoneal mesothelioma is less common and usually presents late, with dull pain, abdominal swelling, weight loss, and ascites. Again, exfoliative cytology may help make the diagnosis.

Currently, the outlook of malignant mesothelioma is poor, with few patients living for 2 years; the time from diagnosis to death is usually about 6 months. As yet, no chemotherapy has been of value, so treatment remains symptomatic. A more hopeful view of therapy will be found in the final chapter of this volume.

Pathologically, the tumor appears to originate in microscopic form in the parietal pleura in cases of diffuse pleural mesothelioma. These nodules exfoliate at an early stage and lead to a seeding of the pleural cavity, mainly affecting the diaphragmatic surface. Nodules in the cardiophrenic angle are particularly difficult to visualize on radiological examination or thoracoscopy. The nodules increase in size until both pleural surfaces are diffusely involved. In some cases, there is extensive papillary growth, with the tips of the papillae breaking off to form morulae of cells, which can be found floating in the pleural fluid. The mesothelial cell can differentiate into either a spindlelike sarcomatous or an epithelial-like cell that forms tubules and papillae, with cystic adenomatous spaces. The epithelial-like cell secretes hyaluronic acid, making the pleural fluid viscid and difficult to aspirate.

The tumor on the parietal pleura tends to invade the chest wall, involving intercostal nerves and causing pain; a tumor on the visceral pleural is likely to invade along the interlobar and intralobar septa and, for the latter, lymphatic spread can penetrate throughout the lung. Penetration can also take place through the diaphragm. General hematogenous spread does occur, but is not common; initially, it was thought that widespread secondary deposits occurred only after surgical intervention, but in the large survey of Elmes and Simpson (6), hematogenous spread had occurred in untreated cases. There is also invasion of the mediastinum and seeding of the opposite parietal and visceral pleural surfaces. At this stage, the two layers on the first affected side often fuse, thereby reducing the effusion and giving the patient a temporary sense of relief. Unfortunately, an effusion may develop in the other side of the thorax. Since the lung on the original side has probably collapsed by this time owing to the constricting effect of the surrounding tumor, the second effusion creates severe respiratory distress, which is often terminal. The pericardium may become invaded, leading to cardiac tamponade, or there may be constriction of the vital structures in the mediastinum.

The origin of the tumor in peritoneal mesothelioma is uncertain, but when an early diagnosis is made, nodules have been observed on both the serosal surface of the gut and the inferior surface of the diaphragm. These spread along the serosal surfaces, creating adhesions between the coils of the intestines, surrounding and constricting the abdominal organs. As in the pleural cavities, an effusion may be the prominent feature and, if it contains hyaluronic acid, it will be difficult to aspirate. Gradually, the whole peritoneal cavity becomes full of tumor which, as a terminal event, may invade through the diaphragm and involve the thorax. Invasion of the gut wall is unusual; the tumor confines itself to the serosa.

Ovarian involvement is usually a surface phenomenon; it is controversial whether or not some of these tumors originate in the ovary, but this is a difficult point to solve. Since the surface of the ovary and parietal peritoneum is continuous, surface tumors of the ovary may be histologically indistinguishable from mesotheliomas and, to add to the problem, some of the ovarian tumors secrete hyaluronic acid. In both pleural and peritoneal tumors, tracking-through to overlying skin is a fairly common event. This may follow the course of needles used for paracentesis, or it may occur quite independently of any intervention.

### III.  Fiber Burden in Lungs and Pleura

In 1967, Gold (11) described a method by which asbestos bodies and those fibers visible under phase contrast optical microscope could be extracted from a known weight of lung tissue and be counted in a manner similar to the assessment of the cells in cerebrospinal fluid. Lung tissue was first dissolved in hot 40% KOH, followed by several washings and centrifugation of the residue, which led to a considerable loss of fiber on the glassware. The method was modified by Ashcroft and Heppleston (12) and is still being used extensively in the estimation of lung fiber burden (13,21,22). In 1973, Langer and Pooley described the identification of single fibers by the use of an electron microscope and electron microprobe (23). These techniques were developed by Sebastien et al. (24) in France, and by Pooley (25) in Great Britain. In 1979, these two laboratories presented a combined paper showing that comparable results could be obtained by using a transmission electron microscope (TEM) with an attached energy-dispersive x-ray analytic system (26). The TEM was necessary to study fibers smaller than 0.1 $\mu$m in diameter. The results were presented as the number of fibers counted per gram dry weight of lung. Obviously, the larger the number of fibers counted, the more reliable will be the total.

### A.   Distribution of Fibers in the Lung and Pleura

There is no agreement on the distribution of asbestos fibers in the lung tissue. Asbestos bodies were described by Thomson as being most frequently found at the base of the lower lobes (16). This has not been confirmed when asbestos fibers have been quantified from various sites in the lungs (27). In fact, there has been considerable variation in adjoining blocks of tissue. Therefore, it is considered that lung parenchyma should be taken from several specific regions and that these should be used for all investigations. The other tremendous advantage was that, by using the energy-dispersive x-ray analytical system, it was now possible to identify the type of fiber in the tissue (20). The only studies of the pleura have been reported by Le Bouffant (28) and Sebastien et al. (29). They found a preponderance of short chrysotile fibers in the parietal pleura (where mesotheliomas usually arise).

### B.   Size of the Fibers

In conjunction with TEM, the size and number of individual fibers could be calculated. The significance of the size of the mineral fibers is based on the studies in animals. These findings are accepted for the human situation, but the results are not clear-cut, and to try and obtain unequivocal proof would be unrealistic. These findings suggest that both pulmonary fibrosis and carcinoma of the lung are associated with long fibers, and that on Timbrell's earlier calculation (30), long fibers of up to 3.0 $\mu$m in diameter can be inhaled and retained in the lung parenchyma. These fibers are more than 8.0 $\mu$m in length. Most workers consider that the development of mesotheliomas are associated with fibers smaller than 0.25 $\mu$m in diameter and more than 8.0 $\mu$m in length. In humans, one of the earlier findings, which was well illustrated in the combined studies of Gaudichet et al. (26), was that numerous fibers other than the commercial forms of asbestos were present in the lungs. The other finding was that all adult human lungs, yet examined, contained mineral fibers. This pinpointed two problems: Which fibers caused significant disease, and how many fibers of a specific type had to be present to cause disease (31)? These two questions have led to considerable controversy. In combination with epidemiologists, it was accepted that all types of asbestos, providing that sufficient fibers were inhaled, cause asbestosis, and the larger the amount of fiber inhaled the more severe was the disease. This also applies to carcinoma of the lung, especially in smokers (32).

Difficulties immediately arose over the amounts of chrysotile and the amphiboles required. If calculated on fiber number, then there was far more chrysotile present than amphibole; on mass calculation, the amount of chrysotile was far less (33). Another difficulty was that, even in distilled water, chrysotile fibers tended to break up by longitudinal splitting into numerous fibrils, at least 100 fibrils of chrysotile being the equivalent mass of 1 amphibole fiber (25). The final difficulty lies in the question: Is it necessary for the fibers to be retained to cause fibrosis and subsequent carcinoma of the lung? There are two opinions among investigators. On the one hand, it is stated that this depends on the long-term retention and durability of the fiber (31,34). On the other, it is that the presence of the fiber for a short period is sufficient, so that, although the chrysotile is rapidly removed from the lung or becomes soluble in the lung tissue, its presence will be sufficient, during this short time, to initiate the process of fibrosis and of malignancy (35,36). Although the chrysotile concentrations level off, indicating an equilibrium between routes of deposition and clearance, that of the (durable) amphibole fiber increases in a linear manner. There is thus a selective retention of amphibole fiber: there is no known explanation for this phenomenon (33).

### C. Chrysotile

Two points should be raised: (1) Deposits are found worldwide in any geological area in which a serpentine outcrop has formed. Therefore, it may be present in the environment, not as a result of direct industrial usage, but as part of the natural background of mineral dust produced by weathering and erosion of serpentine masses. (2) It is generally considered that uncontaminated chrysotile fibers will not cause mesotheliomas.

### D. Tremolite and Chrysotile

The whole situation becomes much more complicated and raises bitter controversy when the problems of mesothelioma of the pleura are considered. This is mainly because among other minerals, chrysotile deposits are contaminated with tremolite (37,38), an amphibole of little commercial value. Examination of the lungs of those exposed to commercial chrysotile reveal that, although the tremolite is usually a 1% contamination of chrysotile, the amount of tremolite found in the lungs of chrysotile miners and manufacturers is far greater than that of chrysotile (14,15,17,18,39,40). This is the prime example of selective retention of amphibole fibers. Does this indicate that tremolite is the cause of pulmonary fibrosis and mesotheliomas in those exposed to chrysotile, or is this an indication that 100 times as much chrysotile was initially inhaled (13,19,40) and that the chrysotile initiated the processes of fibrosis or malignancy (36)? A further facet to the problem of mesotheliomas is that when the parietal pleural is examined for fiber content (28,29), even in cases of mesotheliomas, the parietal pleural contained more chrysotile than amphibole and, occasionally, amphibole was not present, and virtually all of these chrysotile fibers were shorter than 5.0 $\mu$m in length and thus, in the light of current knowledge, unlikely to cause mesotheliomas. However, it has been pointed out that most mesotheliomas appear to arise from the parietal pleura (28,29).

### E. Tremolite

There are numerous geological forms of tremolite, from very fine, long fibers to thick flakes, which are only considered as fibers because of a breadth/length ratio of more than 3. In our animal experiments, it was only the very fine tremolite longer than 8.0 $\mu$m and smaller than 0.25 $\mu$m in diameter that caused mesotheliomas (41). In addition to this animal data, there is widespread contamination and deposition of tremolite in an area from East Turkey to Austria. In these regions, most of the tremolite seems to be of the coarse variety, causing massive pleural calcification, but it is of the correct size to cause mesotheliomas in only a few rare situations; for example, in Turkey, Cyprus, and in the asbestos mines in Quebec.

### F. Mesotheliomas with Amphibole

It is considered by most investigators that these tumors are associated with the retention and durability of these fibers (31). Considering the biological effects of the amphiboles, we put forward the following hypotheses (42):

1. The total count of amphiboles of 1 million/g dry weight of lung is the highest level that can be accepted for a nonoccupational or paraoccupational exposure.
2. Mesotheliomas will occur when the fiber concentration is more than 1 million/g dry weight of fibers longer than 5.0 $\mu$m and a diameter smaller than 0.25 $\mu$m.
3. Definite asbestosis will occur at a count of more than 100 million. Severe asbestosis will occur from 1 billion/g dry weight. The highest count that we have observed was in an amphibole asbestos mixer, with a count of 17 billion, who worked in a factory in London.

## IV.   Historical Evidence for the Existence of Mesotheliomas

According to Wolff (43), the first reference to tumors of the pleura was made by Joseph Lieutaad, in 1767. According to Robertson (44), a clear description of primary pleural tumors was that of Laennec, in 1819 (45). Actually, it is Wagner's report in 1870 (46) of a single case that is generally accepted as the first description of the pathology, with mention of the lymph channels crowded with tumor cells; 15 years later, the first case was recorded in Britain by Colliers (47). In 1890, the first case recorded in the United States by Biggs (48) was termed "endothelioma of the pleura." It was Engelbach, in 1891 (49), who first considered whether these endotheliomas of the pleura arose from the lymphatics or from the cells lining the serous surfaces, and these tumors were frequently described in the European literature (1870–1895) by most of the well-known pathologists, with considerable controversy over whether there was such an entity as primary tumors of the pleura. A review by Glockner, in 1897 (50), accepted 75 cases as being primary endothelioma of the pleura, adding his own 16 further cases of either the pleura or peritoneum. By the end of the century there were more than a 100 cases, with a thesis by Bloch (51) giving an extensive review of the subject. He accepted two types of primary tumors of the pleura, endothelioma and sarcoma.

Later, the term *mesothelioma* was used first by Eastwood and Martin in 1921 (52). Since then, primary diffuse pleural mesotheliomas have been described by numerous authors: Klemperer and Rabin in 1931 (53); then successively in the 1950s by Campbell (54) and Leibow (55) in the United States; Tobiassen in Sweden (56); Belloni and Boro in Italy (57); Godwin in the United States (58); McCaughey in Britain (59); and Poulson and Sorenson in Denmark (60).

Robertson (44) wished to establish whether such tumors were primary, and if they were endothelial in origin. He stated that "This review apparently proves that only the sarcoma can be classified as primary malignant tumours of the pleural tissues and that all other growths are secondary, representing extensions, implantations, or metastases from an unrecognised or latent primary source, usually the lungs." Willis, in the successive edition of his treatise (61), considered all pleural tumors to be secondary in origin. Those that would not accept the primary nature of this tumor were influenced by the variegated histological pattern. This was remarked on by Klemperer and Rabin (53). Why such variation occurs is appreciated when the multipotentiality of the cells lining coelomic cavities is considered. This was demonstrated in studies on tissue by Maximow, in 1927 (62). Novak, in 1931 (63), stated that the mucosa of all parts of the mullerian canal and the germinal epithelium were derived from these multipotent cells. Then Stout and Murray, in 1942 (64), showed that cells derived from mesothelioma would present both sarcomatouslike cells and epithelial-like cells in tissue culture. Campbell (54) considered the presence of both epithelial and mesenchymal cells a diagnostic feature. Leibow (55) stated that "the more usual microscopic picture resembles carcinomatous tissue, at times in combination with a sarcomatous pattern, or on occasion a pure sarcomatous pattern. The former may be of the simplex, epidermoid or glandular type." In describing the histology of these tumors, McCaughey (59) demonstrated that either the epithelial or mesenchymal element might be preponderant. This has now been confirmed in our experimental studies (65). In view of this confirmed biphasic potentiality of the mesothelial cell, Robertson's objection (44) to the epithelial-like tumors, reported by Glockner and the other authors, is no longer valid. This would endorse the fact that more than 100 diffuse mesotheliomas had been observed in human cases before the year 1900. It is most unlikely that these cases had been exposed to asbestos dust or erionite (34). This would add further support to the contention that malignant mesotheliomas can occur without exposure to mineral dusts.

## V. The Association Between Exposure to Crocidolite Asbestos and the Development of Diffuse Mesotheliomas

An association between a case of pleural mesothelioma had been described by Wedler in Germany in 1943 (66), and further cases were mentioned by Paul Cartier during the discussion at a meeting in Canada, in 1952 (67). Van der Schoot (69) had seen several cases of this nature in Holland and, in 1958, stated that the possibility of mesotheliomas occurring in asbestos workers should be investigated. We had seen our first case in South Africa in 1956 and, by 1960, had a series of 33 cases, which we published (69). In the same year, Konig (70) published the description of several cases from Hamburg, and Keal (71) wrote up a few cases from an East London factory. Keal, unfortunately, had come under the influence of Willis and, thus, his cases were not fully described until 1963, when they were fully investigated by Entiknap and Smithers, in 1964 (72). In the same year, with Sluis-Cremer, I explained that the South African cases were definitely associated with blue asbestos (crocidolite), and that we could find no evidence of cases of mesotheliomas occurring among the miners and millers in South Africa who had been exposed to only chrysotile or amosite (73).

As chrysotile accounted for 95% of the world asbestos production, it became important to establish whether this type of fiber was implicated in the causation of these particular tumors. In 1965, the world production of chrysotile was about 5 million tons. About 2 million tons were produced both by Canada and the former USSR, and the rest was mined in southern Africa, Cyprus, and Italy, with small quarries in many other countries (74).

As the South African evidence had shown that these diffuse mesotheliomas were highly malignant, could occur following short exposures after a long latent period, and were inevitably fatal (69), it thus became urgent to undertake epidemiological studies. Such investigations were directed by McDonald in North America in 1980 (75), and by Kogan in Russia (76). These studies have confirmed that mesotheliomas are exceedingly rare in Canada and have not been observed in the mines and mills in Russia.

## VI.  Mesotheliomas in Humans and Experimental Animals

In considering the use of experimental animals in the assessment of risk to humans, it is paramount that the interest remains with the possible effects on humans and that precise interpretation of the fate of the animal must be considered in this light. Therefore, it is essential to use the epidemiological evidence that has been obtained from human exposure in known situations to calibrate the results obtained experimentally. When human evidence is lacking, we are fortunate in having an endpoint against which other fibers can be assessed. This material is a form of zeolite, known as erionite. Where this material occurs in the form of fine fibers (i.e., smaller than 0.25 $\mu$m in diameter and longer than 5.0 $\mu$m), it causes an extremely high rate of mesotheliomas in humans, as reported by Baris et al. (77,78). In experimental studies in rats and mice with this type of fiber, intrapleural inoculation resulted in 100% mesotheliomas (79,80) and 100% by inhalation (79).

When these results with erionite in humans and experimental animals are compared with the other mineral fibers, the effects of the latter are far less severe.

### A. Mineral Fibers Other Than Asbestos

It is here that our major interest lies, as we are looking for ways of predicting the possible hazard associated with exposure to these fibers, which can be grouped as follows:

*Natural Mineral Fibers*

There are few natural mineral fibers of possible economic value.

1. Wollastonite: There is no evidence of human disease.
2. The absorbent clays: These are palygorskite, attapulgite, and sepiolite. There is no evidence of human disease.

*Synthetic Fibers*

The synthetic fibers include

1. The man-made mineral fibers (vitreous) (MMVF): slag wool, and rock wool; glass is produced in three forms, wool, filament, and microfibers.
2. Refractory fibers, which include those with ceramic, aluminum, or zirconium base.

There is little evidence that any of the other fibers have an effect on humans. There is some evidence that, in the 1930s, exposure to a certain form of rock wool was associated with subsequent development of carcinoma of the lung, but this occurred on a small scale, and the findings are far from conclusive.

### B. Conclusions from Human Evidence

It is on these asbestos substitutes that further evidence is required, in spite of the fact that most have not been shown to be dangerous, and there has been a reasonable epidemiological follow-up. It is unlikely that fibrosis and subsequent carcinoma of the lung are going to be a danger in the future, providing the principles of good housekeeping are applied, and exposure to straight fibers is less than five fibers per cubic centimeter. It is most important to discourage smoking. This leaves us with the problem of diffuse malignant mesotheliomas. There is no evidence that any of the aforementioned fibers have caused these tumors in humans. However, it can still be argued that, in some cases, the exposure has not been long enough, as the follow-up should be at least 50 years. Novel fibers will continue to be developed that will require testing.

### C. Testing Fibers for Possible Association with Mesotheliomas

If the fiber is larger than 0.5 $\mu$m in diameter and shorter than 5 $\mu$m in length, then such fibers are not going to produce mesotheliomas.

It must be remembered that there is a natural incidence of mesotheliomas of the pleura and the peritoneum in both humans and experimental animals (81).

#### Inhalation Method

All the authorities have agreed when assessing the biological effects of dusts in experimental animals that the inhalation procedure is the only satisfactory method of study. These experiments are complex to set up, extremely expensive to run, and long-term, with no significant results for 3 years. However, the results, when available, will provide evidence of the fibrogenicity and carcinogenicity of the fiber. This latter would include both carcinomas and possibly mesotheliomas. The low rate of mesotheliomas produced in the inhalation studies correlates with the human experience, providing the known background incidence is taken into consideration.

#### Intratracheal Injection

The intratracheal injection method was developed as a possible alternative, cheaper method of exposure than inhalation and as a means of obtaining more rapid results. This is not a satisfactory method of exposure, particularly when studying fibrous dusts. The distribution in the lung varies greatly, with the fibers blocking the air passages and causing obstructive nonspecific disease.

#### Intraserosal Implantation or Injection

When I first developed the intrapleural method for exposing animals to asbestos fibers, my hypothesis was that: "Asbestos fibres, if present in the pleural cavity, will cause mesotheliomata." It was never considered that this should be used as a method for calibrating the carcinogenic effect, for as a method it is unnatural, bypassing all the lung's defense mechanisms. At all possible doses, there is an intense localized exposure that is far greater than would ever happen in humans.

The results from intraperitoneal studies have indicated that the peritoneal cavity of experimental rats is far more reactive and produces such a high rate of mesotheliomas so that the results become nonspecific, as even particulate nonfibrous materials can produce mesotheliomas.

## VII. Conclusions

It is hoped that there will be very few situations in the future in which workers are exposed to such large amounts of asbestos dust capable of initiating asbestosis and carcinoma of the lung. The more likely risk is from the development of diffuse mesotheliomas following exposure to relatively small amounts of amphibole asbestos fiber or erionite dust. The fibers, being acicular in shape, durable, and of a length longer than 5 $\mu$m and a diameter smaller than 0.25 $\mu$m, are the ones likely to cause trouble. The amount of fibers inhaled should be sufficient to produce a residuum in the lung parenchyma that, on analysis, reveals the presence of at least 1 million fibers of the aforestated size. The presence of these fibers in commercial materials can be demonstrated in the laboratory, without resort to biological assay.

The only satisfactory manner in which mineral fibers can be tested in experimental animals is by inhalation. This procedure is very expensive and time-consuming. It is hoped that the elucidation of the basic mechanisms of the biological effects of exposure to mineral fibers will come from in vitro studies. The in vitro studies can be confirmed by animal inoculations.

Finally, it is essential to remember that spontaneous or, more correctly, cryptogenic, diffuse mesotheliomas do occur in humans and in animals (82).

## References

1. Wagner JC. In: Sluyser M, ed. Asbestos and related cancers. Chichester: Ellis Horwood, 1991:9.
2. Wagner JC. In: Brown RC, Hoskins JA, Johnson NF, eds. Mechanisms in fibre carcinogenesis. NATO ASI Series, New York: Plenum Press, 1991:452.
3. Wagner JC. In: Henderson DW, Shilkin L, Suzanne P, Langlois P, Whitaker D, eds. Malignant mesothelioma. New York: Hemisphere Publishing, 1992: XVII.
4. Wagner JC. Br J Ind Med 1991; 48:399.
5. Wagner JC. In: Jaurand MC, Bignon J, Brochard P, eds. Mesothelial cells and mesothelioma, past, present and future. Eur Respir Rev 1993; 3:9.
6. Elmes PC, Simson MJC. Q J Med 1976; 427:179.
7. Harries PG. Report on the effects and control of diseases associated with exposure to asbestos in Devonport dockyard. C.R.W.P./71. Gosport, England: Inst Naval Med, 1970.
8. Parkes WR. Occup Lung Disord 1982; 9:255.

9. Stephens M, Gibbs A, Pooley FD, Wagner JC. Thorax 1987; 42:583.
10. Wagner JC, McConnochie K. Physician 1983; 1:397.
11. Gold C. J Clin Pathol 1967; 20:674.
12. Ashcroft T, Heppleston AG. J Clin Pathol 1973; 26:224.
13. Case BW, Sebastien P, McDonald JC. Arch Environ Health 1988; 2:178.
14. Case BW, Sebastien P. Ann Occup Hyg 1988; 32:171.
15. Churg A. Am Rev Respir Dis 1986; 134:125.
16. Thomson JG. Ann NY Acad Sci 1965; 135:196.
17. Churg A, Wiggs B. Am J Ind Med 1986; 9:143.
18. Churg A, Wright JL, De Paoli L, Wiggs B. Am Rev Respir Dis 1989; 134:891.
19. Churg A. Chest 1988; 93:621.
20. Gaudichet A, Janson X, Monchaux G, Dufour G, Sebastien P, De Lajarte G, Bignon J. Ann Occup Hyg 1988; 32(suppl 1):213.
21. Oldham PD. In: Bogovsky P, Gilson JC, Timbrell V, Wagner JC, eds. Biological effects of asbestos. IARC Scientific Publication No. 8; 1973:45.
22. Whitwell F, Scott J, Grimshaw M. Thorax 1977; 32:377.
23. Langer A, Pooley FD. In: Bogovsky P, Gilson JC, Timbrell V, Wagner JC, eds. Biological effects of asbestos. IARC Publication No. 8; 1973:119.
24. Sebastien P, Billon MA, Janson J, Bonnaud G, Bignon J. Arch Mal Prof (Paris) 1978; 39:229.
25. Pooley FD. Br J Ind. Med 1972; 29:146.
26. Gaudichet A, Sebastien P, Clark NJ, Pooley FD. In: Biological effects of mineral fibres. IARC Sci Publ 1980; 30:61.
27. Bossard E, Stolkin I, Spycher MA, Ruttner JR. In: Biological effects of mineral fibres. IARC Sci Publ 1980; 30:35.
28. Le Bouffant L. Rev Fr Mal Respir 1976; 4:121.
29. Sebastien P, Janson X, Bonnard G, Riba G, Masse R, Bignon J. In: Lemon R, Dement JM, eds. Dust and disease. Park Forest, IL: Pathotox Publ 1979:65.
30. Timbrell V. Ann NY Acad Sci 1965;135:255.
31. Wagner JC. Cancer 1986; 57:1905.
32. Selikoff IJ. JAMA 1968; 204:106.
33. Pooley FD, Wagner JC. Ann Occup Hyg 1988; 32:187.
34. Mossman BT, Bignon J, Corn M, Seaton A, Gee JBL. Science 1990; 247:294.
35. Nicholson WJ, Perkel G, Selikoff IJ. Am Ind Med 1982; 3:259.
36. Nicholson WJ. In: Nonoccupational exposure to mineral fibres. IARC Sci Publ 1989; 90:239–261.
37. Pooley FD. Environ Res 1978; 12:281.
38. Rowlands N, Gibbs GW, McDonald AC. Ann Occup Hyg 1982; 26:411.
39. McDonald JC, Armstrong B, Case BW, Doell D. Cancer 1989; 63:1544.
40. Churg A, DePaoli L. Exp Lung Res 1988; 14:567.
41. Wagner JC, Chamberlain M, Brown RC. Br J Cancer 1981; 45:352.
42. Wagner JC. Progress in etiopathogenesis of respiratory disorders due to occupational exposure to mineral and organic dusts. 7th Internationl Pneumoconiosis Conference, Pittsburg, 1990:22–24.
43. Wolff A. Die lehre von der krehakrand 1911:834.
44. Robertson HE. J Cancer Res 1924; 8:317.

45. Laennec RTH. Traité de l'auscultation médicale. 1819:368.
46. Wagner E. Arch Klin Exp Ohren Nasen Kehlopfheild 1870; 2:495.
47. Colliers W. Lancet 1885; ii:945.
48. Biggs H. Proc NY Pathol Soc 1890; pp. 119.
49. Engelbach O. Inang-Diss Frieborg. 1891.
50. Glockner A. Z Heilk 1897; 18:209.
51. Bloch M. Les néoplasmes malins primitifs de la plèvre. Thèse, Paris, no 414, 1905.
52. Eastwood EH, Martin JP. Lancet 1921; 1:172.
53. Klemperer P, Rabin CB. Arch Pathol 1931; 11:385.
54. Campbell WN. Am J Pathol 1950; 26:473.
55. Leibow AN. Atlas Tumour Pathol 1952; 17:176.
56. Tobiassen G. Acta Pathol Microbiol Scand 1955; 105:198.
57. Belloni G, Boro G. Acta Med. Patavina 1957; 17:1.
58. Godwin MC. Cancer 1957; 10:298.
59. McCaughey WTE. J Pathol Bacteriol 1958; 76:517.
60. Poulson T, Sorenson B. Acta Radiol 1959; 188:216.
61. Willis RA. Pathology of tumours. London: Butterworth, 1948, 1953, 1966.
62. Maximow A. Arch Exp Zellforschen 1927; 4:1.
63. Novak E. Am J Obstet Gynecol, 1931; 22:820.
64. Stout AP, Murray MR. Arch Pathol 1942; 34:951.
65. Wagner JC, Johnson NF, Brown DG, Wagner MMF. Br J Cancer 1982; 46: 294.
66. Wedler HW, Med Wochhenschr 1943; 69:575.
67. Cartier P, Smith WE. Arch Ind Hyg Occup Med 1952; 5:262.
68. Van Der Schoot HC. Ned Tijdschr Geneeskd 1955; 105:1988.
69. Wagner JC. Br J Ind Med. 1960; 17:260.
70. Konig A. Arch Gewebepathol 1960; 18:15.
71. Keal EE. Lancet 1960; 2:1211.
72. Entiknap JB, Smithers WJ. Br J Ind Med 1964; 21:20.
73. Wagner JC, (a) and (b), Sluis-Cremer GK, Wagner JC. Asbestos dusts and malignancy. Proc 14th int conf occup health, Madrid, 1963:1066–1067; 609.
74. Hendry NW. Ann NY Acad Sci 1965; 132:12.
75. McDonald AD, McDonald JC. Cancer 1980; 46:1650.
76. Kogan FM, Troitsky SK, Gulevskaya MR. Gig Tr Prof Zabo 1966; 8:28.
77. Baris Y, Sahin A, Ozesmi M, et al. Thorax 1978; 33:181.
78. Baris I, Simonato I, Artvinli M, et al. Int J Cancer 1987; 39:10.
79. Wagner JC, Skidmore JW, Hill RJ, Griffiths DM. Br J Cancer 1985; 51:727.
80. Maltoni C, Minardi F, Morisi L. Environ Res 1982; 29:238.
81. Ilgren EB, Wagner JC. J. Reg. Toxicol 1990; pp 27.
82. Wagner JC. Biological effects of short fibres. Proc 7th int pneumoconiosis conf, Pittsburgh. Washington: NIOSH 90-108, National Institute of Occupational Safety and Health, 1990:835–840.

# 2

## Environmental Mesothelioma

**NICHOLAS DE KLERK**

University of Western Australia
Perth, Western Australia, Australia

## I. Introduction

*Environmental mesothelioma* is usually understood to mean malignant mesothelioma that has been caused by contamination of the nonoccupational environment with asbestos or asbestiform fibers. It also includes mesothelioma caused by contamination of the occupational environment that is involuntary or unknowing. Thus, the major concern about asbestos today is the possibility of asbestos-related disease, particularly malignant mesothelioma, arising out of such environmental exposure to fibers from the large amounts of asbestos-based products in the general environment. The size of the possible risk is uncertain; it has been the subject of several major conferences and review committees (1-3), and it is still the source of much controversy (4).

One of the many problems in estimating this risk is that the extent of past or even existing mesothelioma resulting from environmental exposure is unknown. First, one needs to discount all cases that have arisen because of occupational exposure and, second, one has to discount all so-called background or spontaneous cases. The existence of a background rate of mesothelioma that is unrelated to exposure to asbestos is generally accepted, although there are some dissenting opinions (5). This is discussed in Chapter 3. In general, however, it is not possible to distinguish background cases from environmental cases.

## II.  Causes of Environmental Mesothelioma

### A.  Definite Environmentally Caused Mesothelioma

That mesothelioma can be caused by nonoccupational exposure to mineral fibers is not in doubt. The highest documented incidence of mesothelioma in the world has been in Karain in Turkey, where naturally occurring erionite, a fibrous zeolite, has been used in building and causes the disease in all sections of the community [see Baris et al. for a recent review (6)]. Similarly, communities built around natural sources of tremolite have also experienced incidence of the disease through nonoccupational exposure (7,8). The importance of tremolite as a cause of mesothelioma worldwide has recently been reemphasized (9).

Crocidolite has probably caused more mesothelioma than any other of the commercially available forms of asbestos. It has contributed to the high rates of mesothelioma in both South Africa and Australia, and workers that have been exposed to crocidolite have the highest rates of any occupationally exposed groups (10). Therefore, it is not surprising that mesothelioma has arisen in people who have lived at Wittenoom in Western Australia, where Australian crocidolite was mined and milled. A follow-up study of nearly 5000 people who had lived at Wittenoom, but had never worked for the mining company Australian Blue Asbestos (ABA), has been started. Most subjects were relatives and friends of ABA employees, and nearly half the cohort were either born at Wittenoom or first went there as children younger than 10 years of age. To the end of 1990, 15 cases of mesothelioma were known to have occurred. Of the 11 female and 4 male cases of mesothelioma thought to have arisen because of environmental exposure, 3 cases occurred in wives and 8 cases in children of ABA workers, 2 in other workers, and 2 in relatives of other workers. The duration of exposure ranged from 1 to 11 years; age at first residence from birth to 51 years; time from first residence to death from 25 to 45 years. The duration of time spent by members of total cohort at Wittenoom ranged from 1 month to 41 years (11).

A similar study has also been piloted in South Africa (12), and it seems that similar problems may be arising in China as well (13).

Mesothelioma and asbestosis have occurred after contact with household members who were occupationally exposed to asbestos (14–18). In a study of mesothelioma in patients aged 40 years or younger, four of the ten cases lived with fathers who worked for long periods with asbestos, and a fifth lived with another relative who worked in an asbestos plant (19). Levels of airborne exposure in this kind of situation have been measured only once, and the results were given in terms of mass of dust not fibers (20). Using conventional mass/fiber conversion factors (21), however, gives an estimate of average exposure of about six fibers per liter, but with a range of up to 150 fibers per liter.

Living in the vicinity of asbestos mines or factories that use asbestos has probably given rise to an increased risk of mesothelioma, particularly in more distant times. In studies that have been able to exclude occupational effects, no excess mortality was found around either an amosite factory (22) or, in a brief preliminary study, around a chrysotile mine where ambient exposures were reported to be very high (23). There was strong evidence that neighborhood exposure from a factory using mainly crocidolite was responsible for 11 of 83 cases of mesothelioma in East London (24). Bohlig and Hain also implicated emissions from an asbestos-processing plant in Hamburg, which used mainly crocidolite, in causing some of 38 nonoccupational mesotheliomas there (25).

In the study of former Wittenoom residents described earlier (11), it has not yet been possible to distinguish whether the exposure of the mesothelioma cases was from household exposure, air pollution from the discharge of extracted dust from the mill into the surrounding air, or from general levels of environmental pollution caused by the widespread use of asbestos tailings for roads, paths, gardens, and so on. No cases have yet arisen in people first exposed after the mine ceased operating in 1966 (11).

A currently more important cause of mesothelioma is indirect occupational exposure to asbestos. Cases of mesothelioma have been reported among people whose work has brought them into contact with asbestos products on occasion: brake mechanics, building custodians, plumbers, and others. These have always been isolated cases among working groups for whom it has been difficult or impossible to assess either their levels of exposure or the statistical significance of their incidence (26,27). So far, this has been true of all the situations described in the foregoing, apart from the incidence among people exposed to erionite in Turkey (6).

### B.   Postulated Environmental Causes of Mesothelioma

The review document from the Health Effects Institute (HEI) (1) was mainly concerned with the effects of asbestos in buildings, and characterized five classes of building occupant. These consisted of (1) occupants; (2) building custodians, who should not have to disturb any asbestos; (3) maintenance workers, who have to disturb asbestos materials; (4) demolition or removal workers, and (5) firemen or emergency workers. Such a categorization can be usefully applied in more general terms, but it is clear from the foregoing discussion that groups 3 and 4 are definitely at risk, whereas estimating the risk of groups 1 and 2 is what chiefly concerns most people today. The HEI report described the risks for group 5 as completely unknown, but of doubtful importance, compared with the other hazards that they faced (1).

The important question concerning possible environmental causes of mesothelioma is the level of contamination with asbestos that is required to significantly increase the risk of disease. Are the amounts of fibers released by the numerous roofs, fences, and other such products, sufficient to cause concern? That is, how do we estimate the risks of mesothelioma for people in group 1 and group 2?

## III. Estimating Risks by Extrapolation from Disease Incidence in Occupationally Exposed Cohorts

To estimate risks of disease after environmental exposure in this fashion, both an exposure–response relation, which describes the way the incidence of disease is related to patterns of exposure, and a measure of the exposure are required.

### A. Exposure–Response Relations

Given data from studies on the former Wittenoom mine and millworkers, the incidence of mesothelioma has been related to the degree of exposure to crocidolite and the time since first exposure (10) according to the formulas:

$$I = k_1 \times F \times [T^4 - (T - D)^4] \qquad [1]$$

or

$$I = k_2 \times F \times [(T - 10)^3 - (T - D - 10)^3] \qquad [2]$$

where $k_1 = 0.14 \times 10^{-8}$, $k_2 = 13.4 \times 10^{-8}$, $I$ is the incidence rate, $F$ is the level of exposure in fibers per milliliter, $T$ is years since first exposed, and $D$ is years of exposure. Both formulas fit the data equally well statistically.

These equations are consistent with dose and time relations from other studies (21,28) and show that there is a greater than exponential increase in the number of cases of malignant mesothelioma with increasing time from first crocidolite exposure. The exponent on time from first exposure is 3 if a minimum lag period of 10 years is assumed and 4 if no such minimum is assumed.

The constant multiplier for degree of exposure has been estimated from other occupational studies for other reviews. The Ontario Royal Commission (21) used Eq. [1] and estimated $k_1$ to be 0.0072 for the Rochdale plant (29), 0.0133 for the North American insulators (30), and 0.213 for the Canadian asbestos–cement manufacturing plant (31). The HEI used Eq. [2] and estimated values of $k_2$ to be 1.0, 1.5, and 12 for the same three studies, with an additional value of 3.2 for the Paterson amosite workers (32). The constants from the Wittenoom data are closer to the Ontario plant than any other, although $k_1$ is smaller for Wittenoom, whereas $k_2$ is larger. For projections, the HEI report used Eq. [2] with a value 1 replacing the 13.4, as being more appropriate for populations exposed mainly to chrysotile asbestos.

### B. Estimates of Environmental Fiber Levels

Even with today's technology, there are still enormous problems in estimating actual levels of environmental exposure to asbestos fibers, mainly because the levels are so low and often at about the detection limits of whatever system is used. In addition, however sensitively or precisely such levels have been measured, they have to be converted to equivalence with the optical microscopy methods used in all the occupational studies for which exposure–response data are available.

Good discussions of all the controversies and problems involved with such measurements can be found in the reviews by Case and Sebastien (33) and by Nicholson (34), and in much more detail throughout the HEI report. Some of the issues are

1.  The use of direct or indirect filter preparation: the direct method probably underestimates fiber concentration, whereas the indirect method overestimates it.
2.  Should counting be restricted to the usual length criterion, longer than 5 $\mu$m, or should all fibers be considered because of the different fiber size distribution found in environmental settings?
3.  Since any exposure is experienced by people moving around, is there any value in using measurements from static area samplers, or should all measurements be made with personal samplers? For example, a survey of the Wittenoom township in 1992 found detectable levels of crocidolite fibers in both personal samplers, but no fibers in all four area samplers (35).

Despite the various difficulties, the HEI produced a range of likely levels of contamination for different situations, based on numerous measurements. They relied mainly on the direct method, because most measurements have been done in this way. Estimates extended from 0.01 fibers per liter in rural areas, through 0.2 fibers per liter as an average in public buildings with asbestos-containing materials, to 5 fibers per liter as the maximum value found in schools with asbestos insulation products. In Western Australia a survey of schools built using asbestos–cement materials found an average concentration of 0.028 fibers per liter with a peak of 0.5 fibers per liter (3). In most nonoccupational settings, fiber concentrations are usually found to be 1 fiber per liter or less.

### C.  Projection of Risks from Current Environmental Exposures

Projected risks are generally calculated in terms of so-called lifetime risks; that is, the probability of contracting mesothelioma in one person's life before a given age (usually 80 or 85). This risk is calculated by applying the theoretical age-specific incidence rates of mesothelioma and the known age-specific death rates from all causes with a hypothetical population of say 1 million people so that the risk is expressed in terms of number of cases per million lifetimes. A more detailed account of the calculation is given in volume 2 of the Ontario Royal Commission Report (21), but it should be remembered that different sets of all-cause death rates will produce different lifetime risks for the same exposure–response equation and the same level of exposure.

Estimates have been made of cumulative risks for nonoccupational exposure and are summarized elsewhere (10). These estimates have been made by several scientists and regulatory bodies, most are about 10–20 per million lifetimes for school-aged exposure (the younger the exposure the higher the lifetime risk). The HEI projections were 6 and 60 for school exposures of 0.5 and 5 fibers per liter. The highest estimate for a background exposure of 1 fiber per liter was that based on the data from Wittenoom, with an estimated 55 cases per million lifetimes, equivalent to an annual rate of less than 1 per million, or less than one case per year in Western Australia. Since the actual concentrations of asbestos fibers in asbestos–cement buildings are probably at least ten times less than this (3), the probable risk is likely to be at least ten times less.

### IV.  Estimating Risks by Observation of Current Data

From the descriptive point of view, there are three kinds of data that could reveal the presence of an appreciable risk of mesothelioma associated with environmental exposure to the products of industrial exploitation of asbestos. First, since women have generally not been exposed occupationally to asbestos, an increase in incidence of mesothelioma in women could be a consequence of environmental exposure. Second, since the latent period from first exposure to asbestos to onset of mesothelioma is probably no fewer than about 15 years and, on average, about 30–40 years, an increase in incidence of mesothelioma in persons younger than about 35 years of age could be due to asbestos in the environment. Third, in most mesothelioma incidence surveillance programs, an attempt is made to classify patients with mesothelioma into those with and those without identified specific exposure to asbestos. Although the accuracy of this classification may not be high, an increasing incidence of mesothelioma in persons without identified exposure to asbestos could indicate an effect of general environmental exposure.

It has been argued that possible risks of mesothelioma from environmental exposure to asbestos, estimated by extrapolation from the experience of occupational cohorts, are not reflected in observed descriptive data. McDonald et al. compared trends in mesothelioma with those expected from risk estimates given in various reviews (36). In none of the populations studied had there been any appreciable increase in incidence (United States or United Kingdom) or mortality (Canada) from mesothelioma. Others have reported similar results (37–39). More recent reviews and estimates of risk from low levels of exposure have predicted, however, a much lower increase in incidence than some predicted in the 1980s, and national incidence figures may not be sensitive enough to detect such small rises.

In contrast with these observations, however, there is evidence that the incidence of mesothelioma has increased in women in both Australia and South Africa (40–45). There appears, however, to have been no appreciable increase in incidence of mesothelioma in Australia in people younger than 35 years of age (41–45). Correspondingly, with many women involved in the asbestos industry in Australia, it would be surprising if their rates had not increased. In Australia there has also been a considerable increase in incidence among people supposedly unexposed to asbestos (Fig. 1).

Since both Australia (specifically Western Australia) and South Africa have produced crocidolite, it is possible that the larger quantities of crocidolite in general use in these countries could have given rise to increasing incidence rates of mesothelioma in persons not exposed occupationally to asbestos, given the high potency of crocidolite in causing mesothelioma (10,46). This might explain the difference from observations in other countries.

### A.  Difficulties in Use of Population Statistics

Various problems have to be considered in the collection and use of mesothelioma incidence and mortality statistics, most of which have been discussed at length elsewhere (e.g., 10,41,43) and will be summarized only briefly here.

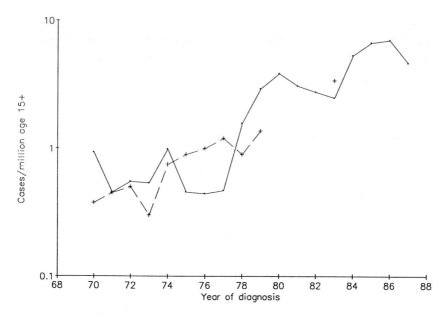

**Figure 1**  Three-year moving average trends in incidence of mesothelioma without identified exposure to asbestos in men and women together in Australia as a whole and in Western Australia, 1969–1988: solid dots, Western Australia; plus signs, Australia. Point for 1983 for Australia from the Australian Mesothelioma Surveillance Programme (44).

The diagnosis of mesothelioma is difficult and, generally, requires the use of a mesothelioma register incorporating a panel of pathologists for accurate diagnoses. With increasing awareness of the disease has come increasing possibility of overdiagnosis, compared with the underdiagnosis of the past when, in some countries, no such disease was supposed to exist, in contrast with others where the diagnosis was much more readily made (39). Mortality statistics have been useful only after the introduction of the eighth revision of the International Classification of Diseases, when a separate code for malignant neoplasms of the pleura was included. In Australia, certainly, this diagnosis is highly specific for mesothelioma, although the sensitivity is low (that is, many cases are missed, but when coded it is usually accurate). In contrast, malignant neoplasms of the peritoneum are of no value in estimating rates of peritoneal mesothelioma.

A further problem in examining rates for persons unexposed to asbestos is in the accurate ascertainment of exposure experienced many years ago. One way of approximately correcting for this in population data is described further in the following. Aside from detailed occupational and environmental questionnaires, only fiber counting in lung tissue has been of any value (45). This is particularly so when exposure has been to the highly durable amphibole fibers, crocidolite and amosite, but is of little value when applied to chrysotile exposure, unless rigorous adjustment for clearance rates is carried out (47,48).

### B. Adjusting Population Rates for Incomplete Ascertainment of Exposure to Asbestos

The process described here was outlined by de Klerk et al. (49) and used Western Australian data from 1980 to 1988, when exposure ascertainment was uniformly thorough. Subjects with unknown exposure status were counted in with subjects with no identified exposure.

Straight lines were fitted by unweighted linear regression to plots of the incidence of mesothelioma in persons without identified exposure to asbestos, for different age groups at diagnosis, as suggested by Peto (50,51).

When information on duration of exposure is unavailable, Eq. [1] is often simplified to

$$I = k \times F \times T^{p'} \tag{3}$$

with $p'$ taken to be between 3 and 4, usually 3.5. $T$ and $F$ are, as before, time from first exposure and fiber concentration.

If grouped data are available, this is then easily plotted as

$$\log(I) = a + p' \times \log T \tag{4}$$

and should be a straight line if both axes are plotted on a log scale, with intercept $a = \log(K) + \log(F)$, and slope $p'$.

The line of best fit to the incidence of mesothelioma in men without identified exposure to asbestos or with unknown exposure status in Western Australia from 1980 to 1988 gave a slope ($p'$) of 5.4 when age at diagnosis was taken as a surrogate for time since first exposure in Eq. [3] (Fig. 2). This slope is far higher than would be expected either in persons truly unexposed to asbestos or with only environmental exposure to asbestos (if this was uniform over the time period of study). A dashed line with the more generally accepted slope of 3.5, in which the age groups younger than 45 years were used to fix the intercept of the line, is also shown in Figure 2. If this line is considered to reflect the true picture, then the numbers of cases that caused the observed values to be above it could be considered more likely to be due to unrecorded occupational exposure (or other specific exposure to asbestos in adulthood) than due to other reasons, or to general environmental exposure. These numbers represent about three-quarters of the cases in men without identified exposure. The crude incidence implied by the fitted line of slope 3.5 was 2.6 per million person

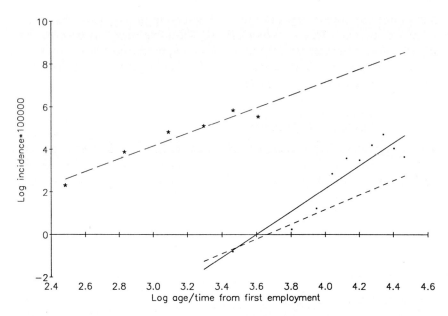

**Figure 2** Incidence of mesothelioma in relation to "time since first exposure" in Western Australian men in 1980–1988 not identified to have had specific exposure to asbestos (age at diagnosis used as a surrogate for time since first exposure) compared with a similar relation in workers exposed to crocidolite at Wittenoom: asterisk, incidence in former Wittenoom workers; dashed line, workers line of best fit, slope 3.1; solid dots, incidence in unexposed ×10; solid line, unexposed line of best fit, slope 5.4; short-dash line, unexposed incidence, slope fixed at 3.5.

years at 15 years of age and older, much less than the observed rate of 9.6, but higher than the figure of 1.6 found for Los Angeles from 1974 to 1978 (50,51). By way of comparison, the same method was used to fit a line to data from workers exposed to crocidolite at Wittenoom in Western Australia (52), but using time from first exposure instead of age at diagnosis in the model.

The corresponding analysis in women in Western Australia between 1980 and 1988 is shown in Figure 3. There were many fewer cases of mesothelioma, and the overall slope for all ages in those with no identified or unknown exposure to asbestos was only 3.7, and 3.5 if the oldest age group only was omitted. The crude incidence shown by the fitted line of slope 3.5 was again 2.6 per million person years at 15 years of age and older, but the total rate (corresponding to the empirical slope of 3.7) was only 3 per million.

There have been increases in the incidence rates of malignant mesothelioma in women, in those without identified exposure to asbestos and, possibly, those younger than 35 years of age in Australia and Western Australia. Although part of the first two increases, at least, may be attributable to specific exposure to asbestos, mathematical modeling of the Western Australian data suggests that there has been about a twofold increase in incidence rates from the 1970s to the 1980s that may be due to increased general environmental exposure to asbestos. The final estimated rate in both men and women in the absence of specific exposure to asbestos was 2.6 per million person years. This rate is higher than the rate of 1.6 per million person years estimated to occur in Los Angeles in the absence of specific exposure (51), a fact that lends support to the suggestion that general environmental exposure to asbestos may have increased mesothelioma rates in Australia. The excess of 1 per million person years over this presumed "background" rate is also, coincidentally, the amount that was estimated as possibly caused by exposure of school children to 1 fiber per liter (as men-

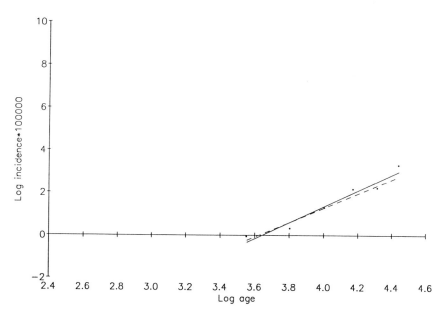

**Figure 3**   Incidence of mesothelioma in relation to age at diagnosis (as a surrogate for time since first exposure) in Western Australian women in 1980–1988 not identified to have had specific exposure to asbestos: solid dots, incidence in unexposed × 10; solid line, unexposed line of best fit, slope 3.7; broken line, unexposed incidence, slope fixed at 3.5.

tioned earlier), a level that might result from use of asbestos-based insulation or other general contamination of the environment with asbestos.

A final consideration in the use of national trend data for estimating environmental effects is the comparison of the likely extrapolated risk from occupational data with the background risk estimated here or from Peto's Los Angeles data. From the Peto paper (50), the incidence of mesothelioma is related to age in the following way:

$$\text{Incidence} = 1.7 \cdot 10^{-12} \cdot (\text{age})^{3.5}$$

which translates to a lifetime risk to age 80 of just over 100 per million people, which is much greater than any of the estimated environmental risks described earlier. An equivalent risk from the adjusted Western Australian data is about 160 per million lifetimes. The question remains as to how these background risks and environmental risks interact. Is the postulated environmental incidence already included in the background incidence, or should the risks be added or even multiplied together? This question is almost certainly unanswerable using epidemiological methods.

## V.  Potential Environmental Problems

Causes of environmental mesothelioma that may arise in the future also have to be considered, and a few examples are presented here.

In demolition and removal of asbestos material, the greatly increased costs of approved procedures will, and do, encourage "quick-and-dirty" removal methods. This may be a danger not only to the removalists, but also to people in the vicinity, as it is well known that fibers will not only be transported all around, but will also persist in the ambient air for some time (53,54).

Other problems may arise owing to the contamination of other mined ores with fibrous materials, such as the tremolite asbestos, found in association not only with chrysotile asbestos, but with vermiculite and talc, or the crocidolite found in some Western Australian deposits of iron ore (55). There is also the possibility that even greater risks could develop from use of alternative fibrous materials that have been inadequately studied.

Finally, despite the overwhelming body of evidence pointing to the considerable risks involved in the use of crocidolite, large quantities of the mineral are still mined, milled, and exported from South Africa to unknown destinations. One can only speculate on the level of information concerning the risks involved that are provided to users and workers.

## VI.  Conclusions

Although Australian data suggest an increase in mesothelioma incidence owing to general environmental exposure to asbestos, it is probably only in situations, as described by McDonald et al. (36), in which there have been no observable increase in rates, that firm conclusions can be drawn from analyses of existing disease rates. Even then, allowance must be made for the latent period (at least 10–15 years) between any increase in environmental exposure and a following possible increase in mesothelioma incidence. It is, perhaps, surprising that mesothelioma incidence rates have not been observed to increase in women in Canada, the United States, and the United Kingdom, since some women have been employed in asbestos production or use in most industrialized countries (at Wittenoom, for example, about 7% of the workforce were women), and many cases of mesothelioma have arisen following household contact with asbestos workers as discussed earlier.

It is doubtful whether epidemiological methods, as described here, could ever be definitive in deciding whether there is an appreciable hazard from general environmental exposure to asbestos (14) or, more importantly, whether the hazard is large enough to justify specific remedial action. A more powerful approach would be by way of population-based case–control studies of mesothelioma, with careful characterization of all possible sources of exposure to asbestos in subjects without occupational exposure. It would be necessary, also, for measurements of asbestos fibers in lung tissue to be included in such studies, as it is only by this means that unrecognized exposure to large amounts of asbestos, particularly amphibole asbestos, can be determined in all subjects (33,45).

The chief cause for concern in Australia and other countries where amphibole asbestos is no longer used in new products, must remain the risk taken by people involved in asbestos removal. There is evidence from the United Kingdom (56) and Holland (57) that protective equipment, even when used correctly, does not work as well as expected, and there always exists the strong chance of the equipment not being used correctly or, indeed, used at all. Dust levels generated in removal work are similar to those experienced in the industry years ago (53). From the existing dose-response relations described in the foregoing, it has been estimated, for example (58), that the risk of a 70-year-old man contracting mesothelioma could be increased more than threefold if he had spent 6 months in demolition work in his 20s using one of the just described respirators. This contrasted with both the small 4% increase in risk from continuous environmental exposure to 0.5 fibers per liter and the 6000-fold increase from working in the Wittenoom mill for the same length of time at the same age.

## References

1. Health Effects Institute — Asbestos Research. Asbestos in public buildings: a literature review and synthesis of current knowledge. Cambridge: HEI-AR, 1991.
2. Landrigan PJ, Kazemi H, eds. The third wave of asbestos disease: exposure to asbestos in place: public health control. New York: New York Academy of Sciences, 1991.
3. Western Australian Advisory Committee on Hazardous Substances. Asbestos cement products. Perth: Health Department of WA, 1990.
4. Stone R. No meeting of the minds on asbestos. Science 1991; 254:928–931.
5. Mark EJ, Yokoi T. Absence of evidence for a significant background incidence of diffuse malignant mesothelioma apart from asbestos exposure. Ann NY Acad Sci 1991; 643:196–204.
6. Baris YI, Simonato L, Saracci R, Winkelman R. The epidemic of respiratory cancer associated with erionite fibres in the Cappadocian region of Turkey. In: Elliott P, Cuzick J, English D, Stern R, eds. Geographical and environmental epidemiology: methods for small-area studies. Oxford: Oxford University Press, 1992:310–322.
7. Baris YI, Bilir N, Artvinli M, Sahin AA, Kalyoncu F, Sebastien P. An epidemiological study in an Anatolian village environmentally exposed to tremolite asbestos. Br J Ind Med 1988; 45:838–840.
8. McConnichie K, Simonato L, Christofides P, Pooley FD, Wagner JC. Mesothelioma in Cyprus: the role of tremolite. Thorax 1987; 42:342–347.
9. Case BW. Health effects of tremolite: now and in the future. Ann NY Acad Sci 1991; 643:491–504.
10. de Klerk NH, Armstrong BK. The epidemiology of asbestos and mesothelioma. In: Henderson DW, Shilkin KB, Langlois SLP, Whitaker D, eds. Malignant mesothelioma. New York: Hemisphere Publishing, 1992:223–250.
11. Hansen J, de Klerk NH, Eccles J, Musk AW, Hobbs MST. Malignant mesothelioma after environmental exposure to blue asbestos. Int J Cancer 1993; 54:578–581.
12. Reid G, Kielkowski D, Steyn SD, Botha K. Mortality of an asbestos-exposed birth cohort: a pilot study. S Afr Med J 1990; 78:584–586.
13. Liu X, Luo S. A study on crocidolite contamination and mesothelioma in Dayao County of Yunnan Province, China [abstr]. Proceedings 8th international conference on occupational lung diseases. Prague, 1992.
14. Gardner MJ, Saracci R. Effects on health of non-occupational exposure to airborne mineral fibres. IARC Sci Publ 1989; 90:375–397.
15. Anderson HA, Lilis R, Daum SM, Fischbein AS. Household-contact asbestos neoplastic risk. Ann NY Acad Sci 1976; 271:311–323.
16. Anderson HA, Lilis R, Daum SM, Selikoff IJ. Asbestosis among household contacts of asbestos factory workers. Ann NY Acad Sci 1979; 330:386–399.
17. Kilburn KH, Lilis R, Anderson HA, Miller A, Warshaw RH. Interaction of asbestos, age and cigarette smoking in producing radiographic evidence of diffuse pulmonary fibrosis. Am J Med 1986; 80:377–381.

18. Kilburn KH, Warshaw R, Thornston JC. Asbestos disease and family contacts of shipyard workers. Am J Public Health 1985; 75:615–617.
19. Kane MJ, Chahinian AP, Holland JF. Malignant mesothelioma in young adults. Cancer 1990; 65:1449–1455.
20. Nicholson WJ, Rohl AN, Weisman I, Selikoff IJ. Environmental asbestos concentrations in the United States. IARC Sci Publ 1980; 39:823–827.
21. Ontario Royal Commission on Asbestos. Report of the Royal Commission on matters of health and safety arising from the use of asbestos in Ontario, vol 2. Toronto: Ontario Ministry of the Attorney General, 1984.
22. Hammond EC, Garfinkel L, Selikoff IJ, Nicholson WJ. Mortality experience of residents in the neighbourhood of an asbestos factory. Ann NY Acad Sci 1979; 339:417–422.
23. Siemiatycki J. Health effects on the general population (mortality in the general population in asbestos mining areas). In: Proceedings of world symposium on asbestos. Montreal, Canada, 25–27 May. Montreal: Canadian Asbestos Information Centre, 1982:337–348.
24. Newhouse ML, Thompson H. Mesothelioma of pleura and peritoneum following exposure to asbestos in the London area. Br J Ind Med 1965; 22:261–269.
25. Bohlig H, Hain E. Cancer in relation to environmental exposure. IARC Sci Publ 1973; 8:217–221.
26. Lilienfeld DE. Asbestos-associated pleural mesothelioma in school teachers: a discussion of four cases. Ann NY Acad Sci 1991; 643:454–458.
27. Anderson HA, Hanrahan LP, Schirmer J, Higgins D, Sarow P. Mesothelioma among employees with likely contact with in-place asbestos-containing building materials. Ann NY Acad Sci 1991; 643:550–572.
28. Gardner MJ. A review of the available evidence for setting occupational exposure limits for asbestos. Paper for WHO Consultation Meeting April 1989 – final version, June 1989.
29. Peto J, Doll R, Hermon C, Binns W, Clayton R, Goffe T. Relationship of mortality to measures of environmental asbestos pollution in an asbestos textile factory. Ann Occup Hyg 1985; 29:305–355.
30. Selikoff IJ, Hammond EC, Seidman H. Mortality experience of insulation workers in the United States and Canada, 1943–1976. Ann NY Acad Sci 1979; 330:91–116.
31. Finkelstein MM. Mortality among employees of an Ontario asbestos–cement factory. Am Rev Respir Dis 1984; 129:754–761.
32. Seidman H, Selikoff IJ, Gelb SK. Mortality experience of amosite asbestos factory workers: dose–response relationships 5 to 40 years after onset of short-term work exposure. Am J Ind Med 1986; 10:479–514.
33. Case BW, Sebastien P. Fibre levels in lung and correlation with air samples. IARC Sci Publ 1989; 90:207–218.
34. Nicholson WJ. Airborne mineral fibres in the non-occupational environment. IARC Sci Publ 1989; 90:239–261.
35. Nevill M, Rogers A. Inquiry into asbestos issues at Wittenoom. Perth: Western Australian Government Internal Report, 1992.
36. McDonald JC, Sebastien P, McDonald AD, Case B. Epidemiological observa-

tions on mesothelioma and their implications for non-occupational exposure. IARC Sci Publ 1989; 90:420–427.

37. Archer VE, Rom WN. Trends in mortality of diffuse malignant mesothelioma of pleura. Lancet 1983; 2:112–113.
38. Enterline PE, Henderson VL. Geographic patterns for pleural mesothelioma deaths in the United States, 1968–81. JNCI 1987; 79:31–37.
39. Andersson M, Olsen JH. Trend and distribution of mesothelioma in Denmark. Br J Cancer 1985; 51:699–705.
40. Zwi AB, Reid G, Landau SP, Kielkowski D, Sitas F, Becklake MR. Mesothelioma in South Africa, 1976–84: incidence and case characteristics. Int J Epidemiol 1989; 18:320–329.
41. Armstrong BK, Musk AW, Baker JE, et al. Epidemiology of malignant mesothelioma in Western Australia. Med J Aust 1984; 141:86–88.
42. Musk, AW, Dolin PJ, Armstrong BK, Ford JM, de Klerk NH, Hobbs MST. The incidence of malignant mesothelioma in Australia 1947–80. Med J Aust 1989; 150:242–246.
43. Xu Z, Armstrong BK, Blunsdon BJ, Rogers JM, Musk AW, Shilkin KG. Trends in mortality from malignant mesothelioma of the pleura, and production and use of asbestos in Australia. Med J Aust 1985; 143:185–187.
44. Ferguson DA, Berry G, Jelihovsky T, et al. The Australian mesothelioma surveillance program 1979–1985. Med J Aust 1987; 147:166–172.
45. Leigh J, Corvalan CF, Grimwood A, Berry G, Ferguson DA, Thompson R. The incidence of malignant mesothelioma in Australia 1982–1988. Am J Ind Med 1991; 20:643–655.
46. Berry G. Epidemiology of mesothelioma. In: Tattersall M, ed. Preventing cancer. Sydney: Australian Professional Publications, 1988:35–44.
47. Berry G, Rogers AJ, Pooley FD. Mesotheliomas – asbestos exposure and lung burden. IARC Sci Publ 1989; 90:486–496.
48. Rogers AJ, Leigh J, Berry G, et al. Dose response relationships between airborne and lung asbestos fibre type, length and concentration and the relative risk of mesothelioma. Ann Occup Hyg (in press).
49. de Klerk NH, Musk AW, Eccles JL, Armstrong BK, Hobbs MST. Mesothelioma and exposure to asbestos in Western Australia. Eur Respir Rev 1993; 3:102–104.
50. Peto J. Dose and time relationships for lung cancer and mesothelioma in relation to smoking and asbestos exposure. In: Fischer M, Meyer E, eds. Zur beurteilung der krebsgefahr durch asbest. Munchen: BGA Schriften, MMV Medizin Verlag 1984; 2/84:126–132.
51. Peto J, Henderson BE, Pike MC. Trends in mesothelioma incidence in the United States and the forecast epidemic due to asbestos exposure during World War II. Banbury Rep 1982; 9:51–69.
52. de Klerk NH, Armstrong BK, Musk AW, Hobbs MST. Predictions of future asbestos-related disease cases among former miners and millers of crocidolite in Western Australia. Med J Aust 1989; 151:616–620.
53. Burdett GJ, Jaffrey SAMT, Rood AP. Airborne asbestos fibre levels in buildings: a summary of UK measurements. IARC Sci Publ 1989; 90:277–290.

54. Chesson J, Hatfield J, Schultz B, Dutrow E, Blake J. Airborne asbestos in public buildings. Environ Res 1990; 51:100–107.
55. Musk AW, de Klerk NH, Cookson WOC, Morgan WKC. Radiographic abnormalities and duration of employment in Western Australian iron ore miners. Med J Aust 1988; 148:332–334.
56. Tannahill SN, Willey RJ, Jackson MH. Workplace protection factors of HSE approved negative pressure full-facepiece dust respirators during asbestos stripping: preliminary findings. Ann Occup Hyg 1990; 34:547–552.
57. Akkersdijk H, Bremmer CF, Schliszka C, Spee T. Effect of respiratory protective equipment on exposure to asbestos fibres during removal of asbestos insulation. Ann Occup Hyg 1989; 33:113–116.
58. de Klerk NH, Musk AW, Eccles JL, Armstrong BK, Hobbs MST. Risk of mesothelioma after environmental exposure to asbestos. Eur Respir Rev 1993; 3:108–110.

# 3

## Mesothelioma: Is There a Background?

**J. CORBETT MCDONALD**

Royal Brompton National Heart and Lung
    Institute
London, England

**ALISON D. MCDONALD**

McGill University
Montreal, Quebec, Canada

## I.  Introduction

Malignant mesothelioma came into prominence, and its existence as a pathological entity was established with publication, in 1958 and the early 1960s, of its frequent occurrence in the crocidolite mining area of South Africa and as a substantial risk for insulation workers and related trades. With hindsight, it is evident that a small number of case reports and small case series with similar work exposure had appeared in the medical literature over the previous 20 or so years. Since then, the full magnitude of the asbestos-related epidemic of mesothelioma has become all too obvious, with incidence continuing to rise in most industrial countries at up to 10% per annum, a trend unlikely to slacken until well into the next century.

In direct consequence of these disastrous events, there is the growing question of whether all cases of mesothelioma have resulted directly or indirectly from the industrial exploitation and use of asbestos. The question has obvious medicolegal importance: if not all cases are so caused, there will always be an element of doubt in attributing a particular case to some specific occupationally related exposure, an idea that plaintiffs' lawyers would like to dismiss and the defense to promote. The question has also much scientific relevance, in that without full understanding of the agents that can cause mesothelioma, it may be difficult to find safe and satisfactory substitutes for the many important uses of asbestos.

In this chapter we review the main evidence now available on whether there is or has been a background incidence of mesothelioma in humans, unrelated to the industrial use of asbestos. Background cases could have resulted from airborne asbestos or other natural mineral fibers liberated by wind and water erosion from the almost ubiquitous distribution of deposits in the earth's surface, or they could have an entirely different etiology. In assessing the evidence, uncertainty over diagnosis is an everpresent problem, especially in earlier times, when the very existence of primary malignant mesothelioma tumors was doubted, and use of the diagnosis was actively discouraged by such eminent pathologists as Willis (1). Even today, far from all cases are confirmed pathologically and, of those that are studied at autopsy and with the most sophisticated histological, biochemical, and immunological tests, the diagnosis in many is left in doubt. Inevitably these problems are particularly acute when the etiological circumstances are unusual as, for example, in childhood cases or in agricultural regions of distant and developing countries.

## II.  Historical Evidence

Asbestos was first mined and milled for industrial purposes in the 1870s, but in only small quantities until after World War I. If one considers that the latent period between first exposure and death is usually 30–40 years, and very seldom less than 20 years, it is reasonable to believe that the case reports and case series of the 1930s and 1940s were possibly asbestos-related, whereas it is quite improbable that cases documented before about 1900 were caused in this way. Among the several early papers, mostly by pathologists, on primary pleural malignancies — usually referred to at that time as pleural endotheliomas — those by Robertson in 1924 (2) and Saccone and Coblenz in 1943 (3) were particularly informative. It is clear from both these sources that, aside from the remarkable, but insufficiently validated, report by Lieutaud in 1767 of two pleural tumors among 3000 autopsies and first recognition of the pathological entity by Wagner in 1870, several large autopsy series published at the end of the last century and from 1900 to about 1920 included cases that cannot easily be attributed to the industrial use of asbestos. The frequency of such cases was approximately 1:1000 autopsies, a proportion that unfortunately cannot be related to any population denominator. It is worth noting, nevertheless, that cases ascertained through pathologists across Canada in the early 1960s, before the present upward trend in incidence was evident, constituted a roughly similar proportion of all autopsies. Other analyses made by Saccone and Coblenz included data from two autopsy series, comprising some 150 cases in Germany, published in 1924 and 1931, and unlikely to have been seriously contaminated by occupational asbestos exposure. These cases showed a male preponderance of 1.7:1 and the following age distribution: younger than 21, 4 cases; 21–40, 26; 41–60, 66; older than 60, 33. Without appropriate denominators these figures cannot really be interpreted, but once again, the pattern is similar to that for Canada in 1960–1968.

## III.  Direct Evidence

The clearest support for the existence of a background unrelated to the industrial use of asbestos is provided by evidence that exposure to other agents or to asbestos fibers in nonoccupational circumstances has also caused the disease. The most compelling indication of this is the extraordinary mortality from mesothelioma in certain villages of Cappadocia, central Turkey, reported by Baris and his colleagues in the 1970s (4). Extensive epidemiological and environmental surveys have strongly supported the hypothesis that the main, but not necessarily the only, causal factor has been exposure from birth to erionite dust, a crystalline fibrous form of the mineral zeolite. In three affected villages, 29 of 125 deaths during a defined period were from pleural mesothelioma, and 4 were from peritoneal mesothelioma (5). The affected villages had higher airborne concentrations of fibers of erionite than an unaffected village. Sheep lungs from the affected villages also had a higher erionite fiber content, although the difference was not statistically significant. Sputum samples from persons living in affected villages contained ferruginous erionite bodies. Age- and sex-specific death rates rose steeply in both sexes, compatible with exposure to a causative agent starting at birth. The youngest case reported in two of the three affected villages was in a man aged 27 years, suggesting that mesothelioma in children, as recorded elsewhere, is unlikely to be due to this type of environmental exposure. There is suggestive, but inconclusive, evidence that erionite deposits in other locations have contributed to mesothelioma incidence. In North America, there was a small, although not statistically significant, excess of cases in proximity to naturally occurring zeolite deposits (6). Also, in a geographic mortality study of pleural mesothelioma in the United States, the authors noted relatively high rates in two Rocky Mountain states and questioned whether these might possibly be explained in this way (7).

Occupational exposure to dust containing fibers in the tremolite series of amphibole minerals has also been associated with a substantial risk of mesothelioma (8). Fibrous tremolite, although very seldom exploited industrially, is nevertheless classifiable as an asbestos fiber, and occupational cases attributable to its commercial production and use cannot be considered as part of any background. The same is true of mesothelioma resulting from occupational exposure in chrysotile mining and milling for which tremolite fiber contamination is suspected of making a disproportionate contribution to the risk. Fibrous tremolite is a common contaminant of various minerals in the earth's crust, some of which are exploited commercially and some not. It is thus conceivable that tremolite fibers liberated by water and wind erosion could contribute to the occurrence of background cases. This possibility is difficult to test, but notably, lung burden analyses, based on 78 Canadian mesothelioma cases and matched controls, showed a significant excess of tremolite fibers (9). Most of this excess may well have resulted from direct or indirect exposure to tremolite contamination of chrysotile in commercial use, but not necessarily all of it. The reality of the latter possibility is demonstrated in northeast Corsica, where general environmental exposure to tremolite and chrysotile fibers has occurred as a result of numerous mineral outcrops in that region (10). A radiographic survey of patients without occupational exposure showed a significantly higher prevalence of bilateral pleural plaques in northeast Corsican residents (3.66%) than in those from the northwest (1.14%), where similar outcrops do not occur. Five cases of pleural mesothelioma were also recorded in patients from the northeast without occupational asbestos exposure, and these were said to have a heavy pulmonary asbestos burden. However, no comparable data were reported for the northwest. Suggestive evidence of a similar nature has also been reported from Cyprus (11) and certain villages in Greece (12), with indications in both that fibrous tremolite could have been responsible.

Over the years, many other chemical, physical, and biological agents have come under suspicion in relation to the sporadic occurrence of mesothelioma in humans and animals, apparently unrelated to asbestos exposure, but the evidence is largely anecdotal and uncontrolled (13). Less easy to dismiss are reports of cases of mesothelioma in sugar cane workers in India (14) and of excess mortality from this cause in southern Louisiana (15). After the harvest the cane is burned off, leading to the formation of long thin respirable silica fibers (16), a process that presumably might also arise in forest fires and other agricultural circumstances. Currently, there are too few epidemiological, experimental, or lung-burden studies to evaluate any of these hypotheses.

## IV. Circumstantial Evidence

### A. Mesothelioma in Children

It is very unlikely that childhood cases could be due to asbestos exposure because the shortest latent period for which there is reasonably firm evidence is 14 years (17), nor is there any indication that the length of the latent period is affected by age. In a critical review, published in 1964, Kaufman and Stout (18) concluded that, after exclusion of dubious cases, there remained ten, ranging in age from a few months to 14 years — seven in boys and three in girls — for which the diagnosis was thought reliable. All ten were pleural and were more frequently fibrous than tubular or tubulopapillary, as are those in adults. The earliest two cases in the series had been published first in 1886 and 1904, respectively. In a recent review of 80 cases of mesothelioma in children reported 1869-1986 (19), including some of the ten just mentioned, 67.5% were pleural, 25% peritoneal, and 7.5% pericardial. Their ages ranged from 1 to 19 years (mean 9.7 years), with a male/female ratio of 1.4. In only 2 of the 80 cases was there a history of possible exposure to asbestos, 1 in a 3-year-old girl, whose father worked in an insulation plant, and the other in a 17-year-old girl possibly exposed at school. The incidence of mesothelioma in children younger than 20 years of age can be roughly estimated from three studies. In our own Canadian survey, 1960-1968, four fatal cases were ascertained by systematic inquiry from all pathologists — a rate of about 0.7:10 million per annum (20). A very similar figure can be derived from the 13 cases identified by Grundy and Miller (21) among death certificates in the United States of America, 1965-1968. Finally, Cooper et al. (22), using data from the Surveillance, Epidemiology, and End Result (SEER) program in the United States of America, 1973-84, estimated the case incidence at 0.5:10 million per annum. As mesothelioma in children may well be underdiagnosed, a conservative estimate for the annual case incidence in North America is likely to be at least 1:10 million per annum, but even so, appreciably lower than any comparable estimate for adults.

### B. Mortality Trends in Men and Women

The short clinical course of mesothelioma from first symptom to fatal outcome, almost always within 2 years, implies that mortality rates closely parallel incidence rates. Mesothelioma has only recently been given a unique code in the International Classification of Diseases, so that, in the past, satisfactory ascertainment was difficult from death certificates. In Canada, annual incidence rates based on cases ascertained through pathologists, when extrapolated backward, suggest that male and female rates were similar at or before 1950, at a level of about 1–2 per million population (23). This pattern is similar to trends found in the SEER cancer surveillance program of the United States of America (24) and for mortality observed in Britain, Finland, Norway, and Denmark (8). The increasing male excess appears due to the much more frequent history of occupational asbestos exposure in men than in women. In the SEER program, regions with higher age-adjusted incidence rates for mesothelioma in white males, presumably attributable to work-related asbestos exposure, had a higher ratio of male to female cases than regions with lower rates. This is illustrated in Figure 1, in which linear extrapolation would suggest that, at the point where the sex ratio is equal, the incidence would be about 5 per million, although with wide confidence limits. In Los Angeles County equal numbers of cases in

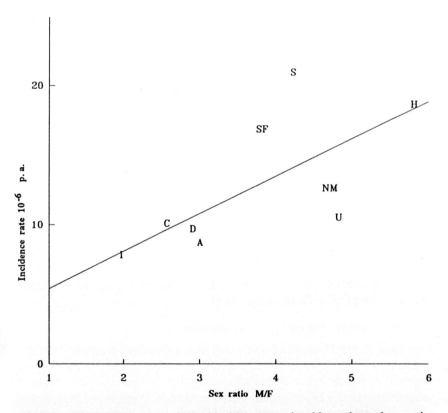

**Figure 1**  Mesothelioma age-adjusted incidence rates in white males and sex ratios by geographic area, United States of America, 1973–1984 (24). A, Atlanta; C, Connecticut; D, Detroit; H, Hawaii; I, Iowa; N, New Mexico; S, Seattle; SF, San Francisco–Oakland. Trend line fitted by least squares.

men and women were without history of exposure to asbestos, suggesting a background incidence of about 2 per million (25). In France, careful inquiry failed to identify any opportunity for asbestos exposure in younger subjects with mesothelioma; these included equal numbers of males and females (26). In all these various studies, efforts to detect causes other than asbestos have been largely unsuccessful, although in a few cases there has been mention of chronic inflammation and exposure to ionizing radiation or beryllium (27).

## V. Analyses of Lung Burden

Evidence of an etiological agent other than asbestos could conceivably have been detected in lung burden analyses. This has not been demonstrated in the few studies yet reported, although these have been confined to the identification and examination of mineral fibers. In two investigations of mesothelioma cases and controls in North America, the first in 1972 (28) and the second in 1979–1984 (9), a substantial excess of amphibole fibers was seen. In the latter study discrimination between cases and controls was almost wholly due to long fibers ($\geq 8$ $\mu$m), which it was estimated could explain about two-thirds of the cases. Altogether, 25 varieties of mineral fiber were recognized by electron microscopy but, apart from the amphibole fiber types, no important difference was observed between cases and controls. In the first of the studies mentioned, based on 99 case–control pairs, in 2, neither amphibole nor chrysotile fiber was detected. In the second study, based on 78 pairs, neither chrysotile nor any amphibole fibers were detected in 1 case; on the other hand, no long asbestos fibers ($> 8$ $\mu$m) were seen in 14 cases. A similar study in the United Kingdom, although not entirely comparable, gave much the same result (29). These three sets of data are thus compatible with a background incidence unrelated to asbestos, but the evidence is weakened by the few cases studied and limits of detectability by the electron microscopic techniques used. There is also the question of the extent to which postmortem analyses adequately reflect exposures that occurred many years earlier.

## VI. Conclusion

All five types of evidence considered in this review point to the existence of a background incidence of primary mesothelial malignancies unrelated directly or indirectly to exposure from the production or industrial use of asbestos, although with varying levels of certainty. The disastrous experience of certain villages in Cappadocia puts the proposition beyond doubt, but there is little to indicate whether or not the fibrous zeolites have caused the disease elsewhere. Indeed, it would appear that the liberation of tremolite amphibole fibers from widespread surface deposits may have a greater potential. The historical evidence is also strong, although subject to a certain degree of uncertainty over diagnosis. It is not that pathologists 50–100 years ago were less competent or discriminatory than they are today, but a few mistakes made when mesothelioma was rare or nonexistent would have a far greater impact on the question in hand than a similar number of diagnostic errors today when the disease is common.

The circumstantial evidence is by nature less conclusive. If mesothelioma in childhood is the same disease as that commonly seen in older men as a result of occupational asbestos exposure, it would strongly support the hypothesis. There is general consensus among pathologists that this is so. The analyses of sex-specific incidence rates in relation to time or region are consistent in pointing to an annual rate of about 1 or 2 per million in both sexes at a time or place when the industrial use of asbestos could have had little influence. However, this evidence depends on extrapolation, an essentially speculative procedure. The weakest evidence is undoubtedly that provided by lung burden analyses, depending as it does on failure to identify an etiological agent at death in a disease of very long latency.

In questions of this kind, analogous to those of cause and effect, certainty is not achievable. In a legal text, *proof* has been defined as "anything which serves immediately or mediately to convince the mind of the truth or falsehood of a fact or proposition." The eminent epidemiologist and statistician Bradford Hill advised the use of the following question: "Is there any other way of explaining the facts before us; is there any other answer equally, or more likely than cause and effect?" By these standards the evidence that there is and has been a background incidence of mesothelioma unrelated to the industrial exploitation of asbestos is quite convincing.

## References

1.  Willis RA. Pathology of tumours, 3rd ed. London: Butterworths, 1960:185–650.
2.  Robertson HE. J Cancer Res 1924; 8:317.
3.  Saccone A, Coblenz A. Am J Clin Pathol 1943; 13:188.
4.  Baris Y, Simonato L, Artvini M, Pooley FD, Saracci R, Skidmore J, Wagner JC. Int J Cancer 1987; 39:10.
5.  Gardner MJ, Saracci R. In: Nonoccupational exposure to mineral fibres. IARC Sci Publ 1989; 90:375.
6.  McDonald AD, McDonald JC. Cancer 1980; 46:1650.
7.  Enterline PE, Henderson VL. JNCI 1987; 79:31.

8. McDonald JC, McDonald AD. In: Liddell FDK, Miller K, eds. Mineral fibers and health. Boca Raton: CRC Press, 1991:147.

9. McDonald JC, Armstrong B, Case B, Doell D, McCaughey WTE, McDonald AD, Sebastien P. Cancer 1989; 63:1544.

10. Boutin G, Viallat JR, Steinbauer J, Dufour G, Gaudichet A. In: Nonoccupational exposure to mineral fibres. IARC Sci Publ 1989; 90:406.

11. McConnochie K, Simonato L, Mafrides P, Christofides P, Pooley FD, Wagner JC. Thorax 1987; 42:342.

12. Langer AM, Nolan RP, Constantinopolous SH, Moutsopoulos HM. Lancet 1987; 1:965.

13. Pelnar P. Scand J Work Environ Health 1988; 14:141.

14. Das PB, Fletcher AG, Deodhare SG. Aust NZ J Surg 1976; 46:218.

15. Rothchild H, Mulvey JJ. JNCI 1982; 68:755.

16. Newman RH. Lancet 1983; 2:857.

17. Browne K. J Soc Occup Med 1983; 33:190.

18. Kauffman SL, Stout AP. Cancer 1964; 17:539.

19. Fraire AE, Cooper S, Greenberg SD, Buffler P, Langston C. Cancer 1988; 62:838.

20. McDonald AD, Harper A, El Attar OA, McDonald JC. Cancer 1970; 26:919.

21. Grundy GW, Miller RW. Cancer 1972; 30:1216.

22. Cooper SP, Fraire AE, Buffler PA, Greenberg SD, Langston C. Pathol Immunopathol Res 1989; 8:276.

23. McDonald JC. Environ Health Perspect 1985; 62:316.

24. Connelly RR, Spirtas R, Myers MH, Percy CL, Fraumeni JF. JNCI 1987; 78:1053.

25. Peto J, Henderson BE, Pike MC. Quantification of occupational cancer. Banbury Rep 1981; 9:51.

26. Hirsch A, Brochard P, De Cremoux H, Erkan L, Sebastien P, Di Menza L, Bignon J. Am J Ind Med 1982; 3:413.

27. Peterson JT, Greenberg D, Buffler PA. Cancer 1984; 54:951.

28. McDonald AD, McDonald JC, Pooley FD. Ann Occup Hyg 1982; 26:417.

29. Wagner JC, Pooley FD, Berry G, Seal RME, Munday DE, Morgan J, Clark NJ. Ann Occup Hyg 1982; 26:423.

# 4

## Is There a Genetic Predisposition to Malignant Mesothelioma?

**HENRY T. LYNCH**

Creighton University School of Medicine
Omaha, Nebraska

**HODA ANTON-CULVER
and TOM KUROSAKI**

University of California
Irvine, California

## I. Introduction

A hereditary etiology has been established for a variable subset of virtually all forms of cancer. This includes cancers that involve a strong environmental effect, such as that which occurs with cigarette smoking in cancers of the lung (1), urinary bladder (2,3), and pancreas (4–8). This same phenomenon applies to asbestos exposure and malignant mesothelioma (9), the subject of this chapter.

When environmental effects are extremely pervasive, as in cigarette smoking and asbestos exposure, it is often difficult to ferret out the importance of genetic factors in the particular tumor's etiology. The significance of genetics in cancer's etiology should not be surprising when considering evidence at the biomolecular level when binding levels of benzo[$a$]pyrene to DNA vary 50- to 100-fold in cultured human tissues and cells (10). There is variation in carcinogen metabolism in humans that may be attributed to the fact that most chemical carcinogens require enzymatic activation and, herein, host factors play a major etiological role in determining variation in such enzyme capability (11). The sum total of these effects led Harris et al. to postulate that the ratio of metabolic activation to deactivation of carcinogens may determine the individual's cancer risk (12). This reasoning is in full accord with the concept of *ecogenetics*, an apt term for describing heritable variation in response to environmental exposures, including carcinogens (13). For asbestos, there is no known enzyme activation required for the expression of its carcinogenic properties.

## II. Classification of Mesotheliomas

Ilgren and Wagner (14) provide a broad classification of mesotheliomas in humans, which are similar to those in experimental animals, and is as follows: "(1) spontaneously occurring; (2) those with a latent period less than 10 years; (3) childhood mesotheliomas; (4) *familial cases* [italics ours]; (5) cases before the 20th century; (6) mineralogically negative mesotheliomas; and (7) mesotheliomas caused by nonasbestiform agents."

## III. Environmental Issues

Huncharek (15) has extensively reviewed the subject of environmental factors in malignant mesothelioma. Malignant mesothelioma, a previously relatively rare tumor, has been increasing in incidence during the past two decades and is becoming a relatively common clinical problem. However, our tumor registry data does not indicate such an increase (see subsequent discussion). In addition to the well-recognized risk among asbestos insulation workers, several additional occupational groups, including brake repair and general automobile mechanics, railroad workers, and members of the differing construction trades, where asbestos-containing materials are employed, have shown an excess of mesothelioma. Indoor asbestos exposure is also of concern. For example, two cases of pleural mesothelioma were observed in school teachers, both of whom were exposed to friable ceiling and pipe insulation over the course of many years (16).

The type of asbestos fibers has been meticulously scrutinized to determine which specific type was more closely linked to cancer occurrence. Crocidolite has been frequently suggested as the preponderant form associated with cancer. However, Huncharek (15) concludes that "available data support the idea that all fiber types are capable of inducing malignancy. Although crocidolite may be more potent than chrysotile, it is not unique in its tumorigenic ability. With the widespread use of chrysotile in a multitude of products and applications, it would seem unwise to ignore the potential health risks of chrysotile."

Cigarette smoking significantly increases the risk for lung cancer among patients exposed to asbestos. However, Muscat and Wynder did not find any association between cigarette smoking and mesothelioma for either men or women (17). It is pertinent that in Huncharek's extensive review (15) of the epidemiology and risk groups associated with malignant mesothelioma, there was no mention whatsoever of the potential etiological importance of host factor susceptibility to malignant mesothelioma among these variously exposed individuals. Therefore, it is of interest that the 1980 WHO report stated that there was no evidence for primary host factor effect in malignant mesothelioma (18). These statements are surprising, given the earlier accounts of familial occurrences of malignant mesotheliomas and the animal data on the subject (19,20).

## IV. Animal Studies: Strain Susceptibility to Carcinogen-Induced Mesothelioma

Rice et al. reviewed animal studies of carcinogen-induced mesotheliomas (20). They had noted that certain strains of mice treated intragastrically with methylcholanthrene developed intraperitoneal mesotheliomas. Intraperitoneal injection of asbestos zeolites was shown to have induced mesotheliomas in the peritoneum of mice. In their own studies, these authors examined female mice of six strains (C3H/He, BALB/c, C57BL/6, DBA/2, Swiss, and AKR) employing 3-methylcholanthrene (MC) intragastrically. Half of these mice were pretreated 24 h before methylcholanthrene administration with intraperitoneal $\beta$-naphthoflavone ($\beta$-NF), a noncarcinogenic inducer of certain cytochrome P-450 isozymes. The remaining mice were given olive oil intraperitoneally in a similar manner in the absence of subsequent exposure to MC. Following sacrifice of the mice 18 months after initiation of treatment, practically all of the mice exhibited peritoneal injury, inclusive of inflammation, necrosis, granuloma formation, and mineralization. However, of particular interest to the genetic epidemiology of mesothelioma was the finding that "Mice of some of the strains also presented peritoneal mesotheliomas in addition to a variety of other tumors. The incidence of unequivocal mesothelioma-bearing mice was 12/31 C3H/He and 9/32 BALB/c mice given only MC. The incidence was low in C57BL/6 (1/31) and DBA/2 (1/26), and no definite mesotheliomas were found in Swiss or AKR mice." Therefore, the C3H/He strain showed the greatest incidence of mesotheliomas (12/31) and, interestingly, this strain also had the highest incidence of peritoneal injury (12/31). The authors concluded that the occurrence of intraperitoneal mesotheliomas was, to a certain extent, *strain-dependent*. Furthermore, the MC-induced mesotheliomas of the

Rice et al. experiment were accompanied by varying degrees of chronic peritoneal injury, which appeared to be secondary to the intraperitoneal injections of $\beta$-NF or oil that preceded the intragastric MC treatment (20). The authors concluded, therefore, that nonspecific injury to the mesothelium likely predisposed to the chemical carcinogen causation of neoplasia. Furthermore, they suggested that

> asbestos and related physical agents are not only carcinogenic to the mesothelium, lung, or other tissues per se, but have a syncarcinogenic or tumor-enhancing effect with chemical agents, thus explaining in part the synergism of cigarette smoking and asbestos or mineral dust exposure on lung cancer. Other sources of injury such as lung disease and peritonitis have been cited as possible contributing factors in human mesothelioma. This hypothetical syncarcinogenesis or tumor enhancement could consist of effects prior to carcinogen exposure, setting the stage for tumor initiation; could act cocarcinogenically during chemical exposures; or could act to provide promotional stimuli after initiated cells are in place. Such a role as a promoter of mesothelioma has been proposed by Browne (21).

Given this interesting hypothesis, it must also be realized that a host factor effect, namely, the occurrence of carcinogen-induced mesotheliomas in certain (susceptible) mouse strains (C3H/He and BALB/c), but not in others (resistant; Swiss or AKR), must be entertained. Extrapolation of this reasoning to humans must be done with great caution. However, this reasoning provides useful fodder for developing hypotheses about differences in susceptibility and resistance to carcinogen-induced cancer in humans, comparable with the findings of Harris et al. (10).

## V.  Childhood and Early-Onset Mesotheliomas

In reviewing the pathology of childhood mesothelioma, Cooper et al. conclude that mesothelioma occurs rarely in children and that its diagnosis is exceedingly difficult to establish (22). They note that the available data do not support an association between childhood mesothelioma and asbestos exposure, although this exposure cannot be categorically excluded, particularly in older children for whom there is a potential for longer duration of exposure and, therefore, the possibility of an induction period. They suggest that "mesothelioma in children, as well as in adults, is likely to have a multifactorial etiology. Radiation, prenatal medications, and genetic factors are all possible etiologic agents in childhood mesothelioma." Importantly, these investigators call attention to the need to not only pursue the patient's environment, including prior radiation and medication exposures, both pre- and postnatally to cancer diagnosis, but moreover, that a *family history* of cancer should be obtained.

Kane et al. described ten patients with malignant mesothelioma, aged 40 years or younger at the time of diagnosis (23). The median latency period, namely, the time between initial asbestos exposure and diagnosis of this disease, was 19 years. They emphasized the significance of nonoccupational exposure to asbestos as a probable causative factor and briefly discussed possible *genetic predisposition.*

## VI. Family Studies

Hammar et al. described two families with multiple cases of mesothelioma (24). In one of the families, three brothers, all of whom worked in the asbestos insulation industry, manifested mesothelioma. In the second family, a father, who was occupationally exposed to asbestos, died from a tubulopapillary peritoneal mesothelioma. The authors concluded that genetic factors appeared to be important in the genesis of some occurrences of mesothelioma.

In reviewing the literature on familial mesothelioma through 1989, Hammar et al. (24) noted five reports in which mesotheliomas occurred in two or more family members (9,19,25–27). Interestingly, in most of these reports, those patients who developed mesotheliomas had either occupational or secondary exposure to asbestos. Hammar et al. also note a report suggesting an association with certain human leukocyte antigens (HLA; 24). Lynch et al. described a family in whom two brothers with prolonged occupational exposure to asbestos manifested malignant pleural mesotheliomas of similar histology (9; Fig. 1).

The pathological characteristics in these two brothers showed striking similarities. This was based on our review of the slides from patient II-1 (see Fig. 1). The slides could not be obtained for this patient's brother (II-2); however, our interpretation of the pathology report on this patient led us to conclude that there were very similar structural lesions of the pleural mesothelium in these two brothers.

In reviewing the literature through 1985, we noted similarity in the histology of malignant mesothelioma within several multicase families (9). Table 1 includes the salient findings in the only previously published familial accounts of malignant mesothelioma that provided descriptive histological appearance of the lesions. This table has been updated with inclusion of the Hammar report, which contained two additional families and the Dawson et al. study (see later). In one of these families in the Hammar report,

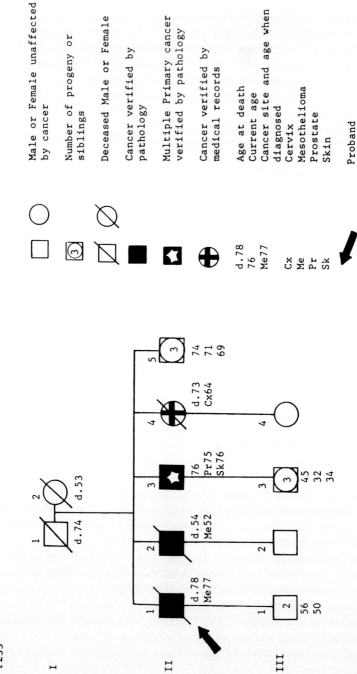

**Figure 1** Pedigree of family showing mesothelioma in two siblings in conjunction with other cancer incidences. (From Ref. 9.)

already mentioned, a father who was occupationally exposed to asbestos died from a tubulopapillary peritoneal mesothelioma and his son died from an identical histological type of peritoneal mesothelioma.

Precerutti et al. described a 40-year-old woman who had not had prior exposure to asbestos and who developed pleural mesothelioma (epithelial type) (28). At thoracotomy, the surgical material, by microscopy, did not contain any asbestos fibers. Of interest was that the patient's father and the father's sister (the patient's paternal aunt) both died from pleural mesotheliomas at the ages of 60 and 65 years, respectively. The patient's paternal grandfather had worked with asbestos and both of his mesothelioma-affected children had been exposed to asbestos, indirectly, during their youth.

Dawson et al. described nine new cases of mesothelioma that clustered in four families (29). Interestingly, all of these families had some degree of exposure to asbestos. Although Lynch et al. (8) and Martensson et al. (24) had suggested that genotypic factors determine host response to the histological pattern of the mesothelioma-prone families, Dawson et al. did not see such an association in their investigation (29). Specifically, their study (which involved transmission electron microscopic examination and energy-dispersive x-ray analysis for quantifying lung mineral content, coupled with a review of the histological diagnosis of their paper to determine whether age of occurrence, site, and histological appearance of mesothelioma occurring in the familial setting differed when compared with non-familial mesotheliomas) failed to show any significant differences either in histological type or in the quantification of long asbestos fiber burden (29).

In addition to the nine new cases that these authors describe, they gathered additional patients from four previously reported families and, thereby, detailed an additional 17 cases of mesothelioma occurring in eight families. This updated the literature to a total of 64 persons with mesothelioma in 27 families. In addition, they reviewed the literature and showed that the "age at which these mesotheliomas occur, their site, and histologic pattern are similar to these characteristics in mesotheliomas occurring in the non-familial setting. We quantified long asbestos fiber burden in 8 cases and found significant levels of amphiboles in them all, despite a potentially misleading history in one case."

In considering similarities and dissimilarities in the histopathology in familial mesothelioma, it is important to realize that environmental factors must be given major consideration. Specifically, familial clustering of any disease, including mesothelioma, may result from pure chance, common environmental exposures or, in certain circumstances, primary genetic factors, or the interaction of environment and genetics in accord with multifactorial etiology. More research will be required to elucidate the relative contributory role of these events in the etiology of mesothelioma.

**Table 1** Familial Mesothelioma

| Author (Ref.) | Relation | Diagnosis | Age at diagnosis | Asbestos exposure Yes/no | Possible source | Duration (yr) | Smoking history Type/amount (per day) | Duration (yr) |
|---|---|---|---|---|---|---|---|---|
| Smith et al. (27) | Brother | Peritoneal mesothelioma (fibromatous type) | 54 | Yes | Application of asbestos lining to piles | 35 | NG/NG | NG |
| | Brother | Peritoneal mesothelioma (fibromatous pattern in some areas and solid epithelial formation in others) | 50 | Yes | Insulation of pipes and boilers with asbestos (exposure to asbestos and its dust) | 36 | NG/NG | NG |
| Li et al. (19) | Father | Pulmonary asbestosis adenocarcinoma of lung | 60 71 | Yes | Pipe insulator (1940–1965) | 25 | Cigarettes, 1–2 packs | 20 |
| | Mother | Mesothelioma of right pleura similar to daughter's | 50 | Yes | From husband's clothing | NG | Nonsmoker | |
| | Daughter | Mesothelioma (mixed pattern of epithelial-type cells with papillary formations) | 34 | Yes | From father's clothing | NG | Cigarettes, 2 | 15 |
| Risberg et al. (26) | Father | Possible "malignant peritoneal mesothelioma" | 61 | Yes | Agricultural worker since "youth," building worker | NG 8 | Cigarettes/ NG | NG |

| | | | | | | | |
|---|---|---|---|---|---|---|---|
| Son | Tubulopapillary mesothelioma | 57 | Yes | Sawmill worker, builder's laborer for rest of life | 2 NG | Cigarettes, 0.5–1 pack | NG |
| Son | Tubulopapillary mesothelioma | 59 | Yes | Builder's laborer, paper industry for "rest of life" | 2 NG | Cigarettes, 0.5–0.75 pack | NG |
| Daughter | Tubulopapillary mesothelioma | 50 | No | | NG | Cigarettes, 0.5–1 pack | NG |
| Son | Tubulopapillary tumor with abundant hyaline stroma | 48 | Yes | Building trade | NG | Cigarettes, 1 pack | NG |
| Hammer et al. (24) Family 1 | | | | | | | |
| Brother | Mesothelioma pleura (mixed papillary epithelial and sarcomatoid appearance) | 66 | Yes | Insulation industry | 46 | Nonsmoker | |
| Brother | Mesothelioma, intra-abdominal (not determined if bowel, pancreas, bile duct, or liver) poorly differentiated epithelial | 54 | Yes | Insulation industry | NG | NG | NG |
| Brother | Mesothelioma, preponderantly sarcomatoid but some epithelial features | 59 | Yes | Insulation industry | NG | NG | NG |

**Table 1** Continued

| Author (Ref.) | Relation | Diagnosis | Age at diagnosis | Asbestos exposure | | | Smoking history | |
|---|---|---|---|---|---|---|---|---|
| | | | | Yes/ no | Possible source | Duration (yr) | Type/ amount (per day) | Duration (yr) |
| | Family 2 | | | | | | | |
| | Father | Peritoneal carcinomatosis, tubulopapillary histology of epithelial mesothelioma; intra-abdominal mesothelioma, diffuse, invading omentum, distinct papillary appearance of a tubulopapillary mesothelioma; no evidence of metastatic renal cell carcinoma | 63 | Yes | Shipyard (had previously resected clear-cell renal carcinoma) | WWII | NG | NG |
| | Son | Intra-abdominal mesothelioma, tubulopapillary histological appearance consistent with epithelial mesothelioma | 40 | NG | NG | NG | NG | NG |
| Precerutti et al. (28) | Daughter | Pleural mesothelioma (epithelial type) | 40 | No | | – | NG | NG |
| | Father | Pleural mesothelioma | 60 | Yes | Father's clothing? | NG | NG | NG |
| | Paternal aunt | Pleural mesothelioma | 65 | Yes | Father's clothing? | NG | NG | NG |

| | Diagnosis | | Asbestos exposure | Occupation | Duration | | |
|---|---|---|---|---|---|---|---|
| **Dawson et al. (43)** | | | | | | | |
| Family A | | | | | | | |
| Brother 1 | Peritoneal epithelial mesothelioma | NG | Yes | Insulation worker | 33 | NG | NG |
| Brother 2 | Peritoneal epithelial mesothelioma | NG | Yes | Insulation worker | NG | NG | NG |
| Family B | | | | | | | |
| Brother 1 | Peritoneal epithelial mesothelioma | NG | Yes | Insulation worker | 5 | NG | NG |
| Brother 2 | Pleural epithelial mesothelioma | NG | Yes | Insulation worker | 5 | NG | NG |
| Brother 3 | Peritoneal epithelial mesothelioma | NG | Yes | Insulation worker | 5 | NG | NG |
| Family C | | | | | | | |
| Brother 1 | Pleural spindle mesothelioma | NG | Yes | Engineer in asbestos factory | 25 | NG | NG |
| Brother 2 | Pleural spindle mesothelioma | NG | Yes | Engineer in asbestos factory | 20 | NG | NG |
| Family D | | | | | | | |
| Brother 1 | Peritoneal epithelial mesothelioma | NG | Yes | Estimator in asbestos factory | 37 | NG | NG |
| Brother 2 | Peritoneal mesothelioma, pattern unknown | NG | Yes | Engineer in asbestos factory | 5 | NG | NG |
| Family E | | | | | | | |
| Brother 1 | Pleural mesothelioma, mixed pattern | NG | Yes | Worker in asbestos factory | 2 | NG | NG |
| Brother 2 | Pleural epithelial mesothelioma | NG | Yes | Toolmaker; parents died of asbestosis | NG | NG | NG |

**Table 1** Continued

| Author (Ref.) Relation | Diagnosis | Age at diagnosis | Asbestos exposure | | | Smoking history | |
| | | | Yes/ no | Possible source | Duration (yr) | Type/ amount (per day) | Duration (yr) |
|---|---|---|---|---|---|---|---|
| **Family F** | | | | | | | |
| Brother | Pleural spindle mesothe-lioma | NG | Yes | Asbestos sheet trim-mer in asbestos-processing plant | 46 | NG | NG |
| Sister | Pleural epithelial meso-thelioma | NG | Yes | Worker in asbestos-processing plant | 8 | NG | NG |
| **Family G** | | | | | | | |
| Father | Pleural mesothelioma, mixed pattern | NG | Yes | Office manager at Wittenoom mine | 10 | NG | NG |
| Son | Pleural epithelial meso-thelioma | NG | Yes | Holidayed at Witten-oom as a child; haulage contractor with asbestos | 3 9 | NG | NG |
| **Family H** | | | | | | | |
| Sister 1 | Pleural spindle mesothe-lioma | NG | NG | NG | NG | NG | NG |
| Sister 2 | Pleural epithelial meso-thelioma | 68 | NG | NG | NG | NG | NG |

NG, not given
*Source:* Ref. 9.

## VII.  Molecular Aspects

Flejter et al. noted recurring loss involving chromosomes 1, 3, and 22 in malignant mesothelioma and, thereby, speculated that these could be potential sites of tumor suppressor genes (30).

Cote et al. examined four mesothelioma cell lines for genetic abnormalities in p53 (31). Their cytogenetic analysis showed that two of the four tumors had abnormalities, within numerical or structural chromosome 17, at the *p53* gene locus. Two tumors had loss of heterozygosity in the region of 17p13. They concluded that " . . . The correlation of chromosomal loss in 17p on the cytogenetic and molecular level along with p53 mRNA expression and DNA sequence data indicate that genetic alterations in p53 could be a feature of malignant mesotheliomas and may reveal an important role of asbestos fibers in tumor suppressor gene inactivation." It would seem prudent to search for genetic alterations in p53 in malignant mesothelioma from familial occurrences of this disease.

## VIII.  A Population-Based Study of Mesothelioma

A population-based study of mesothelioma was conducted using data from the Cancer Surveillance Program of Orange County (CSPOC). Established in 1983, CSPOC was developed as the model registry for implementing the California State legislation that made cancer a reportable disease throughout the state. By California law, any cancers diagnosed among the 2.4 million residents of Orange County at any facility in California must be reported to CSPOC. A description of CSPOC and epidemiological studies that have used these cancer data have been reported (32–35). The total number of cases of mesothelioma ascertained in Orange County from 1984 to 1991 was 145 (122 males and 23 females). During this same 8-year period the total number of invasive lung cancer cases was 9105, and the total number of cases with invasive cancer of all types was 61,132. The annual age-adjusted incidence rate of mesothelioma was 1.67:100,000 in males and 0.24:100,000 in females. There was no time trend in the age-adjusted incidence rate during the study period.

### A.  Tumor Characteristics

Most mesothelioma were located in the pleura (72%), but in 13% of cases, the tumor was in the peritoneum and, in 11% of cases, in the lung. In the remaining 3% of cases, tumors were located in other sites. The histological distribution of mesothelioma was: 70% malignancy, not otherwise specified; 14% epithelial carcinoma; 10% fibrous carcinoma; and 6% biphasic carcinoma.

The anatomical and histological distributions of mesothelioma by gender are shown in Table 2. There was no difference in the anatomical distribution of mesothelioma in males compared with that in females. In patients with epithelial mesothelioma, the proportion of females was greater than that in patients with other histological types of mesothelioma, but this difference was not statistically significant.

Almost all epithelial tumors were located in the pleura (20 of 21, or 95%). For the other histological types of mesothelioma, approximately 70% were located in the pleura. The relation between anatomical site and histological type was statistically significant at $p < 0.01$. In 35 (24%) patients, the stage of disease was localized or with direct extension only. There was regional spread involving lymph nodes in 5 (3%) patients. Metastatic disease was seen in 58 (40%) patients. Cancer was not stageable in 47, or 32%, of cases. In patients with cancer of the lung, the distribution of stage of disease was 22% localized disease or direct extension only, 14% regional disease involving lymph nodes, 45% metastatic disease, and 19% not stageable. In patients with cancer of all types, the distribution of stage of disease was 49% localized disease or direct extension only, 14% regional disease involving lymph nodes, 24% metastatic disease, and 13% not stageable. The majority of mesothelioma and lung cancer cases were diagnosed at advanced stages of disease.

Females were diagnosed at an earlier stage of disease than males. In

**Table 2**  Anatomical and Histological Distributions of Mesothelioma by Gender, Orange County, California 1984–1991

|  | Males ($n = 122$) | Females ($n = 23$) |
|---|---|---|
| Anatomical site |  |  |
| Pleura | 88 (72%) | 17 (74%) |
| Peritoneum | 16 (13%) | 3 (13%) |
| Lung | 14 (11%) | 2 (9%) |
| Other Site | 4 (3%) | 1 (4%) |
| Histological type |  |  |
| Epithelial | 16 (13%) | 5 (22%) |
| Fibrous | 12 (10%) | 2 (9%) |
| Malignant, NOS | 87 (71%) | 15 (65%) |
| Biphasic | 7 (6%) | 1 (4%) |

**Table 3** Ethnic Distribution of Patients with Mesothelioma, Lung Cancer, and Cancers of All Types, Orange County, California 1984-1991

| Ethnic group | Mesothelioma ($n = 145$) | Lung cancer ($n = 9,105$) | All cancers ($n = 61,132$) |
|---|---|---|---|
| Non–Hispanic | 128 (88%) | 8,359 (92%) | 54,010 (88%) |
| Hispanic | 7 (5%) | 320 (4%) | 3,771 (6%) |
| Asian/Pacific Islander | 8 (6%) | 259 (3%) | 2,158 (4%) |
| Other | 2 (1%) | 167 (2%) | 1,193 (2%) |

males 20% (25 of 122) were diagnosed with localized disease or direct extension only. In females, however, 43% (10 of 23) were diagnosed with localized disease or direct extension only. The association between gender and stage of disease was statistically significant, $p < 0.018$.

### B. Ethnicity

The ethnic distribution of patients with mesothelioma, lung cancer, and cancers of all types is shown in Table 3. The ethnic distribution in mesothelioma cases is similar to the ethnic distribution of all cancer patients and of lung cancer cases. The mesothelioma cases are representative of the total population of cancer in Orange County.

### C. Age

The age distribution of mesothelioma cancer cases is shown in Table 4. Included also are the age distributions of cases of lung cancer and of patients with cancers of all types. These data show the age distribution of

**Table 4** Age Distribution of Patients with Mesothelioma, Lung Cancer, and Cancers of All Types

| Age | Mesothelioma | Lung cancer | All cancers |
|---|---|---|---|
| <25 | 0 (0%) | 6 (0%) | 1,326 (2%) |
| 25–34 | 2 (1%) | 46 (1%) | 2,331 (4%) |
| 35–44 | 9 (6%) | 210 (2%) | 4,023 (7%) |
| 45–54 | 15 (10%) | 956 (10%) | 6,841 (11%) |
| 55–64 | 39 (27%) | 2,505 (28%) | 13,061 (21%) |
| 65–74 | 40 (28%) | 3,140 (34%) | 17,370 (28%) |
| 75–84 | 38 (26%) | 1,821 (20%) | 12,161 (20%) |
| 85+ | 2 (1%) | 421 (5%) | 4,019 (7%) |

mesothelioma cancer cases to be similar to that of all cancer patients and of lung cancer cases in the population.

Eight of 23, or 35%, of female patients were diagnosed before age 60, whereas in males, 35 of 122, or 29%, were diagnosed before age 60. However, the mean age at diagnosis and standard deviation were 65.0 + 12.5 in men and 64.9 + 13.6 in women.

Ethnic minorities (nonwhites) tended to have disease at a younger age than non-Hispanic whites. Only 27% of non-Hispanic whites were diagnosed at younger than 60 years of age compared with 43% of nonwhites. The mean age at diagnosis and standard deviation were 65.8 + 12.1 in non-Hispanic whites and 59.4 + 15.5 in nonwhites; the difference in means was statistically significant at the 0.0489 level.

Among patients younger than 60 years of age, the proportion having either localized disease or direct extension only was 33% (14 of 43). In patients 60 years of age or older, the proportion having "early" disease was 21% (21 of 102). This difference was not statistically significant.

### D.  Occupation

The distribution of occupation in patients with mesothelioma, lung cancer, and cancers of all types are shown in Table 5. It is of interest that the occupational distributions show a greater proportion of blue-collar and service workers among the mesothelioma cases than seen in the lung cancer cases and in all cancer patients. Perhaps the similarity seen in the distributions of occupation between lung cancer cases and all cancer patients may be because smoking is a major risk factor for lung and other malignancies in both occupational groups. On the other hand the increased proportion of blue-collar and service workers in mesothelioma cases may indicate the importance of occupation as a risk factor for mesothelioma, and that smoking plays a much smaller role in its etiology.

The proportion of women patients among cases who were employed in white-collar occupations was 12% (5 of 43) compared with 2% (1 out of 44) among cases who were employed in blue-collar and service occupations. This difference was marginally significant ($p < 0.085$).

**Table 5**  Distribution of Occupation in Patients with Mesothelioma, Lung Cancer, and Cancers of All Types

|                       | Mesothelioma | Lung cancer   | All cancers    |
| --------------------- | ------------ | ------------- | -------------- |
| White-collar          | 43 (49%)     | 2,443 (62%)   | 16,937 (73%)   |
| Blue-collar or service | 44 (51%)     | 1,471 (38%)   | 6,357 (27%)    |

**Table 6** Explicit Statement of "Exposure to Asbestos" in the Medical Chart of Mesothelioma Patients

| Statement | Male | Female |
|---|---|---|
| "Exposure to asbestos" | 52 (43%) | 2 (9%) |
| "No asbestos exposure" | 12 (10%) | 3 (13%) |
| No mention of asbestos exposure | 58 (48%) | 18 (78%) |

Information relating to asbestos exposure was abstracted from hospital medical charts as part of the cancer patient abstract. The results of reviewing cancer abstracts of all mesothelioma cases are shown in Table 6. In the majority of female cases, data on asbestos exposure was not in the hospital medical chart. In male mesothelioma cases, however, there was an explicit statement of asbestos exposure in 52 cases, and in 12 there was an explicit statement of no asbestos exposure.

### E. Smoking

Twenty-eight percent of mesothelioma cases were nonsmokers, with 72% having a positive smoking history (23% current and 49% former smokers). This contrasts with the smoking history of lung cancer cases—only 7% were nonsmokers and the proportions of current and former smokers were 66 and 27%, respectively. The distribution of smoking in all cancer patients was 40% nonsmokers, 39% current smokers, and 21% former smokers. Risk of mesothelioma is associated with smoking, however, to a far lower degree than the risk of lung cancer from smoking.

Surprisingly, a greater proportion of women with mesothelioma (83%, or 15 of 18) had a history of cigarette smoking than male mesothelioma patients (69%, or 51 of 74); however, the difference in proportions was not statistically significant.

Smoking was more prevalent in patients with mesothelioma of the peritoneum (89%) and lung (83%) compared with those with mesothelioma of the pleura (68%). The association between smoking and anatomical site was not statistically significant. Although the frequency of nonsmokers in patients with epithelial mesothelioma (35%) was greater than that in patients with either fibrous (12%) or unspecified malignancies (25%), this difference was not statistically significant. Stage of disease was not associated with smoking history: in nonsmokers the proportion diagnosed with localized disease or direct extension only was 19% (5 of 26) compared with 29% (19 of 66) in patients who were either current or former smokers.

### F.  Family History of Cancer

In 27 of 63 mesothelioma patients (43%) there was a positive history of a primary invasive cancer of all types in one or more first-degree relatives. Among the 12 female cases, there were 5 patients (42%) in whom cancer was reported in one or more first-degree relatives. In the 51 male cases, there were 22 patients (43%) in whom cancer was reported in one or more first-degree relatives. Lung cancer in a first-degree relative was reported in 4 of the 51 male probands (8%). Lung cancer in a first-degree relative was not reported in any of the 12 female patients. Family history of mesothelioma was not found in any of the 63 cases for whom a family history of cancer was ascertained. Data on a family history of cancer in patients with mesothelioma, lung cancer, and cancers of all types are shown in Table 7. Among lung cancer probands, 41% reported a history of cancer in a first-degree relative, whereas 10% reported a history of lung cancer in a first-degree relative. In Orange County patients who were diagnosed with cancer of all types, 40% reported a positive family history of any cancer, and 6% reported a family history of lung cancer in a first-degree relative.

### G.  Family History of Cancer and Its Relation to Tumor Characteristics and Other Risk Factors

Twenty-seven of 63 mesothelioma patients (43%) reported a positive history of primary invasive cancer of all types in one or more first-degree relatives.

The proportion of cases of mesothelioma of the pleura who had a positive family history of cancer in at least one first-degree relative was 42% (20 of 48). Among cases of mesothelioma of the peritoneum, the proportion of such cases was 62% (5 of 8). These data are shown in Table 8.

Table 8 also shows the distribution of mesothelioma cases who have one or more first-degree relatives with cancer by histological type. In patients with epithelial mesothelioma, there was an increased proportion who had a positive family history of cancer compared with that of patients

**Table 7**  Family History of Cancer in Patients with Mesothelioma, Lung Cancer, and Cancers of All Types, Orange County, California 1984–1991

| Cancer in first-degree relatives | Mesothelioma | Lung cancer | All cancers |
|---|---|---|---|
| Any cancer | 27/63 = 43% | 1287/3121 = 41% | 5398/13,544 = 40% |
| Lung cancer | 4/63 = 6% | 307/3121 = 10% | 764/13,544 = 6% |
| Mesothelioma | 0/63 = 0% | 1/3121 = 0.03% | 4/13,544 = 0.03% |

**Table 8** Distribution of Mesothelioma Cases
with One or More First-Degree Relatives with
Cancer and Histological Type

|  | Proportion of familial mesothelioma |
|---|---|
| Anatomical site | |
| Pleura | 20/48 = 42% |
| Peritoneum | 5/8 = 62% |
| Lung | 2/6 = 33% |
| Other sites | 0/1 = 0% |
| Histological type | |
| Epithelial | 6/9 = 67% |
| Fibrous | 3/8 = 38% |
| Malignant, NOS | 18/42 = 43% |
| Biphasic | 0/4 = 0% |

with all other histological types of mesothelioma, but the difference in proportions was not statistically significant.

In patients with a family history of cancer the disease was not diagnosed at an earlier stage than in those with a negative family history of cancer. Family history of cancer and the age which it was diagnosed were not associated. The distributions of stage of disease and age at diagnosis by family history of cancer was shown in Table 9.

Among the 15 patients who were nonsmokers, the proportion who had a family history of cancer was 33% (5 of 15). In the 45 patients who were either current or former smokers, 21 (47%) had a positive family history of cancer. The difference in proportions of those who had a family history of cancer was not statistically significant.

**Table 9** Stage of Disease and Age at Diagnosis in Relation to Family
History of Cancer

| Family history of cancer | Stage of disease (proportion of localized disease or direct extension only) | Age at diagnosis (proportion younger than 60 years of age) |
|---|---|---|
| No family history | 9/36 = 25% | 10/36 = 28% |
| Positive family history | 6/27 = 22% | 7/27 = 26% |

## IX.  Discussion

The etiological link between asbestos exposure and mesothelioma was firmly established in 1960 by Wagner et al. (36). This was based on 33 cases of diffuse pleural mesothelioma from the North Western Cape Province of South Africa. All 33 patients had contact with asbestos. The crocidolite type of asbestos is mined in this area of South Africa. Two years following this report, mesothelioma was found to be associated with asbestosis in Western Australia (37) where crocidolite asbestos is mined. Subsequently, Selikoff et al. reviewed the relation between exposure to asbestos and mesothelioma in a study of 307 consecutive deaths (1943–1964) among asbestos insulation workers in New York and New Jersey (38). They found ten deaths caused by mesothelioma of the pleura (four cases) or peritoneum (six cases). They concluded that " . . . mesothelioma must be added to the neoplastic risks of asbestos in insulation showing lung cancer (53 of 307 deaths) and probably cancer of the stomach and colon (34 of 307 deaths) as a significant complication of such industrial exposure in the United States." However, family histories were *not* reported in these early studies.

Domestic exposure to asbestos among women residing in the same houses as asbestos workers was described by Lillington et al. (39). In one such example, there was a case of connubial mesothelioma. Herein, the husband developed mesothelioma following industrial exposure to asbestos, and his wife's mesothelioma was attributed to asbestos exposure that occurred from washing her husband's dusty clothes. Similar domestic exposure to asbestos, with subsequent mesothelioma among household contacts, was described by Anderson et al. (40).

Ottee et al. described three members of a family (father, mother, son) who died of mesothelioma secondary to exposure from an asbestos cement product that was manufactured in their home (41). In addition, Driscoll et al. described five patients with malignant mesothelioma who were members of a Native American pueblo of 2000 persons wherein asbestos had been routinely used in the production of silver jewelry (42).

Baris et al. described endemic malignant mesotheliomas in two villages in Turkey, namely Karain and Tuzkoy (43). Clumps of asbestiform fibers were found in the water from the old wells of Karain. Interestingly, 11 of 18 deaths in Karain during 1974, when the population was only 604, were due to malignant pleural mesothelioma. The investigators found fibers of respirable sizes in rock samples and field soils of Karain. The fibers were found to be erionite-type zeolite through x-ray diffraction and analytic transmission electron microscopy studies. Interestingly, a pedigree referred to as the Sencan family, which included a sister (age 52) and a brother (age 44) with pleural mesothelioma, was described. The brother's spouse had mesothelioma at age 54. Unfortunately, details on the pathology of these lesions were not provided.

In the second town (Tuzkoy), there were reportedly 1125 individuals older than 25 years. Endemic cases of calcified plaques and pleural thickening or fibrous pleuritis, as well as clustered cases of pleural and peritoneal mesothelioma and other types of cancers were observed. These diseases were not found in a control village 5 km from Tuzkoy. As in Karain, many fibers of respirable sizes were found in the rock samples, street, and field soils, which were erionite-type zeolite. Significantly, these fibers were found in the lung tissues of a patient diagnosed with fibrous pleuritis. Finally, the authors called attention to positive family histories of malignant pleural mesothelioma and other neoplastic diseases among residents of Karain and Tuzkoy. However, with the exception of the single pedigree (Sencan family), details on this subject were lacking.

Lynch et al. were the first to call attention to the familial similarity in the histological types of malignant mesotheliomas, examples of which are found in Table 1 (9). It will be important to gather more data on the pathology of malignant mesotheliomas in families to test the hypothesis of histopathological specificity of the gene in certain of the familial occurrences of mesothelioma.

### Acknowledgments

I deeply appreciate the excellent typing of the manuscript and all of the technical assistance provided by my secretary, Bonnie Adamson.

Cancer incidence data have been collected under subcontract 050H-8710 with the California Public Health Foundation. The subcontract is supported by the California Department of Health Services as part of its statewide cancer-reporting program, mandated by Health and Safety Code Section 210 and 211.3. The ideas and opinions expressed herein are those of the authors, and no endorsement of the State of California, Department of Health Services, or the California Public Health Foundation is intended or should be inferred. The authors wish to thank all staff of the Cancer Surveillance Program of Orange County (CSPOC) for their contributions to the collection and processing of cancer incidence data.

### References

1. Lynch HT, Kimberling WJ, Markvicka SE. Cancer 1986; 57:1640.
2. Lynch HT. Cancer genetics. Springfield, IL: Charles C Thomas, 1976.
3. Lynch HT, Kimberling WJ, Lynch JF, Brennan K. Cancer Genet Cytogenet 1987; 27:161.

4. Danes BS, Lynch HT. JAMA 1982; 247:2798.
5. Lynch HT, Voorhees GJ, Lanspa SJ, McGreevy PS, Lynch JF. Br J Cancer 1985; 52:271.
6. Lynch HT, Fitzsimmons ML, Smyrk TC, Lanspa SJ, Watson P, McClellan K, Lynch JF. Am J Gastroenterol 1990; 85:54.
7. Lynch HT, Fusaro RM. Pancreas 1991; 6:127.
8. Lynch HT, Fusaro L, Lynch JF. Pancreas 1992; 7:511.
9. Lynch HT, Katz D, Markvicka SE. Cancer Genet Cytogenet 1985; 15:25.
10. Harris CC, Mulvihill JJ, Thorgeirsson SS, Minna JD. Ann Intern Med 1980; 92:809.
11. Khouri RE. Genetic differences in chemical carcinogenesis. Boca Raton: CRC Press, 1978.
12. Harris CC, Autrup H, Stoner G. In: T'so PO, Gelboin HV, eds. Polycyclic hydrocarbons and cancer: chemistry, molecular biology, and environment. New York: Academic Press, 1981:331.
13. Mulvihill JJ. JNCI 1976; 57:307.
14. Ilgren EB, Wagner JC. Regul Toxicol Pharmacol 1991; 13:133.
15. Huncharek M. Cancer 1992; 69:2704.
16. Huncharek M, Muscat J. Thorax 1987; 42:897.
17. Muscat JE, Wynder EL. Cancer Res 1991; 51:2263.
18. Hirayama T, Waterhouse JAH, Faumeni JF. Cancer risks by site, vol 41. Geneva: UICC technical report series.
19. Li FP, Lokich J, Lapey J. JAMA 1978; 240:467.
20. Rice JM, Kovatch RM, Anderson LM. J Toxicol Environ Health 1989; 27: 153.
21. Browne K. Arch Environ Health 1983; 38:261.
22. Cooper SP, Fraire AE, Buffler PA, Greenberg SD, Langston C. Pathol Immunopathol Res 1989; 8:276.
23. Kane MJ, Chahinian AP, Holland JF. Cancer 1990; 65:1449.
24. Hammar SP, Bockus D, Remington F, Freidman S, Lazerte G. Hum Pathol 1989; 20:107.
25. Martensson G, Larsson S, Zettergren L. Eur J Respir Dis 1984; 65:179.
26. Risberg B, Nickels J, Wagermark J. Cancer 1980; 45:2422.
27. Smith PG, Higgins MCR, Park WD. Br J Surg 1968; 55:681.
28. Precerutti JA, Mayorga M, Dalurzo L, Pallotta G, de la Canal A. Hum Pathol 1990; 21:983.
29. Dawson A, Gibbs A, Browne K, Pooley F, Griffiths M. Cancer 1992; 70: 1183.
30. Flejter WL, Li FP, Antman KH, Testa JR. Genes Chrom Cancer 1989; 1:148.
31. Cote RJ, Jhanwar SC, Novick S, Pellicer A. Cancer Res 1991; 51:5410.
32. Anton-Culver H, Culver BD, Kurosaki T, Osann KE, Lee JB. Cancer Res 1988; 48:6580.
33. Anton-Culver H. J Am Coll Toxicol 1989; 8:933.
34. Anton-Culver H, Bloss JD, Bringman D, Lee-Feldstein A, DiSaia P, Manetta A. Am J. Obstet Gynecol 1992; 166:1507.

35. Anton-Culver H, Lee-Feldstein A, Taylor TH. Am J Epidemiol 1992; 136:89.
36. Wagner JCJ, Sleggs CA, Marchand P. Br J Ind Med 1960; 17:260.
37. McNulty JC. Med J Aust 1962; 2:953.
38. Selikoff IJ, Churg J, Hammond EC. N Engl J Med 1965; 272:560.
39. Lillington GA, Jamplis RW, Differding JR. N Engl J Med 1974; 291:583.
40. Anderson HA, Lilis R, Daum SM, Fischbein AS, Selikoff I. Ann NY Acad Sci 1976; 270:311.
41. Ottee KE, Sigsgaard TI, Kjaerfulff. Br J Ind Med 1990; 47:10.
42. Driscoll RJ, Mulligan WJ, Schultz D, Candelaris A. N Engl J Med 1988; 318: 1437.
43. Baris YI, Artvinili M, Sahin AA. Ann NY Acad Sci 1979; 330:423.

# 5

## Clinical Diagnosis of Pleural Malignancies

**CHRISTIAN BOUTIN, J.-R. VIALLAT, FRANÇOISE REY, and PHILIPPE ASTOUL**

Hôpital de la Conception
Marseille, France

## I. Introduction

Malignant mesothelioma is a disease for which no treatment has been effective (1,2). Death usually occurs within about 1 year after diagnosis. Perhaps because of this poor prognosis, early screening has incited little interest. This pessimistic view omits the fact that certain forms may have a better prognosis when diagnosed early and treated by radio-, chemo-, or immunotherapy.

Diagnosis depends mostly on histological findings. In the past, histologists were reluctant to advance a diagnosis without an autopsy report to bolster their findings. Nowadays, with the increased incidence of this disease and the availability of immunolabeling, pathologists are more forthcoming, although they still hide their incertitudes behind the cover of a "panel."

The factors influencing prognosis have been elucidated by statistical analysis of survival data from several large series. As a result, practitioners now have the ability to classify and follow-up mesothelioma patients.

## II.  Diagnosis of Malignant Mesothelioma of the Pleura

### A.  Symptoms and Signs

The mean age at diagnosis of mesothelioma is 60 years. However, onset as early as the fourth decade can be observed in subjects with a history of exposure to asbestos during childhood.

Asbestos exposure has been reported in 20–90% of cases (mean: 70%). This wide range of variation is due to differences in the occupational or environmental criteria used in various studies and to the importance of industrial use of asbestos in the regions where these studies were conducted. Calcified plaques have rarely been observed. Previous radiotherapy has sometimes been noted (3), as in two cases in our series.

The incidence of mesothelioma is much higher in men. This is probably because exposure to asbestos at the worksite is less common in women.

At the onset of the disease, functional or general manifestations are nonspecific. Pleural effusion is not especially large or painful at the beginning and, in many cases, radiography fails to detect any mass. In nonpleural tumoral forms, localized pain, which is often moderate, is the most frequent first symptom.

Since mesothelioma has no characteristic clinical manifestations, this diagnosis should always be considered in any patient with signs in the pleural region. Negative histological findings do not rule out mesothelioma. Systematic screening allowed detection of 3% of the patients in the Ruffie et al. series (4). In our series of 180 patients, 88% had chronic pleurisy, 2% had purulent pleurisy, 1% had spontaneous pneumothorax, and 9% had unproductive nodular pleural images.

When pleural fluid is present at the onset, the specificity of a computed tomography (CT) scan is limited. A CT scan is more precise if the fluid is removed, but it is most useful for subsequent follow-up. The CT scan images are variable. In our series, 40% had fibrohyalin or calcified plaques. Up to double this amount has been reported by other authors. Pleural effusion is a frequent finding, but at first it is not especially large and is indistinguishable from that accompanying other types of pleurisy.

A decrease in the diameter of the affected hemithorax is frequent with mesothelioma, but this finding is also associated with infectious pleurisy. Mediastinal changes are more specific: uneven, nodular thickening of the mediastinal pleura, pericardial pleura, hilus, and its lymph nodes. As will be discussed further on, mediastinal status is an important factor in staging the disease. Mediastinal changes develop at an advanced stage of mesothelioma and are a highly unfavorable prognostic feature.

Needle biopsy under CT scan control is of limited sensitivity, since sample volume is usually too small for histological assessment. Moreover, this examination often leads to tumoral invasion of the chest wall.

### B. Diagnostic Criteria

Biopsy is the most reliable diagnostic method; however, it is highly dependent on the method of sample collection. The reported sensitivity of pleural fluid cytology ranges from zero to 64%. Likewise, the sensitivity of needle biopsy varies from 6 to 38%. Herbert and Gallacher claimed that the value of both these methods was limited and advocated surgical biopsy (5). With thoracoscopy we have achieved results similar to those of surgery and better than cytology or Abrams biopsy (Table 1) (6).

Regretfully, thoracoscopy, which is a simple and safe examination, is not used more often for diagnosis of mesothelioma. In terms of the reliability of histological diagnosis, the tissue specimens obtained by thoracoscopy are as valuable as those obtained by thoracotomy, which is far more invasive. Thoracoscopy is indicated in practically every suspected case of mesothelioma. In most of the patients in our series, the pleura was free or presented only localized fibrous adhesions that did not hamper thoracoscopy. In only nine patients were adhesions so extensive that thoracotomy was required to establish diagnosis.

In 85% of cases, endoscopy revealed nodes or masses ranging from a few millimeters to 10 cm in diameter. In most patients these nodules and masses were associated with thickening of the pleura by as much as several centimeters. In one of five patients the nodules were small (i.e., 1-5 mm).

The typical endoscopic appearance of a mesothelioma mass is a clear or yellowish white, translucent, smooth pedunculated or sessile nodules, 5-20 mm in diameter. However, this so-called grapelike aspect is not absolutely specific, since it has also been observed in 3% of metastatic pleural tumors.

**Table 1** Diffuse Malignant Mesothelioma
Sensitivity of Diagnostic Methods[a]

| Method | No. patients (%) | |
| --- | --- | --- |
| Fluid cytology | 35/152 | (23) |
| Abrams needle biopsy | 33/135 | (24) |
| Thoracoscopy | 148/157 | (93) |
| Surgery | 9/9 | (100) |

[a]Thoracoscopic biopsy was positive in every case in which it was feasible. Thus, sensitivity was 100 in 148 patients. Thoracoscopy was unfeasible in nine cases, and surgery was necessary to establish diagnosis.

In 10–15% of patients, thoracoscopy revealed no distinctive macroscopic lesions, but rather, a simple inflammation of the pleural cavity. Inflammation was sometimes associated with lymphangitis.

An important diagnostic criteria is the status of the visceral pleura and lung, which can be visualized through the thoracoscope. Involvement of the visceral pleura, especially at the onset of the disease, is always much more limited than that of the parietal pleura. Nodules in the visceral pleura are always fewer and smaller. In 23 patients the visceral pleura appeared macroscopically normal, and the results of systematic biopsy were negative.

### C.  Preventive Local Radiotherapy

To prevent spreading along the pathway of the trocar or drain, we wait 10–12 days to allow the incisions to heal and then perform radiotherapy at 12.5–15 MeV on the chest wall: 21 Gy are applied over a 48-h period in three sessions, average penetration is 3 cm. The sides of the field are 4–12 cm at the site of the drain and puncture.

We assessed this preventive treatment in a series of 40 patients with mesothelioma who were randomly distributed into two equal groups. One group underwent radiotherapy after thoracoscopy and the other did not. Of the 20 treated patients, none developed nodules along the pathway of the drain or trocar: of the 20 untreated patients, 9 developed such nodules. Following this study we began performing preventive radiotherapy systematically after diagnostic thoracoscopy in mesothelioma patients and have not observed any nodules since then.

### III.  Prognosis of Mesothelioma

Prognosis depends on numerous factors that have been studied separately or in multiple correlation studies (Cox model).

### A.  Histological Type

The histological type appears to be important. Epithelial or mixed forms have a better prognosis than fibrosarcomatous forms. Mean survival is 10–17 months for the former patients and 4–7 months for the latter.

### B.  Disease Stage

Disease staging is useful, not only to establish prognosis, but also to allow evaluation of the effectiveness of treatment. The first classification was that of Butchart et al. (7) that includes four stages (Table 2). Survival and prognostic factors published by others are given in Tables 2 and 3 (2,7–13).

**Table 2** Survival According to the Staging of Mesothelioma

| | Butchart (7) | | Antman (8) | | Brenner (9) | | Alberts (2) | |
|---|---|---|---|---|---|---|---|---|
| Stage | n | Survival (mo) | n | Survival (mo) | n | Survival (mo) | n | Survival (mo) |
| Stage I<br>Localized tumor in the homolateral pleura | 13 | 17 | 31 | 16 | 62 | 13 | 202 | 11 |
| Stage II<br>Involvement of mediastinal organs or of the wall or of the contralateral pleura | 4 | 11 | 4 | 9 | 52 | 11 | 35 | 8 |
| Stage III<br>Subdiaphragmatic extension | 2 | 9 | 5 | 5 | 7 | 4 | 13 | 7 |
| Stage IV<br>Remote metastasis | 0 | | 2 | 4 | 0 | | 12 | 2 |

Only patients in the first stages are eligible for treatment. In stage II, the chest wall or mediastinum is involved, with or without mediastinal adenopathy. In all classification systems, late-stage mesothelioma is fatal in from a few weeks to 4 or 5 months.

Although a coherent classification system is difficult to design and is of little clinical value for advanced stages of the disease, we propose the following stages (14):

*Stage I:*   A. Unilateral involvement of the parietal or diaphragmatic pleura
        B. Additional involvement of the visceral pleura on the same side
*Stage II:*  A. Homolateral involvement of the chest wall or mediastinum, or both
        B. Contralateral involvement of the pleura or mediastinum, or both
*Stage III:* Extrathoracic involvement, subclavicular lymph nodes, transdiaphragmatic peritoneal involvement
*Stage IV:* Remote involvement and metastasis

We stage all our patients according to this classification. Thoracoscopy is used to demonstrate involvement of the visceral pleura, which can

**Table 3**  Prognosis of Pleural Mesothelioma (Multifactorial Analysis): Favorable Prognostic Factors

| | Chahinian (10) | Alberts (2) | Antman (11) | Calvrezos (12) | Spirta (13) | Ruffie (4) |
|---|---|---|---|---|---|---|
| Year | 1982 | 1988 | 1988 | 1988 | 1988 | 1989 |
| Number of cases | 57 | 262 | 136 | 93 | 1137 | 118 |
| Sex | | | | | F | |
| Age | <65 yr | | <50 yr | <50 yr | <50 yr | |
| Sl-Dg[a] | | >6 mo | >6 mo | | | |
| Histology | Epithelial | | Epithelial | Epithelial | | |
| Stage | | I | I | I | Localized | I |
| PS[b] | | 0–1 | 0–1 | 0–1 | | |
| Chest pain | | | Absent | Absent | | |
| Previous exposure to asbestos | | | | | | Absent |
| Platelets | <400 000 | | | | | <400 000 |
| Race | | White | | | | |

[a]Delay between first sign and diagnosis.
[b]Performance status.

be clearly visualized. Until the CT scan became available in 1976, front radiographic views were used to assess the chest wall and mediastinum. Classification into stages III and IV poses no particular problem.

The mean survival for patients in stage IA was 30 months compared with only 8 for patients in stage IB; thus, involvement of the visceral pleura (and lung) is an unfavorable prognostic factor. In stage II patients with involvement of the mediastinum, survival is practically the same as in stage IB. This suggests that mediastinal involvement appears rapidly after involvement of the lung or even without involvement of the lung.

The advantage of thoracoscopy over CT scan is to accurately detect visceral pleura involvement at the onset of the disease and to allow early differential diagnosis. Conversely, a CT scan is more effective for detection of involvement of the mediastinal pleura and for follow-up. These two examinations are complementary for prognostic classification of patients.

### C.  Other Prognostic Factors

Several other prognostic factors have been assessed by multifactorial analysis (see Table 3). Most are of little clinical value. However, it is noteworthy that survival does appear to be longer in women older than 50 years who have not been exposed to asbestos. Survival is also longer in subjects with no previous medical history, no chest pain, and no elevated platelet level.

## IV. Conclusions

The incidence of malignant mesothelioma is increasing. Prognosis is poor, average survival after diagnosis being about 12 months. Survival might be longer if diagnosis is made early. This possibility raises several questions. How can early diagnosis be achieved in these patients who account for 10% of all patients with cancer-related pleural effusion? Can therapy really prolong survival at this stage of the disease? Are surgery, chemotherapy, and immunotherapy effective at the onset of the disease?

## V. Summary

Early diagnosis of mesothelioma depends on simple clinical findings, including recent pleuritis; previous asbestos exposure; chest pain, weight loss (usually moderate), and advancing radiographic abnormalities. The sensitivity of laboratory tests is low: 23% for pleural fluid cytology and 24% for Abrams needle biopsy. Thoracoscopy is conclusive in 93%, failing only in patients with adhesive pleuritis or having undergone symphysis.

In general prognosis is better in female patients younger than 50, with no history of asbestos exposure, in good overall condition, and without chest pain.

## References

1. Chahinian AP. In: Chretien J, Hirsch A, eds. Diseases of the pleura. New York: Masson, 1983:224.
2. Alberts AS, Falkson G, Goedhals L, Vorobiof DA, Van Der Merwe CA. J Clin Oncol 1988; 6:527.
3. Antman KH, Corson JM, FP. J Clin Oncol 1983; 1:695.
4. Ruffie P, Feld R, Minkin Q, Cormier Y, Boutan-Laroze A, Ginsberg R, Ayoub J, Shepherd FA, Evans WK, Figueredo A, Pater JL, Pringle JF, Kreisman H. J Clin Oncol 1989; 7:1157.
5. Herbert A, Gallagher PJ. Thorax 1982; 37:816.
6. Boutin C, Viallat JR, Rey F. In: Antman K, Aisner J, eds. Asbestos related malignancy. New York: Grune & Stratton, 1986:301.
7. Butchart EG, Ashcroft T, Barnsley WC, Holden MP. Thorax 1976; 31:15.
8. Antman KH. N Engl J Med 1980; 303:200.
9. Brenner J, Sordillo PP, Magill GB. N Engl J Med 1980; 49:2431.
10. Chahinian AP, Pajak TF, Holland JF, Norton L, Ambinder RM, Mandel EM. Ann Intern Med 1982; 96:746.

11. Antman K, Shemin R, Ryan L, Klegar K, Osteen R, Herman T, Lederman G, Corson J. J Clin Oncol 1988; 6:147.
12. Calavrezos A, Koschel G, Husselmann H, Taylessani A, Heilmann HP, Fabel H, Schmoll HJ, Dietrich H, Hain E. Klin Wochenschir 1988; 66:607.
13. Spirtas R, Connelly RR, Tucker MA. Int J Cancer 1988; 41:525.
14. Boutin C, Rey F, Gouvernet J, Viallat JR, Astoul P, Ledoray V. Cancer 1993; 72:394.

# 6

## The Pathogenesis of Malignant and Nonmalignant Serosal Lesions in Body Cavities Consequent to Asbestos Exposure

**JOHN E. CRAIGHEAD**

University of Vermont
Burlington, Vermont

**AGNES B. KANE**

Brown University
Providence, Rhode Island

## I. Natural History of Human Malignant Mesothelioma

Malignant mesothelioma (MM) is a unique, uncommon tumor of mesenchymal origin. Although most tumors occur in the pleural and peritoneal cavities, MM occasionally develops in the pericardial sac and tunica vaginalis (1,2). These lesions are morphologically diverse. Malignant mesothelioma usually presents clinically when the tumor mass is bulky and has spread widely to encompass the organs of the body cavity. At this time, symptomatic effusions of serous or serosanguinous fluid accumulate. Recent studies strongly suggest that a vascular leakage factor (3,4), generated by the tumor cells, contributes to the formation of effusions (unpublished data). Most of the tumors in major body cavities result from exposure to asbestos, but roughly 20–40% develop spontaneously and are of unknown etiology, or are consequent to therapeutic irradiation (5). Our attention in this review will focus on the pathogenesis of the asbestos-induced lesions since little is known about the cause of the remaining tumors.

Epidemiological studies of workers and family members exposed to asbestos provide clues to the origin of this tumor. Presumably, MM can develop from a single or limited exposure to asbestos fibers, but the prevalence of tumors increases in rough proportion to the duration and intensity of exposure. Characteristically, MMs have a long latency period, ranging from 15 to 50 years. However, it is impossible to estimate how long the tumor has been present before it becomes clinically apparent. Circumstantial observations suggest that the lesions may require many years to develop to the point of clinical recognition, as is true with many types of cancer. There is no correlation between the presence of asbestosis and the development of MM. Indeed, fewer than half the patients with these tumors have asbestosis, and it is not uncommon for MM to occur in persons having no histological evidence of asbestos bodies in the lung. In contrast to bronchogenic carcinomas, which are more common in smokers exposed to asbestos, there is no association between MM and cigarette smoking.

Malignant mesotheliomas are believed to develop from mature mesothelial cells, or from the progenitors of these cells, in the serosal lining of the chest or abdomen (6–8). We have presented elsewhere observations that argue for an origin of these tumors in a mesothelial cell progenitor element, but this concept is not universally accepted. Indeed, the hypothetical progenitor cell has not been clearly identified as a morphological entity. It is appropriate to ask whether or not MMs are unifocal in origin and spread to involve and encompass the organs of a body cavity from one site of origin, or whether they develop at multiple sites nearly simultaneously. There is no objective evidence to permit us to argue vigorously for one or the other of these alternatives, but it seems likely that a lesion develops at a localized site and spreads by pleural lymphatics, centrifugal surface growth, or implantation metastases to multiple sites in a body cavity. Thus, in this review, our discussion will focus first on the mechanisms whereby these tumors develop at a localized site and, second, on the events that hypothetically contribute to metastasis and spread of the tumor over the surfaces of organs.

In considering the pathogenesis of MM, it is necessary to address the events that occur during the latency period from exposure to the time when symptoms of disease first appear. Unfortunately, we possess no information concerning biological events during this period, and observations using experimental models are limited. With rare exceptions, latency extends over a period of 20 or more years, with an average of longer than 30 years, although some patients have apparent latency periods as long as 40 or 50 years. Continuous exposure to asbestos during this period is not required, and MMs often occur in individuals who experienced an exposure for a finite period early in life. When, then, does malignant transformation occur? And, to what extent do tumor cells in the preclinical stages of their evolution undergo cumulative genetic change during the course of their growth and spread to become clinically evident lesions? We will consider in the following the experimental evidence that provides insights into the question.

## II. Properties of Mineral Fibers Relevant to Disease

The relative pathogenicity of the different mineralogical types of asbestos in the causation of MM is discussed elsewhere in this monograph. Suffice it to state that all, or the great majority, of these tumors develop in individuals heavily exposed to the commercial amphibole asbestos types, crocidolite and amosite, and occasionally the noncommercial amphibole, tremolite (9). Malignant mesotheliomas also develop in inhabitants of the Anatolian region of Turkey, where environmental exposure to the mineral erionite, a fibrous aluminum silicate, occurs. This observation indicates that the physical form of the fibrous particle, not only its chemical composition, is a critical consideration in the development of this tumor.

Fiber dimensions influence the deposition, clearance, and translocation of fibers in the lungs (10). Inhaled fibers have been shown to migrate to the pleura after depositing elsewhere in the lung parenchyma (11,12). Fiber length also determines clearance from the pleural and peritoneal spaces. Those fibers longer than 8 $\mu$m are trapped at the mesothelial lining because the openings of lymphatic channels draining these spaces are 8–12 $\mu$m in diameter (8). Long amphibole fibers are engulfed by phagocytes, but are incompletely phagocytosed, an event that may uniquely stimulate release of cytokines and active oxygen species by macrophages (13,14). These observations provide an anatomical explanation for the hypothesis advanced by Stanton and his colleagues many years ago. These, and later workers, found that asbestos preparations that comprise fibers longer than 8 $\mu$m and smaller than 0.25 $\mu$m in diameter were more carcinogenic in the pleural cavities of rats than preparations of shorter fibers (15–17). Cations within the crystal lattice also contribute to the toxicity of mineral fibers. Magnesium ($Mg^{2+}$) ions on the surface of chrysotile asbestos are important in cytotoxicity and carcinogenicity in experimental animals; acid-leached fibers are less active than native fibers (18). The $Fe^{2+}$ and $Fe^{3+}$ content of amphibole fibers is important because these cations catalyze the Fenton or Haber–Weiss reactions, generating highly toxic and potentially mutagenic reactive oxygen species (19,20). Chemical modification of the surface of the amphibole fiber amosite greatly reduces its carcinogenicity (21). These physicochemical properties of mineral fibers also contribute to their persistence at the target site. In the lungs, short fibers are more easily cleared than long fibers. Chrysotile asbestos fibers fragment more readily and gradually dissolve, whereas amphibole persists in the lungs for a lifetime (22,23). This feature no doubt is an important consideration in the relative carcinogenicity of the two different fiber types. It is reasonable to hypothesize that neoplastic transformation requires the presence of nondestructable, long, thin fibers at a site adjacent to or within target mesothelial cells or their progenitors during the latency period of this cancer.

A small percentage of fibers, principally amphiboles, become coated with an iron–protein coagulum to form asbestos bodies within the lungs. These coated fibers are histological markers of prior asbestos exposure (24). It is unknown whether coated fibers are more or less toxic than uncoated fibers. In the lungs, the lack of an inflammatory reaction associated with these bodies argues that they are no longer pathogenic.

What cellular and molecular events transpire to result in the development of lesions after fiber deposition? Is there a threshold of exposure under which cancer will not occur? And, if the answer is affirmative, can we hypothesize that a single amphibole fiber may possess the potential to initiate malignant transformation? Although answers to these questions are not forthcoming, observations accumulated in experimental animal systems provide some insight.

### III.  Animal Models of Malignant Mesothelioma

Malignant mesothelioma can be reproduced in rodents by direct intrapleural or intraperitoneal injection (17) or by aerosol exposure to mineral fibers (25–27) (Fig. 1). The prolonged latency, variable histological appearance, growth pattern, and natural history of rodent MM are identical with the human disease. A clear dose–response relation, with a relatively high threshold, has been demonstrated in rats (28). Genetic factors are also important; for example, our studies have shown that susceptibility to tumor development differs among various inbred strains of mice (29). However, animal models are not useful for identifying the physical and chemical properties of mineral fibers relevant to the production of MM in humans. For example, fibers that have little or no carcinogenic role in humans (anthophyllite, chrysotile, fiberglas) readily cause these tumors in rats, on intracavitary injection.

Rodent models have several other shortcomings that limit their application for human risk assessment. A major criticism is that inhalation exposure, not direct intrapleural or intraperitoneal injection, more closely resembles the human experience. After inhalation of asbestos fibers by rodents, the latency period of the tumors is prolonged and relatively few animals develop tumors (27). A second criticism is the experimental use of a single, large dose (10–40 mg) of fibers to induce MM, whereas humans

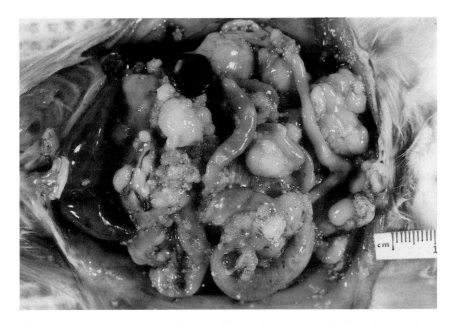

**Figure 1** Abdominal cavity of a rat with a malignant mesothelioma induced by a single injection of crocidolite asbestos. Note the tumor deposits of varying size and configuration located on and over the loops of intestine, the spleen, and the serosal surface of the peritoneum. Lesions of this type develop 6-18 months after a single inoculation of asbestos (Ref. 26, published with permission).

usually are exposed repeatedly to substantially smaller amounts of asbestos, often over decades. To reproduce human occupational exposure, one of us (AK) developed a new model using weekly intraperitoneal injections of 200 $\mu$g (5.8 $\times$ $10^8$ fibers) of crocidolite asbestos fibers in male mice. The MM occurred in 30-40% of animals after a latency period of 30-60 weeks. Major differences exist between this model and previously described rodent models of the disease (7,25). In the earlier animal work, rats received a single implant or injection of asbestos fibers. The fibers accumulated into massive conglomerates of fibers sequestered in the omentum and other intraperitoneal sites, surrounded by a granulomatous fibrous tissue (7,30) (Fig. 2a-c). In contrast, the much smaller dosages of fibers used in our murine model are cleared through lymphatic channels on the inferior surface of the diaphragm (31). The target site of asbestos fibers in this murine model is the parietal mesothelium, covering the inferior surface of the diaphragm. After inhalation of fibers by humans, fibrous plaques commonly develop on the parietal pleural lining in the intercostal region and

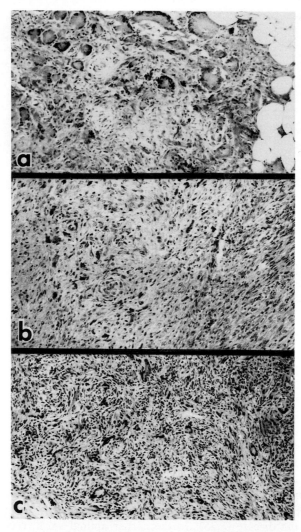

**Figure 2**   Granulomatous lesions developing in the parietal pleura of a rat exposed to crocidolite asbestos. The multinucleate giant cells seen in (a) are a response to the presence of the long fibers of asbestos. Note the numerous multinucleate giant cells in (b) and (c). One can observe the proliferation of dense fibrous tissue, the accumulation of chronic inflammatory cells, such as histiocytes and lymphocytes, and the overall cellular response (c). It is hypothesized that microscopic tissue sections of a similar nature give rise to MM. However, the lesions would be of a different order of magnitude, since the granulomata depicted here encase numerous asbestos fibers. It is likely that only a few fibers at localized sites may give rise to the tumors. Thus, the granulomatous response would be more subtle than that illustrated.

on the superior surface or dome of the diaphragm. The location of these fibrous plaques corresponds to sites of lymphatic clearance from the pleural space. The distribution of lymphatic channels on the superior or pleural surface of the diaphragm mirrors the location of lymphatics on the inferior or abdominal surface (31). Early lesions and MM arise at sites of lymphatic clearance in our murine model.

The early tissue response to these accumulations of asbestos is a circumscribed granuloma that comprises abundant numbers of macrophages and multinucleated giant cells accompanied by neovascularization (32) and the deposition of collagen by fibroblasts. Interestingly enough, these lesions develop in the subserosal tissue and do not involve the mesothelial cells directly. What events then transpire within these granulomatous lesions?

## IV. Oxidants, DNA Damage, and Genetic Alterations

Specific information from in situ studies in animal models is limited, but a substantial body of experimental data has accumulated using cultured cells. Phagocytosis of mineral fibers by macrophages leads to generation of reactive oxygen metabolites and release of lysosomal enzymes, neutral proteases, arachidonic acid metabolites, cytokines, and growth factors (reviewed in Ref. 33). Macrophages and other potential target cells exposed to asbestos in vitro are killed by an oxidant-dependent mechanism (13). Exogenously administered superoxide dismutase, catalase, and hydroxyl radical scavengers prevent cell death in these model systems. It is hypothesized that iron catalyzes the formation of hydroxyl radicals from superoxide anion and hydrogen peroxide by a modified Fenton reaction. This hypothesis is supported by the observation that chelation of iron by coating fibers with deferoxamine decreases asbestos fiber toxicity in vitro (13). Asbestos-induced injury to mesothelial cells in vivo is mediated by a similar mechanism. Production of superoxide anion by macrophages localized around fiber clusters can be demonstrated in situ (34). Intraperitoneal injection of superoxide dismutase or catalase conjugated to polyethylene glycol prolongs the half-life of these scavenging enzymes and, in turn, decreases mesothelial cell injury. Deferoxamine-coated crocidolite asbestos fibers are also less toxic than native fibers in vivo (34).

Generation of highly reactive hydroxyl radicals by asbestos fibers is especially relevant to asbestos carcinogenesis because these molecules can modify and damage cellular DNA (35). Asbestos and other mineral fibers produce oxidized bases in DNA in a cell-free system in the presence of hydrogen peroxide (36). We and others have shown that long, thin amphibole asbestos fibers are unusually effective in stimulating release of reactive oxygen species from macrophages (37) and cause DNA damage in cultured fibroblasts (38) and macrophages (39). Ineffectual repair of this oxidative base damage may lead to point mutations or to DNA strand breaks. Asbestos fails to induce mutations in assays using bacterial or mammalian cells. We have detected DNA injury and repair in macrophages and in mouse embryo fibroblasts and Chinese hamster ovary (CHO) cells exposed to crocidolite asbestos in vitro (unpublished data). This damage is prevented by oxidant-scavenging enzymes, deferoxamine-coated fibers, and inhibitors of poly-ADP ribose polymerase (39). Recently, Hei et al. reported that exposure of the AL human–hamster hybrid cell line to crocidolite or chrysotile asbestos fibers produces large, multiloci deletions in the human marker chromosome 11, but no point mutations at the hypoxanthine–guanine phosphoribosyltransferase (HGPRT) locus (40). Experiments using our murine model of MM have shown that partial deletions and structural changes (not point mutations) develop at the *p53* tumor suppressor gene locus. These types of genetic lesions could be induced indirectly by oxidants or directly by physical interference with the mitotic apparatus (41,42). Asbestos and other mineral fibers interfere with chromosome segregation at anaphase, leading to aneuploidy and formation of micronuclei. This mechanism may explain the multiple chromosomal changes that are commonly found in human and rodent MM (38,43–47).

Numerous cell lines have been established from human and rodent MM. Specific marker chromosomal alterations have not yet been identified, although almost all malignant mesothelial cell lines have numerous cytogenetic alterations. Thus far, there is no evidence for point mutations in activated protooncogenes that are commonly involved in human carcinomas. A histochemical search for *p21*, the protein product of the activated *ras* oncogene, failed to detect expression in human MM, although it was expressed in bronchogenic carcinomas (48). Direct transfection of the activated human EJ-*ras* oncogene into a normal human mesothelial cell line stimulated continuous growth in vitro independent of epidermal growth factor (EGF), but did not lead to growth in soft agar or tumorigenicity in nude mice (49). Barrett transfected DNA from human malignant mesothelial cell lines into NIH 3T3 cells and obtained transformants (41). He detected an apparently unique oncogene that has not yet been characterized; it is not a member of the *ras* gene family. Normal or hyperplastic mesothelial cells would be more appropriate recipients of putative MM oncogenes than the standard NIH 3T3 cell assay.

Point mutations in the *p53* or *Rb* tumor suppressor genes are also rare in human (50,51) and murine MM cell lines. However, reduced expression and rearrangements of the *p53* tumor suppressor gene were found in our murine neoplastic mesothelial cell lines (52).

The relevance of these in vitro observations to the evolution of MM in vivo is uncertain. Additional research, using both human surgical and autopsy specimens and rodent models, is required to identify the multiple cellular and molecular alterations responsible for the development of MM. In situ hybridization; combined with immunohistochemical assays for expression of specific cytokines and growth factors, will provide a link between in vitro and in vivo studies. These advances will certainly provide new insights about the mechanisms leading to the development of MM.

## V.  Cytokines and Growth Factors

Phagocytosis of asbestos by macrophages results in other events, specifically, the release of multiple chemotactic factors, cytokines, and growth factors. We and others have shown that exposure of macrophages to asbestos fibers triggers release of several growth factors, including transforming growth factor (TGF)-$\beta$1, a homologue of platelet-derived growth factor (PDGF) and insulin-like growth factor-1 (IGF-1) and cytokines, including tumor necrosis factor-alpha (TNF-$\alpha$). Direct exposure of mesothelial cells to asbestos fibers or to macrophage-derived cytokines also stimulates expression and release of additional inflammatory mediators and cytokines, specifically, fibronectin (53), interleukin-8 (IL-8; neutrophil-activating peptide-1) (54,55), IL-1$\beta$, IL-6, granulocyte colony-stimulating factor (G-CSF), and granulocyte–macrophage colony-stimulating factor (GM-CSF) (19). Mesothelial cells are unusual because they elaborate or respond to a wide range of growth factors including PDGF, TGF-$\beta$1, EGF, fibroblast growth factor (FGF), IL-$\alpha$, IL-1$\beta$, interferons (IFNs), and TGF-$\alpha$ (57–61). The mechanisms by which mineral fibers induce expression of cytokines and growth factors by macrophages, mesothelial cells, and fibroblasts is an important question under investigation in several laboratories. However, the role of cytokines and growth factors in asbestos-induced disease is as yet only speculative. These factors may amplify the inflammatory and fibrogenic response and serve as autocrine or paracrine growth factors for mesothelial cells at sites of injury (62).

## VI.  Tumor Latency and Progression

Over the long latency period of the MM, one might envision that the interaction of asbestos fibers with phagocytic cells could result in repetitious injury to the DNA of MM progenitor cells with macrophage-derived growth factors enhancing the proliferation of the surviving genetically altered cellular elements (Fig. 3). Cumulative events of this type might be expected to

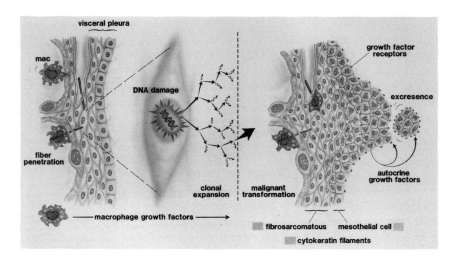

**Figure 3**  Hypothetical construct depicting a possible mechanism for the development of malignant mesothelioma in the pleura. One envisions that macrophages phagocytosing asbestos fibers deposited adjacent to the pleural mesothelial cells or their progenitors. As a result, the macrophages elaborate active oxygen species that have the potential to damage DNA of the target cell. Concomitantly, macrophage growth factors are generated. The proliferation of cells stimulated by the growth factors increases the outgrowth of damaged clones of progenitor cells; perhaps the proliferating cells have an increased sensitivity to the oxygen radicals. Events such as this, occurring over an extended period, could lead to the development of autonomous malignant clones of cells in an occasional asbestos-exposed individual. Malignant transformation results in the proliferation of mesothelial cells, which have the capacity to form spheroids as exhibited in the illustration. Spheroid formation may be under the control of growth factors and influenced by the density of cell surface receptors. Thus, an autocrine or paracrine method of growth stimulation results. The illustration also depicts the development of fibrosarcomatous elements from the progenitor cells of the mesothelium and of epithelioid mesothelial cells from a more mature cellular element.

result ultimately in the selection of clones of neoplastically transformed cells (see Fig. 1), with the ability to proliferate autonomously. But do asbestos fibers in the tissue continue to provoke a response throughout the long latency period of the tumors? We just do not know. Anchorage-independent growth of cultured cells has been demonstrated within a week after exposure to asbestos (41,63,64). These morphological events suggest that biological transformation could occur shortly after the interaction of asbestos with target cells. Clastogenic effects on the chromosomal makeup of cells in short-term culture have been repeatedly demonstrated using in vitro experimental systems (65,66). Animal experiments supporting this concept were carried out several years ago by Brand and his associates, who used nonbiodegradable materials to stimulate carcinogenesis (67). These workers found a marker of chromosomal changes in preneoplastic, reactive cells that accumulated adjacent to the foreign body many months before tumors developed. One must ask whether or not a clone of neoplastic cells could develop from the deposition of a single asbestos fiber adjacent to progenitor cells. The question most probably will never be answered. However, it seems reasonable to hypothesize that premalignant lesions may evolve at multiple sites in the same asbestos-exposed person, with clinical disease resulting from a single focus that grows faster than the others. Similar considerations are believed to influence the development of a clinical bronchogenic carcinoma from one of multiple sites of preneoplastic change in the airways of the cigarette smokers.

## VII. Development of Tumors in Body Cavities

Malignant mesotheliomas developing in body cavities grow progressively and spread to encompass major organs. Assuming a unifocal origin of these lesions, we must inquire into the mechanism(s) involved. Direct microscopical examination of human experimental animal specimens supports three possible, but not mutually exclusive, routes. Spread of tumor in subserosal lymphatic channels is one (Fig. 4), and centrifugal surface spread of tumor over the serosa from an initial nidus of neoplastic change is a second. Finally, tumor originating in the papillary excrescences that commonly develop on the surfaces of these lesions (Fig. 5) may be disseminated by implantation metastasis. The common presence of tumor "spheroids" in effusions that accompany epithelial tumors provides support for this concept (Fig. 6). In our view, the widespread dissemination of these tumors at the time of clinical presentation is consistent with this latter mechanism.

Malignant mesotheliomas often grow on the surface of body organs, without obvious evidence of invasion of the subjacent tissue. Although the lesions may be 1-cm thick, or more, they rarely exhibit arterial vascularization, an observation suggesting that the tumor tissue may be nurtured, in whole or in part, by the fluid that forms in the body cavities surrounding them (Fig. 7).

The concept of tumor progression dictates that cumulative, often spontaneously occurring, alterations in the genetic makeup of a tumor cell results in changing biological characteristics of the neoplasm with time. Initially, MM growth is restricted to the surface of organs, but later in the clinical course of the patient, these lesions become invasive or metastasize

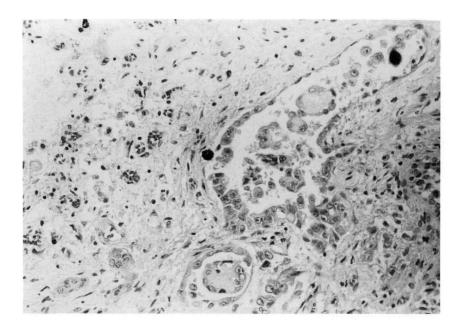

**Figure 4**  Malignant mesothelioma cells growing in a lymphatic channel in the pleura of the lung. The pleomorphism of the cells and the formation of spheroids is evident, even in the vessel lumen. On the right margin of the photomicrograph, one can see pleural mesothelial cells. It is uncertain whether or not this is a significant means whereby tumor spreads throughout the pleural cavity.

widely. This phenomenon confounds the work of the investigator focusing on the study of human lesions, for the features described in a particular clinical sample may reflect only one stage in an evolutionary process.

Growth factors may play an important role in the spread of MM in body cavities. Human MM cells have been found to express the c-*sis* protooncogene and secrete a PDGF-like mitogen extracellularly (59,60). We have demonstrated by immunohistochemistry several different growth factors (EGF, FGF, IGF-1, and TGF-$\beta$) in cells of human tumors and EGF, TGF-$\beta$, and IGF-1 in lesions developing in asbestos-inoculated rats. In our work (JC), cultured cells from rat MM elaborated IGF-1 and the various isotypes of TGF-$\beta$. Production was demonstrated by cells from some, but not all, of the tumors studied. Of particular interest was the finding of IGF-1 and other mitogenic proteins in the ascitic fluids of rats that developed lesions after intraperitoneal asbestos inoculation. We conclude, at least preliminarily, that polypeptide growth factors play a seminal role

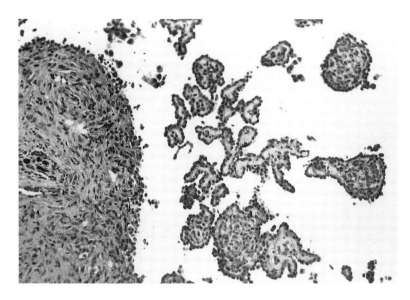

**Figure 5** Papillary excrescences of a MM developing in a rat inoculated with crocidolite asbestos (Ref. 26, published with permission).

in sustaining the growth and spread of MM by autocrine or paracrine mechanisms.

Characteristically, MM comprise a heterogeneous mixture of epithelial and mesenchymal cellular elements in a complex montage of patterns. The factors influencing tumor cell differentiation remain to be defined. Two fundamental cellular mechanisms might account for the unique features of these tumors. First, clonal differentiation from a common stem cell into cells having differing growth patterns and morphological features is a plausible explanation (68). However, experimental evidence to support this notion is limited and unconvincing. Alternatively, macrophage-derived cytokines, or growth factors elaborated by tumor cells, may influence changes in the biology and differentiation of cells. Recently, we showed that differentiation of rat MM cells in vitro could be influenced by products of tumor cells. In these experiments, conditioned medium from tumor cell cultures was shown to mediate a morphological change in epithelial tumor cells to fibroblastoid cells (unpublished data). One could envision a combination of cytokines and growth factors generated by the intact tumor in vivo influencing cellular growth and differentiation in a seemingly helter-skelter manner. Obviously, much remains to be learned about this interesting phenomenon.

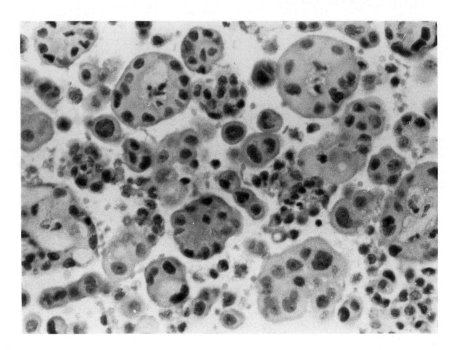

**Figure 6**   Spheroids and morulalike structures in sedimented pleural fluid from a patient with an epithelial MM. One can observe the pleomorphism of the cells, but with the relative lack of mitotic activity. It is hypothesized that cellular accumulations of this type may serve as an effective means for metastasis by means of implantation.

## VIII.   Fibrosis and Benign Tumors of the Pleura

Irregular, but well-circumscribed, plaques of dense collagenous tissue are commonly found on the inner aspect of the chest wall adjacent to ribs and on the dome of the diaphragm in asbestos-exposed men and women. These lesions are sensitive markers of long-term exposure; they occur in individuals who develop no other stigmata of exposure. Less often, the visceral pleura of those exposed to asbestos is diffusely thickened into a layer of dense fibrous tissue that occasionally encapsulates the lungs (69). Often, these thick layers of fibrous tissue fold and are twisted into masses that simulate malignant lesions radiologically (70). We envision the visceral pleural thickening and the typical asbestos-induced plaques of the parietal pleura to be the benign counterpart of MM. The plaques appear to develop in the parietal pleura where fibers accumulate at the stoma of the lymphatic

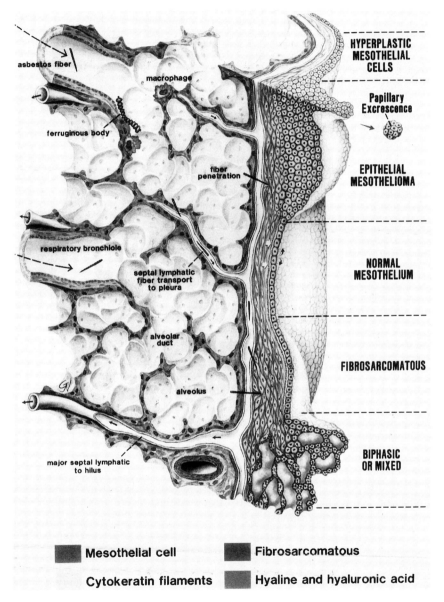

**Figure 7** A hypothetical construct for the overall development of mesotheliomas from the visceral pleura of an asbestos-exposed individual. Asbestos fibers enter the pleura from the subjacent air spaces, either by penetration or through the lymphatics. At this site, they initiate changes in the mesothelial progenitor cells that ultimately result in neoplasia. The proliferating mesothelial cells take several forms.

channels adjacent to the ribs in the chest wall (31) (Fig. 8). At these sites, phagocytosis of asbestos is hypothesized to provoke the release of cytokines and growth factors by the macrophages, stimulating the deposition of the fibrous tissue masses so typical of these lesions (Fig. 9). Similar events may follow the deposition of fibers adjacent to the visceral pleura. Here, the persistent release of macrophage-derived growth factors and cytokines may affect the proliferation of pleural cell elements. Interestingly, the parietal pleural plaques are common in asbestos-exposed persons, whereas visceral pleura thickening occurs sporadically.

Benign fibrous tumors of the visceral pleura (occasionally termed benign mesotheliomas) develop in the absence of a history of exposure to asbestos (Fig. 10). Although these rare, sporadically occurring lesions have not been subject to critical biological study, one might hypothesize that they represent clonal proliferation of submesothelial fibrous tissue at a localized site of the pleura, ultimately resulting in a neoplasmlike mass in the pleural space. These tumors may be a benign counterpart of an MM.

## IX. Concluding Remarks

Malignant mesotheliomas are unique tumors of the serosal surfaces of humans and lower animals. The factors influencing their development and the differentiation of the component cells are unknown. Amphibole asbestos is etiologically responsible for most of these lesions. Experimental evidence strongly suggests that interaction of the asbestos fibers with macrophages elicits the elaboration of active oxygen species that have the capacity to alter the DNA of tumor progenitor cells, and have clastogenic effects. This may occur shortly after exposure to asbestos and long before tumors appear clinically. If so, the subsequent events that led to the development of the MM are unknown. Although the multistage concept of MM progression is appealing, experimental evidence to support this concept is largely lacking. The molecular events responsible for progression of this tumor are unknown.

---

**Figure 7** Continued.
Some tumors are fibrosarcomatous, whereas others are glandular and resemble adenocarcinomas, as depicted. Commonly, both elements are found together; a representation of the so-called biphasic MM. Sheets of malignant mesothelioma cells can also form papillary excrescences and the spheroids that are so typical of the cells found in the pleural cavity of individuals with MM. The formation of spheroids is a typical feature of hyperplastic mesothelial cells, and it is often prominent in overt tumors.

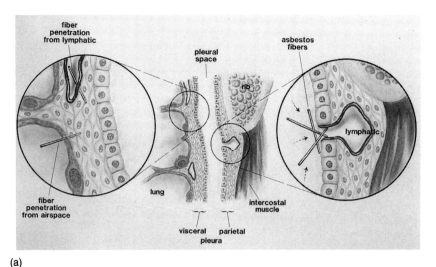

(a)

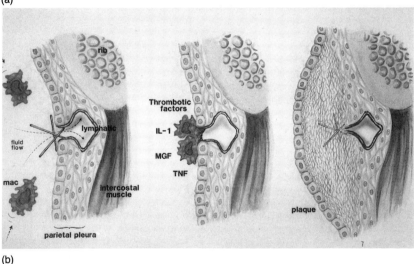

(b)

**Figure 8** Hypothetical mechanism for the formation of pleural plaques from asbestos deposited in the lung. The steps occur as follows: (a) Asbestos enters the pleura adjacent to the mesothelial cells or their progenitors by direct penetration of the lymphatics. The fibers then enter the pleural cavity and are transported in pleural fluid to the stomata of lymphatics subjacent to the ribs in the parietal pleural surface. Because of their size and complexity, the fibers tend to lodge at this site. (b) The presence of asbestos fibers in and at the orifice of the stomata of the lymphatics attracts macrophages, which elaborate cytokines and growth factors. The macrophage response serves as the basis for the proliferation of fibrous tissue, possibly in a stroma of fibrin. This concept was first advanced by Hillerdal (71). Plaques typically develop adjacent to the ribs and over the dome of the diaphragm adjacent to lymphatics. Experimental models tracing the development of pleural plaques have not yet been perfected.

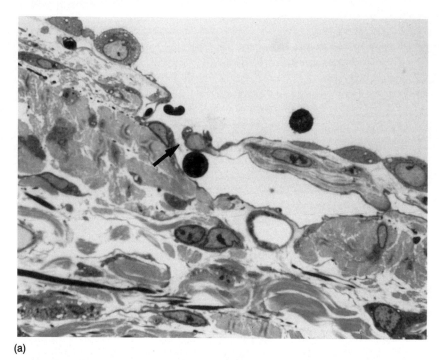

(a)

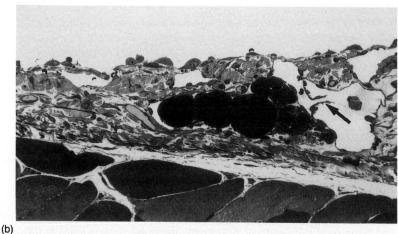

(b)

**Figure 9**  The stoma of lymphatic channels on the parietal pleural surface of a rabbit. Note the erythrocytes at the orifice in (a) after experimental introduction of the red blood cells into the pleural cavity; (b) these cells have accumulated in the lacuna adjacent to the stoma of the lymphatics. The arrow points to a valve in the lymphatic system. (Courtesy of NS Wang.)

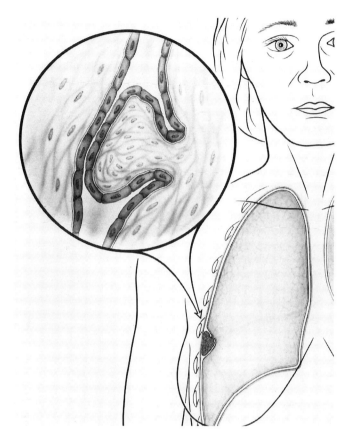

**Figure 10** A localized fibrous pleural tumor developing from the submesothelial connective tissue. Typically, these lesions develop on stalks and serve as a foreign body within the pleural cavity. Note that the proliferation of mesenchymal cells does not involve the surface mesothelium but occurs subjacent to it (Ref. 7, published with permission).

The MMs would appear to develop from a single focus in the pleural or peritoneal serosa and spread to invest the internal organs with an avascular "peel" of tumor. In this review, we have proposed that cytokines and growth factors, elaborated by macrophages and the tumor cells, may influence autocrine or paracrine mechanisms of tumor growth and spread, as well as the differentiation of tumor cells. Although the concept is appealing, proof is lacking. Much remains to be learned about the biology of these intriguing lesions and their possible benign counterparts, the pleural plaques, the benign fibrous tumors of pleura, and visceral pleural thickening. Radiation and chemotherapy of MM are uniformly ineffectual, and aggressive surgery has failed to reverse the clinical course of the disease in most patients. New approaches to treatment undoubtedly will require interventions that depend on a better understanding of the biology of these universally fatal cancers.

## References

1. Japko L, Horta AA, Schreiber K, Mitsudo S, Karwa GL, Singh G, Koss LG. Malignant mesothelioma of the vaginalis testis: report of first case with preoperative diagnosis. Cancer 1982; 49:119–127.
2. Kahn EI, Rohl A, Barrett EW, Suzuki Y. Primary pericardial mesothelioma following exposure to asbestos. Environ Res 1980; 23:270–281.
3. Dvorak HF, Nagy JA, Dvorak JT, Dvorak AM. Identification and characterization of the blood vessels of solid tumors that are leaky to circulating macromolecules. Am J Pathol 1988; 133:95–109.
4. Senger DR, Perruzzi CA, Feder J, Dvorak HF. A highly conserved vascular permeability factor secreted by a variety of human and rodent tumor cell lines. Cancer Res 1986; 46:5629–5632.
5. Pelnar PV. Further evidence of nonasbestos-related mesothelioma. A review of the literature. Scand J Work Environ Health 1988; 14:141–144.
6. Bolen JW, Hammar SP, McNutt MA. Reactive and neoplastic serosal tissue. A light-microscopic, ultrastructural, and immunocytochemical study. Am J Surg Pathol 1986; 10:34–47.
7. Craighead JE. Current pathogenetic concepts of diffuse malignant mesothelioma. Hum Pathol 1987; 18:544–557.
8. Moalli PA, MacDonald JL, Goodglick LA, Kane AB. Acute injury and regeneration of the mesothelium in response to asbestos fibers. Am J Pathol 1987; 128:426–445.
9. McDonald AD, McDonald JE, Pooley FD. Mineral fibre content of lung in mesothelial tumours in North America. Ann Occup Hyg 1982; 26:417–422.
10. Lippman M. Asbestos exposure indices. Environ Res 1988; 46:86–106.
11. Morgan A, Evans JC, Holmes A. Deposition and clearance of inhaled fibrous minerals in the rat. Studies using radioactive tracer techniques. In: Walton WH, ed. Inhaled particles IV. Oxford: Pergamon Press, 1977:259–274.
12. Viallat JR, Raybuad F, Passarel M, Boutin C. Pleural migration of chrysotile fibers after intratracheal injection in rats. Arch Environ Health 1986; 41:282–286.
13. Goodglick LA, Kane AB. Role of reactive oxygen metabolites in crocidolite asbestos toxicity to mouse macrophages. Cancer Res 1986; 46:5558–5566.
14. Mossman BT, Marsh JP, Shatos MA. Alteration of superoxide dismutase activity in tracheal epithelial cells by asbestos and inhibition of cytotoxicity by antioxidants. Lab Invest 1986; 54:204–212.
15. Davis JMG, Addison J, Bolton RE, Donaldson K, Jones AD, Smith T. The

pathogenicity of long versus short fibre samples of amosite asbestos administered to rats by inhalation and intraperitoneal injection. Br J Exp Pathol 1986; 67:415–430.

16. Stanton MF, Layard M, Tegeris A, Miller E, May M, Kent E. Carcinogenicity of fibrous glass: pleural response in the rat in relation to fiber dimension. JNCI 1977; 58:587–603.

17. Stanton MF, Layard M, Tegeris A, Miller E, May M, Morgan E, Smith A. Relation of particle dimension to carcinogenicity in amphibole asbestoses and other fibrous minerals. JNCI 1981; 67:965–975.

18. Monchaux G, Bignon J, Jaurand MC, Lafuma J, Sebastien P, Masse R, Hirsch A, Goni, T. Mesotheliomas in rats following inoculation with acid-leached chrysotile asbestos and other mineral fibers. Carcinogenesis 1991; 2:229–236.

19. Weitzman SA, Graceffa P. Asbestos catalyzes hydroxyl and superoxide radical release from hydrogen peroxide. Arch Biochem Biophys 1984; 288:373–376.

20. Zalma R, Bonneau L, Guignard J, Pezerat H. Formation of oxy radicals by oxygen reduction arising from the surface activity of asbestos. Can J Chem 1987; 65:2338–2341.

21. Brown RC, Carthew P, Hoskins JA, Sara E, Simpson CF. Surface modification can affect the carcinogenicity of asbestos. Carcinogenesis 1990; 11:1883–1855.

22. Bellman B, Konig H, Muhle H, Pott F. Chemical durability of asbestos and of man-made mineral fibers in vivo. J Aerosol Sci 1986; 17:341–345.

23. Morgan A, Holmes A. Solubility of asbestos and man-made fibers in vitro and in vivo: its significance in lung disease. Environ Res 1986; 39:475–484.

24. Craighead JE, Abraham JL, Churg A, Green FHY, Kleinerman J, Pratt PC, Seemayer TA, Vallyathan V, Weill H. The pathology of asbestos associated diseases of the lungs and pleural cavities: diagnostic criteria and proposed grading schema. Report of the Pneumoconiosis Committee of the College of American Pathologists and the National Institute for Occupational Safety and Health. Arch Pathol Lab Med 1982; 106:542–597.

25. Bolton RE, Davis JMG, Donaldson K, Wright A. Variations in the carcinogenicity of mineral fibres. Ann Occup Hyg 1982; 26:569–582.

26. Craighead JE, Akley NJ, Gould LB, Libbus BL. Characteristics of tumors and tumor cells cultured from experimental asbestos-induced mesotheliomas in rats. Am J Pathol 1987; 129:448–462.

27. Wagner JC, Berry G, Timbrell V. Mesotheliomata in rats after inoculation with asbestos and other materials. Br J Cancer 1973; 28:173–185.

28. Davis JMG, Bolton RE, Miller BG, Niven K. Mesothelioma dose response following intraperitoneal injections of mineral fibres. Int J Exp Pathol 1991; 72263–274.

29. Craighead JE, Richards SA, Calore JD, Fan H. Genetic factors influence MM development in mice. Eur Respir Rev 1993; 3:118–120.

30. Friemann J, Muller KM, Pott F. Mesothelial proliferation due to asbestos and man-made fibers. Pathol Res Pract 1990; 186:117–123.

31. Courtice FC, Simmonds WJ. Physiological significance of lymph drainage of the serosal cavities and lungs. Physiol Rev 1954; 34:419–448.

32.  Branchaud RM, MacDonald JL, Kane AB. Induction of angiogenesis by intra-peritoneal injections of asbestos fibers. FASEB J 1989; 3:1747–1752.

33.  Sibille Y, Reynolds HY. Macrophages and polymorphonuclear neutrophils in lung defense and injury. Am Rev Respir Dis 1990; 141:471–501.

34.  Goodglick LA, Kane AB. Cytotoxicity of long and short crocidolite asbestos fibers in vitro and in vivo. Cancer Res 1990; 50:5153–5163.

35.  Floyd RA. The role of 8-hydroxyguanine in carcinogenesis. Carcinogenesis 1990; 11:1447–1450.

36.  Leanderson P, Soderkvist P, Tagesson C, Axelson O. Formation of 8-hydroxyguanosine by asbestos and man-made-mineral fibers. Br J Ind Med 1988; 45:309–311.

37.  Hansen K, Mossman BT. Generation of superoxide from alveolar macrophages exposed to asbestiform and nonfibrous particles. Cancer Res 1987; 47: 1681–1686.

38.  Libbus BL, Craighead JE. Chromosomal translocations with specific breakpoints in asbestos-induced rat mesotheliomas. Cancer Res 1988; 48:6455–6461.

39.  Goodglick LA, Kane AB. Membrane perturbation by asbestos fibers and disease. In: Ohnishi ST, Ohnishi T, eds. Cellular membrane: a key to disease processes. Boca Raton: CRC Press, 1993:123–140.

40.  Hei TK, Piao CQ, He ZY, Vannais D, Waldren CA. Chrysotile fiber is a strong mutagen in mammalian cells. Cancer Res 1992 (in press).

41.  Barrett JC, Lamb PW, Wiseman RW. Multiple mechanisms for the carcinogenic effects of asbestos and other mineral fibers. Environ Health Perspect 1989; 81:81–89.

42.  Wang NS, Jaurand MC, Magne L, Kheuang L, Pinchon MC, Bignon J. The interactions between asbestos fibers and metaphase chromosomes of rat pleural mesothelial cells in culture: a scanning and transmission electron microscopic study. Am J Pathol 1987; 126:343–349.

43.  Frierson HF, Mills SE, Legier JF. Flow cytometric analysis of ploidy in immunohistochemically confirmed examples of malignant epithelial mesothelioma. Am J Clin Pathol 1988; 90:240–243.

44.  Hagemeijer A, Versnel MA, Van Drunen E, Moret M, Bouts MJ, van der Kwast TH, Hoogsteden HC. Cytogenetic analysis of malignant mesothelioma. Cancer Genet Cytogenet 1990; 47:1–28.

45.  Popescu NC, Chahinian AP, DiPaolo JA. Nonrandom chromosome alterations in human malignant mesothelioma. Cancer Res 1988; 48:142–147.

46.  Stenman G, Olofsson K, Monsson T, Hagmar B, Mark J. Chromosomes and chromosomal evolution in human mesotheliomas as reflected in sequential analyses of two cases. Hereditas 1986; 105:233–239.

47.  Tiainen ML, Tammilehto L, Mattson K, Knuutila S. Nonrandom chromosomal abnormalities in malignant pleural mesothelioma. Cancer Genet Cytogenet 1988; 33:251–274.

48.  Lee I, Gould VE, Radosevich JA, Thor A, Ma Y, Schlom J, Rosen ST. Immunohistochemical evaluation of *ras* oncogene expression in pulmonary and pleural neoplasm. Virchows Arch [B] 1987; 53:146–152.

49. Tubo RA, Rheinwald JG. Normal human mesothelial cells and fibroblasts transfected with EJ-*ras* oncogene become EGF-independent, but are not malignantly transformed. Oncogene Res 1987; 1:407–421.

50. Cote RJ, Jhanwar WC, Novic S, Pellicer A. Genetic alterations of the *p53* gene are a feature of malignant mesotheliomas. Cancer Res 1991; 51:5410–5416.

51. Metcalf RA, Welsh JA, Bennet WP, Seddon MB, Lehman TA, Pelin K, Linnainmaa K, Tammielehto L, Mattson K, Gerwin BI, Harris CC. *p53* and Kirsten-*ras* mutations in human mesothelioma cell lines. Cancer Res 1992 52: 2610–2615.

52. Cora EM, Kane AB. Alterations in a tumor suppressor gene, *p53*, in mouse mesotheliomas induced by crocidolite asbestos. Eur Respir Rev 1993; 3:148–150.

53. Kuwahara M, Kuwahara M, Bijwaard KE, Gersten DM, Diglio CA, Kagan E. Mesothelial cells produce a chemoattractant for lung fibroblasts: role of fibronectin. Am J Respir Cell Mol Biol 1991; 5:256–164.

54. Boylan AM, Ruegg C, Kim KJ, Hebert CA, Hoeffel JM, Pytela R, Sheppard D, Goldstein IM, Broaddus VC. Evidence of a role for mesothelial cell derived interleukin 8 in the pathogenesis of asbestos-induced pleurisy in rabbits. J Clin Invest 1992; 89:1257–1267.

55. Goodman RB, Wood RG, Martin JR, Hanson-Painton O, Kinasewitz GT. Cytokine-stimulated human mesothelial cells produce chemotactic activity for neutrophils including NAP-1/IL-8. J Immunol 1992; 148:457–465.

56. Demetri GD, Zenzie BW, Rheinwald JG, Griffin JD. Expression of colony-stimulating factor genes by normal human mesothelial cells and human malignant mesothelioma cell lines in vitro. Blood 1989; 74:940–946.

57. Bermudez E, Everitt J, Walker C. Expression of growth factor and growth factor receptor RNA in rat pleural mesothelial cells in culture. Exp Cell Res 1990; 190:91–98.

58. Gabrielson EW, Gerwin BI, Harris CC, Robert AB, Sporn MB, Lechner JF. Stimulation of DNA synthesis in cultured primary human mesothelial cells by specific growth factors. FASEB J 1988; 2:2717–2721.

59. Gerwin BI, Lechner JF, Reddel RR, Roberts AB, Robbins KC, Gabrielson EW, Harris CC. Comparison of production of transforming growth factor $\alpha$ and platelet-derived growth factor by normal human mesothelial cells and mesothelioma cell lines. Cancer Res 1987; 47:6180–6184.

60. Versnel MA, Hagemeijer A, Bouts MJ, van der Kwast TH, Hoogsteden HC. Expression of c-*sis* (PDGF $\alpha$-chain) and PDGF $\beta$-chain genes in ten human malignant mesothelioma cell lines derived from primary and metastatic tumors. Oncogene 1988; 2:601–605.

61. Walker C, Everitt J, Barrett JC. Possible cellular and molecular mechanisms for asbestos carcinogenicity. Am J Ind Med 1992; 21:253–273.

62. Kelley J. Cytokines of the lung. Am Rev Respir Dis 1990; 141:765–788.

63. Hesterberg TW, Barrett JC. Dependence of asbestos- and mineral dust induced transformation of mammalian cells in culture of fiber dimension. Cancer Res 1984; 44:2170–2180.

64. Hesterberg TW, Butterick CJ, Oshimura M, Brody AR, Barrett JC. Role of

phagocytosis in Syrian hamster cell transformation and cytogenetic effects induced by asbestos and short and long glass fibers. Cancer Res 1986; 46: 5795–5802.

65. Huang SL, Saggioro C, Michelmann H, Malling HV. Genetic effects of crocidolite asbestos in Chinese hamster lung cells. Mutat Res 1978; 57:225–232.

66. Sincock AM, Delhanty JDA, Casey G. A comparison of the cytogenetic response to asbestos and glass fibre in Chinese hamster and human cell lines. Demonstration of growth inhibition in primary human fibroblasts. Mutat Res 1982; 101:257–268.

67. Rachko D, Brand KG. Chromosomal aberrations in foreign body tumorigenesis of mice. Proc Soc Exp Biol Med 1983; 172:382–388.

68. Brown DG, Johnson NF, Wagner MMF. Multipotential behaviour of cloned rat mesothelioma cells with epithelial phenotype. Br J Cancer 1985; 51:245–252.

69. Stephens M, Gibbs AR, Pooley FD, Wagner JC. Asbestos induced diffuse pleural fibrosis: pathology and mineralogy. Thorax 1987; 42:583–588.

70. Hillerdal G. Rounded atelectasis: Clinical experience with 74 patients. Chest 1989; 95:836–841.

71. Hillerdal G. The pathogenesis of pleural plaques and pulmonary asbestosis: possibilities and impossibilities. Eur J Respir Dis 1980; 61:129–138.

# 7

# Immunohistochemical Diagnosis of Mesothelioma

**JACQUES F. LEGIER**

Riverside Regional Medical Center
Newport News and
Eastern Virginia Medical School
Norfolk, Virginia

**JOHN C. MADDOX**

Riverside Regional Medical Center
Newport News, Virginia

## I. Introduction

The use of immunoperoxidase stains in the diagnosis of malignant mesothelioma has become common in the past few years. Although ultrastructural examination is still considered by many as the gold standard of diagnosis of epithelioid mesotheliomas, it is limited in its practical application by expense and convenience. Immunoperoxidase stains present a less costly and less time-consuming alternative method of diagnosis.

Mesothelioma is often a difficult tumor to diagnose because of the many different patterns that it may assume. At one end of the spectrum is the relatively well-differentiated tubulopapillary epithelioid pattern, and at the other is the collagen-rich desmoplastic sarcomatoid mesothelioma. There are several combinations and variations, as well as smaller degrees of differentiation between these two extremes. When the tumor presents with a biphasic pattern or a tubulopapillary pattern alone, the diagnosis is readily suggested. However, when there is a less-differentiated epithelioid tumor or a spindle cell sarcomatoid tumor, other possibilities need to be considered and excluded. Experts on the United States and Canadian Mesothelioma Panel experienced the most difficulties when addressing the differential diagnosis between fibrous pleuritis and sarcomatous mesothelioma (1).

With epithelioid tumors, the basic diagnostic challenge is to distinguish between a primary mesothelioma and carcinoma of the lung. More specifically, poorly differentiated peripheral adenocarcinomas of the lung may be histologically indistinguishable from the less-differentiated epithelioid mesotheliomas. Rarely, other kinds of tumor (i.e., melanoma, metastatic adenocarcinoma) may mimic a poorly differentiated mesothelioma. Traditional histochemical-staining reactions are helpful to a limited extent in some situations. If the tumor contains intracytoplasmic vacuoles, characterization of the type of secretion present is of diagnostic value. Acid mucopolysaccharide secretions that are susceptible to hyaluronidase can be found in mesothelioma, but are usually absent in adenocarcinoma. Conversely, the presence of neutral epithelial mucins that stain with periodic acid-Schiff (PAS)/diastase (or less specifically with Mayer's mucicarmine) can be demonstrated in many mesotheliomas. These staining techniques are not particularly useful when the tumor lacks cytoplasmic vacuoles.

With sarcomatoid tumors, the differential diagnosis includes mainly the spindle cell group of fibrosarcoma, malignant fibrous histiocytoma, the recently described malignant fibrous tumor of pleura, and dedifferentiated sarcomas. It must be remembered that mesotheliomas possess the potential for sarcomatous metaplasia of the chondroid, osseous, or lipoid type, so finding such areas does not necessarily exclude a diagnosis of mesothelioma if more standard mesotheliomatous features can be demonstrated elsewhere in the tumor. There are also certain types of benign fibrous tumors of mesothelial or submesothelial origin that need to be considered and excluded (2).

With peritoneal tumors in women, the distinction between extraovarian serous surface papillary carcinoma and malignant mesothelioma can be very difficult. This has been the subject of comprehensive review (3,4).

Primary peritoneal serous carcinoma, ovarian serous tumors, and peritoneal mesothelioma share a common coelomic cell of origin and, as expected, are hard to differentiate by immunohistochemical means. A study by Khoury et al. (5) applied a battery of antibodies to such tumors and found 85% of nonovarian tumors to express Leu-M1, carcinoembryonic antigen (CEA), and B72.3. Vimentin and human milk-fat globulin (HMFG) 2 had no discriminatory value. Some peritoneal and ovarian tumors may mimic mesothelioma in their lack of expression of CEA and other antigens that readily label adenocarcinoma from other sites. Furthermore, some primary peritoneal tumors fail to stain with all three markers or, when positive, stain in a focal pattern; thus, negative results must be interpreted with caution. Even other ancillary procedures, such as mucin stains and ultrastructural examination, may fail to establish a precise diagnosis.

With cytological specimens, many of the morphological clues to diagnosis are lost, and immunoperoxidase staining becomes even more important in providing objective evidence of differentiation.

## II. Strategy

The goal of immunochemical stains is the demonstration of cellular antibodies that are specific for malignant mesothelioma, yet differ from those found on carcinomatous or sarcomatous cells. This goal has not yet been achieved and may never be realized, since new antibodies repeatedly fail in attaining specificity for mesothelioma. There is no limit to the inventiveness of investigators who bring out new antisera and publish comparative results of updated panels tested on mesotheliomatous, carcinomatous, and reactive mesothelial conditions. As yet, there is no positive mesothelioma marker that has been proved completely specific through enough conclusive field tests. Therefore, this diagnosis remains one of exclusion, after negative results are obtained with a panel of antibodies that reliably decorate carcinoma cells and leave neoplastic mesothelial cells unstained (Table 1).

## III. Pitfalls

There are several cautions when attempting immunoperoxidase confirmation of mesothelioma. The quality of preservation of antigenic sites is important and may vary greatly depending on the method of tissue fixation. In general, frozen sections that have been fixed with acetone or alcohol show the least antigenic alteration; however, they may not show the same pattern of reactivity as formalin-fixed tissues. Conversely, some antibodies may show absent or nonspecific binding when used on formalin-fixed, paraffin-embedded sections.

Overfixation in formalin undoubtedly contributes to weakened or absent immunohistochemical reactions. Delayed fixation (as with autopsy tissue) is usually not a significant problem. Prolonged enzymatic digestion for uncovering antigenic sites before immunostaining can contribute to either false-positive or false-negative results, depending on the antigen.

As with any antibody reagent, the working titers should be tested and adjusted to maximize specificity, without loss of sensitivity.

Pleural needle biopsies contain only a small volume of tissue. Consequently, they are particularly prone to drying artifact, which causes false-positive staining at the edges of the section. There is also the inherent problem of tumor diversity (i.e., viewing a nonrepresentative area of the tumor). This can be manifested as either a nonstaining, nonviable, or an

**Table 1**  Summary of Immunoperoxidase Stains

| Markers of | Reactive mesothelium | Malignant mesothelioma | Adeno-carcinoma | Comments |
|---|---|---|---|---|
| Proven value | | | | |
| CEA | Neg | Gen neg | Gen pos | |
| LEU-M1 | Neg | Neg | Pos | |
| Intermediate value | | | | |
| EMA–HMFG1 | Rare + | Gen pos | Pos | Monoclonal serum |
| VIMENTIN | Gen pos | Gen pos | Gen neg | |
| HMFG2 | Neg | Com pos | Pos | Cytoplasmic pattern |
| KERATIN | Pos | Pos (2 +) | Pos (1 +) | |
| B72.3 | Neg | Gen neg | Gen pos | |
| Promising markers | | | | |
| AUA1 | Neg | Neg | Pos | |
| K1 | Pos | Pos | Neg | |
| BER-EP4 | Neg | Neg | Pos | |
| DONNA | Pos | Pos | Neg | |
| HEA-125 | Neg | Neg | Pos | |
| BMA-120 | Gen pos | Gen pos | Wk pos | Strong in ovar. CA |
| BCA-225 | Neg | | Pos | |
| OV-632 | Neg | Pos | Neg | Pos in ovar CA Some lung CA |

Com, Commonly; Gen, Generally ; Neg, Negative; Pos, Positive; Wk, Weakly.

antigen-poor location of actual tumor, or as misleading positive reactions in lung parenchyma overrun by tumor.

Foci of tumor necrosis will nonspecifically bind immunoreagents, particularly polyclonal antisera and antisera with relatively concentrated working dilutions. Leu-M1 shows distinct staining with granulocytes and monocytes that may infiltrate tumor tissues, and the endogenous peroxidase of eosinophils may rarely cause false-staining reactions when prior blocking agents are not used.

## IV.  Results

The Donna antibody comes close to being a specific positive marker for mesothelioma (6). This antibody was raised against a protein isolated from the cytoplasm of mesothelioma and has shown substantial promise for mesotheliomatous confirmation. All 16 mesotheliomas arising in diverse body cavities decorated with the antibody. In contrast, none of a series of adenocarcinoma reacted. The antibody correctly identified some unusual metaplastic variants of mesothelioma that produced mucinous secretions or contained components of mesenchymal differentiation. The antibody was highly efficient and yielded clear and strong reaction with both benign (reactive) and malignant mesothelial cells. It was tested on formalin-fixed, paraffin-embedded tissues. This antibody merits further testing and potential commercial marketing. An additional antibody, derived from an established mesothelioma cell line labeled HB-ME, stains most formalin-fixed epithelial mesotheliomas, often with a distinct membranous pattern that highlights the microvilli. However, again, it stained a few adenocarcinomas and needs further evaluation (7).

A monoclonal antibody K1 was generated by immunizing mice with OV-CAR3, an ovarian tumor cell line, derived from a poorly differentiated adenocarcinoma of the ovary. This antibody reacted with 67% of nonmucinous carcinoma of the ovary and with 73% of esophageal squamous carcinomas. Reactions were very uncommon with normal human tissues other than serosa. The antigen that reacts with this K1 antibody is designated CAK1. It is a 40-kDa cell surface protein that is released by the action of phospholipase C. The K1 antibody was tested against 23 mesotheliomas, and it consistently reacted strongly with pure epithelioid or biphasic mesotheliomas. However, it did not react with any of the sarcomatous mesotheliomas (8). All 23 control adenocarcinomas remained unstained. This antibody thus shows great promise as a specific marker for the epithelioid components of mesothelioma, even though it is not a sensitive marker of sarcomatoid types. Its effectiveness on paraffin-embedded tissue remains to be proved, since past results pertain to frozen-section material and tumor cell culture lines.

Most important among the negative markers is the carcinoembryonic antigen (CEA). The first investigation of its diagnostic usefulness in the exclusion of mesothelioma was by Wang in 1979 (9). This rule has stood the test of time in numerous subsequent studies. The CEA is a complex glycoprotein of unknown function which, even when purified, displays a molecular heterogeneity. There are numerous antigenic epitopes with structural similarities to CEA, foremost among which are variants of nonspecific cross-reacting antigen (NCA) such as NCA95, NCA55, NCA, CEA "low," biliary glycoprotein 1, and normal fecal antigen 1. Anti-CEA serum can be purified by absorption with granulocyte or lyophilized hepatic and splentic tissue, sources rich in NCA. Carcinoembryonic antigen is a complex molecule, with over 50% carbohydrate content by weight. This allows extensive sugar substitution, with resulting heterogeneity in the biochemical structure of the antigen and in the specificity of the different antibodies against it. Unlike mesothelioma, most carcinomas readily decorate with anti-CEA, the frequency depending on the site of origin. Carcinoma of the lung and gastrointestinal tract are decorated with high frequency, whereas neoplasms of the ovary and breast uncommonly express the antigen.

On occasion, pleural and peritoneal mesotheliomas react positively, a phenomenon attributed to cross-reaction with NCA. Most such positive results were obtained with the use of polyclonal sera. Indeed, the highest frequency of anti-CEA staining in mesotheliomas (45%) was reached with unabsorbed polyclonal serum; however, these reactions persisted even after absorption with splenic tissue. Furthermore, some monoclonal anti-CEA sera, even those known to obtain granulocytes, may still mark mesotheliomas. Some investigators have found an even higher rate of mesothelial staining (1) with monoclonal antibodies than with purified rabbit antiserum. A survey of published results spanning the years 1983 through 1990 lists aggregate positive results of 6% for polyclonal and 1% for monoclonal anti-CEA sera (10) in mesothelioma. Usually, the decoration is weak and focal, but cannot be denied. Some studies are handicapped by the lack of a quantitative score for evaluation of weak peroxidase reactions. A modified-grading system (11) is recommended classifying positively stained cells on a scale of negative to 3+ (neg, staining absent; 1+, fewer than 5% positive cells; 2+, fewer than 50% positive cells; 3+, more than 50% positive cells). Most positive CEA readings in mesothelioma turn out to be low–grade-staining reactions. Because of these findings, a weakly positive anti-CEA stain alone cannot serve to rule out mesothelioma, unless supported by other data. This also points to the need of further molecular research in the antigenic nature of the CEA complex and its relation to NCAs.

In addition, the factor of observer variation may explain the divergence of results, since necrotic tissue may take up the stain and both entrapped pulmonary epithelial remnants or admixed granulocytes–macrophages may be misread as marked mesothelial cells. Tumor with a high hyaluronic acid content may lead to a false-positive CEA interpretation (12).

False-positive monoclonal CEA staining was recently (13) classified in two patterns: one consists of a coarsely granular cytoplasmic staining, concentrated in the perinuclear cytoplasm; it is moderate to strong in intensity and cannot be duplicated with polyclonal antibody. It is thought to be similar to the punctate staining of the Tn antigen in glandular epithelium occurring in the Golgi apparatus. The second is sporadic, linear cytoplasmic staining, which also occurs with polyclonal serum. Such granular- or linear-staining patterns contrast with the diffuse finely granular cytoplasmic staining accentuated at the cytoplasmic border, typically seen in carcinoma.

AUA₁ is an epithelial antigen found in many normal epithelia, in adenocarcinomas, in some squamous carcinomas, and in small-cell carcinomas. It appears to be more useful than CEA, being more commonly distributed in neoplasms. A monoclonal antibody against this 34-kDa cell surface glycoprotein, which is coded for by a gene on chromosome 2, decorates a wide range of adenocarcinomas. It was tested (14) in a series of benign and malignant mesotheliomatous and carcinomatous conditions. It faithfully remained negative in mesothelioma and reactive mesothelial effusion, but was positive in all but 1 of 14 adenocarcinomas, thereby achieving better results than CEA in this small study.

Other tumor-related antigens have been studied. Similar to CEA, the glycoprotein EGP-34, also known as HEA-125, a 34-kDa epithelial glycoprotein, was reported as not expressed by mesothelioma, but frequently present in adenocarcinoma. Earlier investigation had shown reactive mesothelial proliferation and mesothelioma to be HEA-125-negative, in contrast with generally positive results seen in metastatic carcinoma. A study of pleural mesotheliomas analyzing the expression of EGP-34 was unable to confirm the diagnostic specificity of this marker, since 8 of 158 mesotheliomas yielded a positive reaction (15). Thus, HEA-125 staining remains unsuitable as a decisive diagnostic test.

The perfect original performance (16) of antiserum against BER-EP4 (also listed as EGP-34/39) has been blemished in a subsequent study. This monoclonal antibody is directed against a partially formalin-resistant epitope on the protein moiety of two 34-kDa and 39-kDa glycopolypeptides of human epithelial cells. The first reports gave spectacular results, with decoration of 142 of 144 carcinomas and no reaction to nonepithelial tumors, mesothelioma, or reactive mesothelial cells. It was thus felt to be useful in differentiation of nonepithelial tumors verus undifferentiated carcinoma, or of hepatocytes versus bile duct cells. The antigen was poorly expressed in hepatocytes, parietal cells, and apical squamous cells. When again investigated in an expanded series of mesothelioma (17), it proved to be excellent for identifying pulmonary adenocarcinoma (87% decoration) and average for breast carcinoma (64% decoration). However, it stained 1 of 115 mesotheliomas, thereby once again bursting the bubble of expected absolute diagnostic discrimination. Our laboratory has experienced similar strong staining in occasional mesotheliomas. The most recent study (18) found reactivity in 86% of adenocarcinomas, mostly of diffuse and membranous character. Pulmonary tumors stained consistently, in contrast with no or weak reactivity in mammary, renal, and ovarian neoplasms. The study concluded that BER-EP4, based on this differential staining and intensity, remains a useful marker in the distinction of pulmonary carcinoma from mesothelioma.

Anti-B72.3 is a murine IgG antibody, generated against a membrane-enriched fraction of human metastatic breast carcinoma, which recognizes a tumor-associated glycoprotein complex of high relative molecular mass ($M_r$). This antibody reacts with significantly more carcinomas (86%) and binds to a greater percentage of tumor cells (47%) when compared with Leu-M1 (57 and 25%, respectively; 19). Its diagnostic value is greatly diminished by frequent staining of mesothelioma cells, seen in anywhere from 7 up to 48% (5,20–22). In other hands, B72.3 has remained negative in mesothelioma (23). Staining reactions are generally weak and focal and could be interpreted as negative if the number of decorated cells falls below the 1+ scale of staining. Focal positivity on a more-limited sample (such as needle biopsy core) may lead to misclassification of a mesothelioma. Pepsin digestion enhances the reactivity of cells by unmasking antibody-binding sites in formalin-fixed tissue, as it does for cytokeratin epitopes. The antigenic pattern is quite stable, and no difference is noted in staining of biopsy and subsequent autopsy samples. It remains a good marker for carcinoma. But, in spite of its value in confirming the epithelial nature of a neoplasm, it has poor discriminatory potency for mesothelioma.

Anti-Leu-M1 is an IgM immunoglobulin specific for the human myelomonocytic antigen Leu-M1, which is found in a high proportion of carcinomas (80–100%), but which may be focally distributed and, therefore, can be missed when smaller samples are examined. Phagocytosed granulocytes constitute a source of false-positivity. No positive pleural mesotheliomas have been reported (24); however, one peritoneal mesothelioma showed focal staining (12). It stains well on routinely processed formalin–paraffin tissues. It rightfully maintains its place in all mesothelioma panels.

Various antibodies against cytokeratin (CK) detect the large family of 19 types of intermediate filaments that range widely in size (40–68 kDa), so prominently visible on electron microscopy of mesothelioma. Low MW cytokeratins are preponderant in glandular and acinar epithelia; high MW filaments are found in complex epithelia (squamous, transitional). Thus, squamous carcinomas contain high MW filaments; adenocarcinoma of breast, lung, biliary tract, and pancreas display both high and low MW filaments; and gastrointestinal adenocarcinoma contains low MW filaments.

The 34-$\beta$-E12 is a prototype of high MW cytokeratin of 57–66 kDa. KL1 (55–57 kDa) is a very efficient mesothelioma marker. Examples of low MW filament reagents include 35-$\beta$ H11 (52–46 kDa), UCD (52 kDa), PKK-1 (54 kDa), and CAM-5.2 (39, 43, and 54 kDa). A CK antibody mixture in common usage is the AE1/AE3 "cocktail" which covers the range of filament size found in mesothelioma. EAB902 is another panepithelial IgM antibody, and it may stain mesothelioma cells more intensively than those of carcinoma. High MW CK is more often selectively present in epithelioid mesothelioma than is low MW CK(25). However, high MW CK is absent in at least 20% of mesotheliomas. In addition, few adenocarcinomas also contain heavy filaments. Sarcomatous mesothelioma displays some low MW cytokeratin; thus, this overlap limits the value of keratin typing when applied to individual instances.

Cytokeratin staining in mesothelioma is usually strong, homogeneous, and cytoplasmic, often with a perinuclear ring, in contrast with the more common peripheral (membranous) or weaker weblike cytoplasmic pattern of adenocarcinoma. These findings were challenged by other investigators, who found no difference in CK staining between tumor types, and they concluded that the pattern of cytokeratin stains did not allow absolute discrimination between adenocarcinoma and mesothelioma (26,27).

The main value of keratin typing lies in proving the epithelioid nature of spindle cell pleural neoplasms and in demonstrating the antigenic preservation of tissue samples, especially when other stains of the panel fail to decorate. A sarcomatous pleural neoplasm, if sampled sufficiently, can be suspected to be of mesenchymal origin when completely lacking in cytokeratins (28). Paraffin-embedded tissue may not be the best substrate for the demonstration of cytokeratins, so the absence of CK staining does not exclude the diagnosis of mesothelioma if the other features are characteristic (29). One must remember that sarcomatous mesotheliomas stain unevenly for CK and may have large areas that do not express CK. Overall, CK-positivity in all types of mesothelioma was found in 470 of 559 cases (84%) gathered from 30 surveys. A CK-positive reaction can also be found in benign processes, since submesothelial cells may acquire CK expression in reactive states (30).

Epithelial membrane antigen (EMA), or human milk fat globulin-(HMFG1) and human milk fat globulin-2 (HMFG2) have been extensively studied in the diagnosis of mesothelioma. The EMA antiserum is a relatively sensitive marker for epithelial and mesothelial malignancy, but insufficient to cinch a diagnosis by itself. The literature reports rare expression of EMA by reactive mesothelial cells, and 50–95% positivity in mesothelioma (31). Some authors have suggested a membranous-staining pattern in mesothelioma, whereas adenocarcinoma more often displays a cytoplasmic pattern. Monoclonal sera selectively stain carcinoma cells (32). MOC-31 is a newly described EMA marker, reported to react with squamous carcinoma, adenocarcinoma, and small-cell carcinoma of the lung. It decorates 20% of mesothelioma and over half of adenocarcinomas, and thus has little usefulness in separating the tumors (31) and serves only as a general marker for malignancy.

The HMFG2 antigen was found in 39% of mesotheliomas, usually membranous, less commonly cytoplasmic, contrasting with a 95% reactivity in pulmonary adenocarcinoma (of combined cytoplasmic and membranous type) (21). The absence of cytoplasmic staining for HMFG2 strongly favors a diagnosis of mesothelioma, according to Sheibani (1). Both EMA/HMFG1 and HMFG2 are generally not expressed in reactive mesothelial proliferation (33,34).

There are several available antisera to vimentin, and these show quite variable reactivity, many being useful only on frozen sections. In multiple series there was expression of vimentin in 40–95% of mesotheliomas, whereas carcinomas expressed the antigen in 0–35%. This expression was strongest in sarcomatoid areas. The value of vimentin testing is limited owing to considerable overlap in positivity in both neoplasms (23). Overall, these figures add little support to the incorporation of vimentin antiserum in the antibody panel used for differentiating adenocarcinoma from mesothelioma. It can be used (like anticytokeratin) to gauge the antigenic integrity of the tissue by observing the required vimentin positivity within stromal tissue components.

Expression of blood group substances has recently been reported in gastrointestinal and pulmonary adenocarcinoma. An "A"-like antigen occurs in various tumors of patients within any blood group. The Tn antigen, which is one of the incompatible A antigens and a precursor of the Thomsen–Friedenreich antigen, has been detected in up to 88% of pulmonary adenocarcinomas (35). Studies with respective antisera have ensued and have shown no expression of surfactant in mesothelioma or reactive mesothelial conditions. The Tn antigen is not expressed in mesothelioma, but appears in most adenocarcinomas. Differences are noted within the Lewis antigen group in which all Lewis antigens (a, b, x, and y) are present in small numbers of mesotheliomas and in virtually all adenocarcinomas (35). Other markers, of limited value are those against ABH substance (15,23), which were regionally or diffusely expressed by a variable number of adenocarcinomas, but not by mesothelioma. Markers for Clara cell components and for surfactant apoprotein (a unique dedifferentiation antigen of the pulmonary alveolar epithelial cells, derived from type II pneumonocyte and probably Clara cells) have also been explored (35) and have not proved to be of practical importance (23).

CA19.9 is a sialylated lacto-*N*-fucopentose, related to the Lewis[a] blood group antigen, known to be expressed in ovarian, pancreatic, and gastrointestinal carcinoma. It was found to be of potential use by Ordonez (22), as it stained 39% of carcinomas, yet it failed to decorate any mesotheliomas thus achieving weak selectivity.

Secretory component is an antigenically distinct protein of secretory IgA, found in external secretions and in a variety of normal epithelial cells and their neoplasms. No consistent results are available on its discriminatory potential, owing to its widely variable expression in mesothelioma (22) and common presence in adenocarcinoma.

## V. Effusions

The subject of immunocytochemical analysis of serous effusions deserves particular scrutiny, being a common source of diagnostic frustration. This is due to more overlap in the cytological diagnostic criteria for reactive, mesotheliomatous, and metastatic carcinomatous process, when compared with histological preparations of those same tissues. Staining reactions that perform well in histological assays may not necessarily carry through as well when applied to cytological smears, where the thickness of the cell layer (contrasted with the split-thickness of a histological cut) may interfere with the evaluation of the pattern of staining (cytoplasmic vs membranous); where HMFG2 is concerned, a membranous pattern would suggest mesothelioma, whereas a cytoplasmic blush would point to adenocarcinomas (1). Good discrimination can be achieved with the standard "mesothelioma panel" in which the very strong expression of vimentin in reactive mesothelial proliferation contrasts with the lesser expression in metastatic carcinomas of diverse origin. A recent cytological cell block study (36) analyzed the staining pattern of reactive mesothelial cells which, as expected was characterized by low (5%) reactivity to EMA, CEA, and Leu-M1/B72.3 and high expression of vimentin (Table 2). Carcinoma cells were EMA-positive, and seldomly expressed vimentin. The clonality of the EMA serum matters, since polyclonal reagent may stain reactive mesothelial cells more strongly. A monoclonal EMA stain had superior discriminatory power, decorating nearly all adenocarcinomas, without decoration of benign or malignant mesothelium (32). The unanticipated small percentage of carcinoma-associated markers found in a small number of benign mesothelial cells is frustrating. This finding must be interpreted with caution, as it

**Table 2** Immunocytochemical Stains for the Identification of Malignant Cells in Serous Effusions

| Stain | Adenocarcinoma | Mesothelioma | Reactive |
|---|---|---|---|
| EMA | + (96%) | − | − |
| CEA | + (77%) | − | − |
| B72.3 | + (58%) | − | − |
| Leu-M1 | + (42%) | − | − |
| AUA$_1$ | + (88%) | − | − |

does not necessarily imply an aberrant-staining reaction, since one could be dealing with a heterogeneous mixture of benign and malignant cells. It is known that mesothelial cell atypia can be incited by underlying broncho-genic carcinoma (37), and this finding should raise the possibility of an occult carcinoma. Kuhlman et al. (38), reviewing malignant cell blocks, found vimentin and cytokeratin expression in mesothelioma as well as in reactive mesothelial conditions, whereas most carcinomatous effusions did not (or only weakly) express vimentin.

An antiserum against BMA-120, an endothelial marker, was over-whelmingly absent or very weakly expressed in all but ovarian carcinomas, yet it was only variably present in reactive and neoplastic mesothelium (completely absent in 15% of mesotheliomas; 38). The authors reach the timid, yet realistic conclusion that a pattern of negative reaction with epi-thelial markers and a positive reaction with BMA-120 is suggestive of a mesothelial process. Simultaneous positivity for endothelial and epithelial markers, therefore, suggests the possibility of a primary ovarian tumor.

A new IgG monoclonal antibody, 443A6, raised against the A549 human pulmonary adenocarcinoma cell line, detects a 40-kDa cell surface antigen associated with glandular differentiation and was the object of an immunochemical analysis of pleural effusions and fine-needle aspirations (39). This antibody identifies adenocarcinoma of pulmonary, mammary, intestinal, and ovarian origin, in contrast with its nonexpression in endo-metrial ovarian serous and renal carcinoma, as well as almost all meso-theliomas (1 of 36 did stain). Large-cell anaplastic carcinoma had a het-erogeneous and variable-staining pattern, whereas pulmonary squamous carcinoma, small-cell anaplastic carcinoma, and other tumors failed to dec-orate.

Another monoclonal antibody thought to be specific for ovarian neo-plasms was recently applied to cytological smears (32) and yielded interest-ing results: OV-632 was moderately expressed in mesothelioma, absent in reactive mesothelial cells and carcinoma of gut and breast, present in all ovarian neoplasms and in one-third of pulmonary carcinoma. OV-632 anti-serum thus seems useful in its ability to cytologically distinguish malignant from reactive mesothelial cells. Cellular decoration suggests mesothelioma or ovarian (uncommonly pulmonary) carcinoma, in contrast with lack of staining in carcinoma of other source.

BCA-225 (Cu-18) is a breast carcinoma-associated glycoprotein iso-lated in T47-D breast carcinoma cell line, shown to be present in a variety of adenocarcinomas. A monoclonal antibody to this antigen has shown great promise in the distinction of reactive from carcinomatous serous effu-sions. The antibody decorated 75–79% of carcinoma cells in both pleural and peritoneal effusions, with (at first) a perfect nonstaining record against reactive mesothelial cells. When further tested, a single traumatic effusion had reactive mesothelial cell staining for the antibody (40), for a false-positive rate below 1%. The BCA-225 antibody reacted with more than 90% of adenocarcinoma of mammary or pulmonary origin and with a moderate percentage of carcinoma of renal, ovarian, endometrial, and cervical origin. Few gastrointestinal carcinomas were decorated. It serves as a near conclusive marker for carcinomatous malignancy (41), shifting the diagnosis away from a reactive mesothelial process.

An antibody to the cell surface antigen $AUA_1$ has been successfully used in histological sections of various epithelia. The corresponding monoclonal antibody was applied to cytological smears of serosal effusions and yielded an overall diagnostic accuracy rate of 94% (42). This allowed investigators to do away with the usual antibody panel and rely exclusively on demonstration of $AUA_1$ in the detection of carcinoma cells in body fluid. Positive reactions were found in 88% of carcinomatous effusions, with negative reactions in 98% of benign effusions. This lack of staining of benign (and malignant) mesothelium promises to improve the diagnostic accuracy of serosal cytological smears.

No decisive pattern emerges from these studies, since specifying which particular type of neoplasm is involved still requires the application of a wide antiserum panel and may not yield a clear answer in individual instances. It calls for judicious weighing of a batch of diverse antigenic results, handicapped by exceptions to virtually every common rule.

The accuracy of cytological analysis of serous effusions, even augmented by latest immunocytochemistry, remains in dispute. It is argued that a cytological workup contributes useful information in most patients with pleural epithelioid mesothelioma (43). Yet the overall figure of 64% specific interpretation by cytological methods, in the best of hands, is underwhelming, particularly when one considers that terms such as "suspicious, atypical, in favor of, adeno vs meso, and so on" were considered positive readings for the purposes of the study. The quandary of the attending physician when faced with such terms was brought up in a critical letter rebutting the author's laudatory claim (44).

Precise and decisive interpretation on cytological material is a goal still to be achieved, in need of the ultimate positive marker for mesothelioma, since the present system relies on exclusion by a set of negative markers. For now, much support can be had from a multisystem panel that combines a limited number of antisera run in concert, the composition of which reflects personal bias. A basic panel should include CEA, Leu-M1, and $AUA_1$. To these, BMA-120, EMA (especially for cytology), BER-Ep4, BCA-225, and OV-632 could be added. A malignant mesothelioma is more probable than a reactive mesothelial condition when positive reactions are noted for HMFG2, EMA, BMA-120, and OV-632, whereas CEA, Leu-M1, and AUA₁ remain nonreactive. All these markers, except BMA-120, are overwhelmingly negative in reactive mesothelial states.

A diagnosis of adenocarcinoma is more likely than mesothelioma when positive reactions are found for CEA, BCA-225, Leu-M1, and BER-Ep4, since such markers are poorly expressed in mesothelioma. Renal cell carcinoma remains cytochemically inert and often gives negative reactions to common markers. Ovarian carcinoma (and also mesothelioma) decorates for OV-632. Either vimentin or cytokeratin staining can be added to test for antigenicity integrity of the material.

## Addendum

Two studies have appeared since completion of the original monograph.

The latest evaluation of immunohistochemical markers in paraffin-embedded tissue to distinguish pleural mesothelioma from pulmonary adenocarcinoma, again assigned the highest value to CEA for sensitivity and specificity (both at 97%). A combination of CEA, Leu-M1, and B72.3 resolves 74% of diagnostic problems (45). The latest immunocytochemical evaluation of pleural effusions selects, through a system of stepwise logistic regression, a panel of three markers (CEA, EMA, and B72.3) for its ability to characterize over 95% of effusions. When all three markers are absent, the diagnosis of adenocarcinoma is extremely unlikely, when two or three are positive, a diagnosis of adenocarcinoma is almost certain (46).

## References

1. McCaughey WT, Colby TV, Battilflora H, Churg A, Corson JM, Greenberg SD, Grimes MM, Roggli VL, Unni KK. Diagnosis of diffuse malignant mesothelioma: experience of a US/Canadian mesothelioma panel. Mod Pathol 1991; 4:342–353.
2. England DM, Hochholzer L, McCarthy MJ. Localized benign and malignant fibrous tumors of the pleura. Am J Surg Pathol 1989; 13:640–658.
3. McCaughey WT. Papillary peritoneal neoplasms in females. In: vol 20, pt 2. Sommers SC, Rosen PP, Fechner RE, eds. Pathology annual. East Norwalk, CT: Appleton & Lange, 1985: 387–404.
4. Bollinger DJ, Wick MR, Dehner LP, et al. Peritoneal malignant mesothelioma vs serous papillary carcinoma. A histochemical and immunohistochemical comparison. Am J Surg Pathol 1989; 13:659–670.
5. Khoury N, Ragu U, Crissman JD, Zarbo RJ, Greenawald KA. A comparative immunohistochemical study of peritoneal and ovarian serous tumors and mesotheliomas. Hum Pathol 1990; 21:811–819.

6.  Donna A, Betta PG, Jones JS. Verification of the histological diagnosis of malignant mesothelioma in relation to the binding of an antimesothelial cell antibody. Cancer 1989; 63:1331–1336.
7.  Sheibani K, Esteban JM, Bailey A, Battofora H, Weiss LM. Immunopathologic and molecular studies as an aid to the diagnosis of malignant mesothelioma. Hum Pathol 1992; 23:107–116.
8.  Chang K, Pai LH, Pass H, Pogrebniak HW, Tsao MS, Pastan I, Willingham MC. Monoclonal antibody K1 reacts with epithelial mesothelioma but not with lung adenocarcinoma. Am J Surg Pathol 1992; 16:259–268.
9.  Wang NS, Huang SN, Gold P. Absence of carcinoembryonic antigen-like material in mesothelioma: an immunohistochemical differentiation from other lung cancers. Cancer 1979; 44:937–943.
10. Mezger J, Lamerz R, Permanetter W. Diagnostic significance of carcinoembryonic antigen in the differential diagnosis of malignant mesothelioma. J Thorac Cardiovasc Surg 1990; 100:860–866.
11. Corson JM, Pinkus GS. Mesothelioma: profile of keratin proteins and carcinoembryonic antigen. Am J Pathol 1982; 108:80–87.
12. Robb J. Mesothelioma vs adenocarcinoma; false positive CEA and Leu-M1 staining due to hyaluronic acid [letter]. Hum Pathol 1989; 20:400.
13. Stirling JW, Henderson DW, Spagnolo DV, Whitaker D. Unusual granular reactivity for carcinoembryonic antigen in malignant mesothelioma [letter]. Hum Pathol 1990; 21:678–679.
14. Soosay GN, Griffiths M, Papadaki L, Happerfield L, Bobrow L. The differential diagnosis of epithelial-type mesothelioma from adenocarcinoma and reactive mesotheliomal proliferation. J Pathol 1991; 163: 299–305.
15. Vortmeyer AO, Preuss J, Padberg BC, Kastendieck H, Schroder S. Immunocytochemical differential diagnosis of diffuse malignant pleural mesotheliomas — a clinicomorphological study of 158 cases. Anticancer Res 1991; 11: 889–894.
16. Latza U, Niedobitek G, Schwarting R, Nekarda H, Stein H. J Clin Pathol 1990; 43:213–219.
17. Sheibani K, Shin SS, Kezirian J, Weiss LM. Ber-Ep4 antibody as a discriminant in the differential diagnosis of malignant mesothelioma vs adenocarcinoma. Am J Surg Pathol 1991; 15:779–784.
18. Gaffey MJ, Mills SE, Swanson PE, Zarbo RJ, Shah AR, Wick MR. Immunoreactivity for BER-Ep4 in adenocarcinomas, adenomatoid tumors and malignant mesotheliomas. Am J Surg Pathol 1992; 16:593–599.
19. Warnock ML, Stoloff A, Thor A. Differentiation of adenocarcinoma of the lung from mesothelioma: periodic acid–Schiff, monoclonal antibodies B72.3 and Leu-M1. Am J Pathol 1988; 133:30–38.
20. Wirth PR, Legier JF, Wright GL. Immunohistochemical evaluation of seven monoclonal antibodies for differentiation of pleural mesothelioma from lung adenocarcinoma. Cancer 1991; 67:655–662.
21. Tuttle SE, Lucas JG, Bucci DM, Schlom J, Primus J. Distinguishing malignant mesothelioma from pulmonary adenocarcinoma: an immunohistochemi-

cal approach using a panel of monoclonal antibodies. J Surg Oncol 1990; 145: 72–78.

22. Ordonez N. The immunohistochemical diagnosis of mesothelioma; differentiation of mesothelioma and lung adenocarcinoma. Am. J Surg Pathol 1989; 13:276–291.
23. Wick MR, Loy T, Mills SE, Legier JF, Manivel JC. Malignant epithelioid pleural mesothelioma vs peripheral pulmonary adenocarcinoma; a histochemical, ultrastructural, and immunohistologic study of 103 cases. Hum Pathol 1990; 21:759–766.
24. Wick MR, Mills SE, Swanson PE. Expression of myelomonocytic antigens in mesothelioma and adenocarcinomas involving the serosal surfaces. Am J Clin Pathol 1990; 94:18–26.
25. Otis CN, Carter D, Cole S, Battifora H. Immunohistochemical evaluation of pleural mesothelioma and pulmonary adenocarcinoma; a bi-institutional study of 47 cases. Am J Surg Pathol 1987; 11:445–456.
26. Adams VI, Unni KK. Diffuse malignant mesothelioma of pleura: diagnostic criteria based on an autopsy study. Am J Clin Pathol 1984; 82:15–23.
27. Cibas ES, Corson JM, Pinkus GS. The distinction of adenocarcinoma from malignant mesothelioma in cell blocks of effusions: the role of routine mucin histochemistry and immunohistochemical assessment of carcinoembryonic antigen, keratin proteins, epithelial membrane antigen, and milk fat globule-derived antigen. Hum Pathol 1987; 18:67–74.
28. Cagle PT, Truong LD, Roggli VT, Greenberg SD. Immunohistochemical differentiation of sarcomatoid mesotheliomas from other spindle cell neoplasms. Am J Clin Pathol 1989; 92:566–571.
29. Henderson D, Shilkin K, Le Langlois S, Whitaker D. Malignant mesothelioma. New York: Hemisphere Publishing, 1992:124.
30. Bolen JW, Hammar SP, McNutt MA. Reactive and neoplastic serosal tissue; a light-microscopic, ultrastructural, and immunocytochemical study. Am J Surg Pathol 1986; 10:34–47.
31. Delahaye M, Hoogsteden HC, van der Kwast TH. Immunocytochemistry of malignant mesothelioma: OV632 as a marker of malignant mesothelioma. J Pathol 1991; 165:137–143.
32. Nance KV, Silverman JF. Immunocytochemical panel for the identification of malignant cells in serous effusions. Am J Clin Pathol 1991; 95:867–874.
33. Marshall RJ, Herbert A, Braye SG, Jones DB. Use of antibodies to carcinoembryonic antigen and human milk fat globule to distinguish carcinoma, mesothelioma, and reactive mesothelium. J Clin Pathol 1984; 37:1215–1221.
34. Ghosh AK, Butler EB. Immunocytochemical staining reactions of anti-carcinoembryonic antigen, CA, and anti-human milk fat globule monoclonal antibodies on benign and malignant exfoliated mesothelial cells. J Clin Pathol 1987; 40:1424–1427.
35. Noguchi M, Nakajima T, Horohashi S, Akiba T, Shimosato Y. Immunohistochemical distinction of malignant mesothelioma from pulmonary adenocarcinoma with anti-surfactant apoprotein, anti-Lewis, and anti-Tn antibodies. Hum Pathol 1989; 20:53–57.

36. Tickman RJ, Cohen C. Varma VA, Fekete PS, DeRose PB. Distinction between carcinoma cells and mesothelioma cells in serous effusions; usefulness of immunohistochemistry. Acta Cytol 1990; 34:491–495.
37. Yokoi T, Mark EJ. Atypical mesothelial hyperplasia associated with bronchogenic carcinoma. Hum Pathol 1991; 22:695–696.
38. Kuhlmann L, Berghauser K-H, Schaffer R. Distinction of mesothelioma from carcinoma in pleural effusions; an immunohistochemical study on routinely processed cytoblock preparations. Pathol Res Pract 1991; 187:467–471.
39. Spagnolo DV, Whitaker D, Carello S, Radosevich JA, Rosen ST, Gould, VE. The use of monoclonal antibody 44-3A6 in cell blocks in the diagnosis of lung carcinoma, carcinomas metastatic to lung and pleura, and pleural malignant mesothelioma. Am J Clin Pathol 1991; 95:322–329.
40. Loy TS, Diaz-Arias AA, Bickel JT. [Letter to the editor.] Mod Pathol 1991; 4:283.
41. Loy TS, Diaz-Arias AA, Bickel JT. Value of BCA-225 in the cytologic diagnosis of malignant effusions: an immunocytochemical study of 197 cases. Mod Pathol 1990; 3:294–297.
42. Kocjan G, Sweeney E, Miller KD, Bobrow L. AUA1: new immunocytochemical marker for detecting epithelial cells in body cavity fluids. J Clin Pathol 1992; 45:358–359.
43. Sherman ME, Mark EJ. Effusion cytology in the diagnosis of malignant epithelioid and biphasic pleural mesothelioma. Arch Pathol Lab Med 1990; 114:845–851.
44. Scamurra DO. Effusion cytology in the diagnosis of malignant epithelioid and biphasic pleural mesothelioma. Arch Pathol Lab Med 1991; 115:210.

# 8

## Cytological Diagnosis of Malignant Mesothelioma

**THEODORUS H. VAN DER KWAST**

Erasmus University Rotterdam
Rotterdam, The Netherlands

**M. DELAHAYE**

Academic Hospital Rotterdam
Rotterdam, The Netherlands

**JOCELYNE FLEURY**

Hôpital Henri-Mondor
Créteil, France

### I. Introduction

Patients with a diffuse malignant mesothelioma frequently present with dyspnea caused by an accumulation of pleural fluid. This effusion may arise as a consequence of obstruction of lymphatic drainage by tumor cells, or of increased vascular permeability caused by interaction of tumor-derived cytokines with endothelial cells (1). The presence of a unilateral pleural effusion is a common chest radiographic finding in malignant mesothelioma patients. Its incidence in patients with malignant mesothelioma varies from 30 to 95% (2,3). This common manifestation of malignant mesothelioma makes exfoliative cytology the most obvious first-line diagnostic procedure. According to most studies, in about 75–95% of patients with a diffuse malignant mesothelioma of the pleura, a sufficient amount of serous effusion can be obtained by a thin-needle pleural puncture to allow an adequate cytological examination (4–6). As most of these patients require drainage of the pleural cavity for relief of their dyspnea, the effusion is readily available for examination, without imposing additional discomfort on them.

When an insufficient amount of pleural effusion is present, it is sometimes possible to perform a fine-needle aspiration of a pleural lesion that is recognizable on radiography or on a computed tomography (CT) scan (7). Rarely, a lymph node metastasis or a subcutaneous thoracic tumor is available for cytological examination. Although the presence of malignant mesothelioma cells in sputum has been described in two case studies (8,9), the peripheral localization of the tumor makes an early diagnosis on this material very improbable. For these reasons this chapter is entirely devoted to the cytological diagnostics of malignant mesothelioma on pleural effusions.

### A. Objectives of Cytological Diagnosis

Cytological examination of a pleural effusion serves to identify malignancy at an early stage, particularly in those patients without previous diagnosis of malignancy. As diffuse malignant mesotheliomas are characterized by their poor prognosis and lack of response to therapy, their rapid diagnosis shortens the time a patient needs to be hospitalized and obviates the requirement of more complicated and more costly diagnostic procedures involved in the search for a primary tumor.

Histologically, malignant mesotheliomas may consist of tumor cells with epithelial morphology, spindle cell (fibroblastic or sarcomatous) morphology, or combinations of both cell types. The incidence of monophasic, sarcomatous malignant mesothelioma is estimated as between 4 and 32% (10). The large variation in reported incidence of monophasic sarcomatous malignant mesothelioma has been attributed to differences in tumor sampling. An increase in the number of samples or the size of the sample available for histological examination from an individual patient is associated with a higher proportion of biphasic malignant mesotheliomas (10). Although according to some (11–13), but not all (14,15) studies, the prognosis of a monophasic sarcomatous mesothelioma may be somewhat better than that of the two other types; the subdivision of malignant mesothelioma into histological subtypes has no therapeutical consequences. In general, only the tumor cells with epithelial morphology are exfoliated in the effusion fluid. Rarely, cells with a spindle cell morphology, characteristic of the sarcomatous component of a malignant mesothelioma, are encountered in serous effusions. If an effusion is present in a monophasic sarcomatous malignant mesothelioma, malignant cells are generally lacking (16). Employment of cytological examination as a single diagnostic tool does not allow distinction between a biphasic malignant mesothelioma and a pure epithelial-type malignant mesothelioma.

Efforts to distinguish metastatic adenocarcinoma from malignant mesothelioma are justified for a few reasons. Although the survival time of patients with a malignant mesothelioma and those with a pleural metastasis of an adenocarcinoma do not differ greatly, their palliative treatment may depend on a different approach. Moreover, patients may obtain financial compensation if they suffer from an occupational disease; therefore, an early and correct diagnosis of malignant mesothelioma is mandatory.

### B. Impediments to the Cytological Diagnosis of Malignant Mesothelioma

It should be realized that—in essence—the cytological diagnosis of malignant mesothelioma in a pleural effusion relies on two basic steps. Both the *malignant* nature of cells present in an effusion should be ascertained and the *mesothelial* features of the malignant cells should be recognized. Both decision-making processes are hampered with difficulties (5). No single criterion exists that serves to distinguish malignant from reactive mesothelial cells, or adenocarcinoma cells from malignant mesothelioma cells. A reliable cytological diagnosis can be made only on technically well-prepared cytological specimens, with a sufficient number of cells. Experience of the technician and cytopathologist greatly adds to the sensitivity and specificity of the diagnosis. Nevertheless, in a considerable proportion of cases, light microscopic examination alone cannot yield a definite diagnosis and ancillary techniques are required.

### C. Outline of the Chapter

In the first part of the chapter, the technical aspects related to cytology of pleural effusions will be discussed and a brief description of the currently employed techniques for conventional staining, (immuno)cytochemistry, and transmission electron microscopy will be given (see Sec. II). The sensitivity of cytological diagnosis of malignant mesothelioma will be compared with that of other diagnostic techniques, and the accuracy of cytological diagnosis of malignant mesothelioma, as reported in the literature, will be highlighted in Section III. Subsequently, the sensitivity and reliability of a set of morphological criteria distinguishing malignant from benign mesothelial cells, on the one hand, and tumor cells with mesothelial differentiation from adenocarcinoma cells, on the other, will be evaluated (see Sec. IV).

Since immunocytochemistry is now frequently being applied to cytological specimens of pleural effusions, and an increasing number of articles are being published on this matter, an overview of current markers and their application is given (see Sec. V). Its influence on improvement of cytology by raising the level of confidence and objectivity will be discussed. In Section VI, particular emphasis will be given to the role of transmission electron microscopy (TEM) in diagnostic cytology of pleural effusions.

The knowledge of molecular biological changes during oncogenesis is expanding rapidly, and probes detecting oncogenes and their products (mRNA, proteins) have become widely available. Section VII of the chapter is devoted to the perspectives of application of DNA-flow cytometry, DNA in situ hybridization, and the use of oncogene-specific probes in cytological diagnostics.

## II. Technical Aspects

### A. Acquisition and Handling of Pleural Effusions

Factors that may adversely affect a proper evaluation of cytological specimens of pleural effusions are poor morphological quality, the cytologist's lack of awareness of the possibility of a malignant mesothelioma and lack of experience with this diagnosis, and inadequate laboratory processing of the sample (17–18).

### Collection and Cleaning of Specimens

The fluid must be collected in containers with an admixture of an anticoagulant factor (19); no fixative should be added (20,21). Preferably, fluid from the first pleural puncture should be used, since second and following punctures often yield an inadequate, bloody sample (18). At least 50 ml of fluid is necessary for adequate preparation of slides. By visual examination the fluid can be clear, hemorrhagic, or flocculent with (fibrin) clots. All larger, floating elements must be removed before further preparation, as they tend to affect the quality of smear preparations of cell sediments and the processing into cell blocks for histological analysis or TEM. To remove flocculated material and clots, the fluid can be passed through a 100-$\mu$m nylon gauze. This gauze allows the passage of dispersed cells as well as smaller and larger cell groups. The result is a rather cloudy, but homogeneous, sample fit for further processing.

### Separation of Blood Cells

If the obtained fluid is hemorrhagic, the contaminating blood cells must be removed; otherwise they will obscure the presence of the tumor cells. Various techniques are available to remove excess erythrocytes. They can be lysed by mixing the hemorrhagic sediment with acetic acid or a detergent (e.g., saponin; 22,23).

Separation techniques based on differences in cellular density may interfere less with the morphological integrity of the tumor cells. The isolation of a buffy coat after centrifugation of the effusion is a simple technique (24). Density-gradient techniques represent more sophisticated procedures to isolate nucleated cells. One can either apply a continuous gradient (20) or discontinuous gradients, based on Ficoll–Isopaque (17,25). These separation fluids are commercially available at a specific gravity of 1.077, and have become very useful for isolation of the nucleated fraction from hemorrhagic pleural fluid samples. After careful deposition of the sample on top of the gradient in a large test tube, centrifugation at 1200 *g* for 20 min will result in the separation of the nucleated cell band from the contaminating erythrocytes. For a more selective separation, a discontinuous gradient can be made using Percoll at a density of 1.055; only the larger nucleated cells remain within the cell band, whereas lymphocytes and granulocytes sediment through the Percoll (26) together with the erythrocytes. The latter procedure may be particularly useful, as pleural fluids of patients with malignant mesothelioma are often very rich in lymphocytes, which may disturb a proper evaluation.

After enrichment of the cell suspension, the cell pellet can be washed in phosphate-buffered saline (PBS), supplemented with bovine serum albumin (BSA; 0.5 v/v%) to preserve the cells' morphological structure. During the process of application of the cells on the glass slide or other carriers, a further cell concentration can be achieved by using natural gravity (27), or by centrifugation on permeable Millipore or Nucleopore membranes. Most European laboratories make cell smear preparations from sediments obtained by centrifugation in a pointed test tube. We prefer centrifugation in 15-ml tubes at 2000 rpm for 10 min; others centrifuge for 5 min at 1500 rpm (19), for 10 min at 3000 rpm, or for 10 min at 2500 rpm (21).

### Embedding in Paraffin or Plastic

Several methods have been described to embed cell pellets in paraffin to obtain cell blocks. Agar is frequently used to fix the cells before the paraffin-embedding procedure (28). A disadvantage of this method is that the cells are exposed to temperatures over 40°C which may lead to morphological deterioration. We prefer the technique described by Kaps (29): briefly, 1 volume of a solution of 12.5% glutaraldehyde is mixed with 5 volumes of 7.0% BSA, and the cell pellet is subsequently mixed in equal volumes. After centrifugation for 20 min, a coagulant containing the admixed cells will be obtained. The cell pellet can be cut in several pieces, and these may be further fixed in formalin or glutaraldehyde. For sections of the paraffin-embedded specimens, light microscopy and immunocytochemistry for several antigens is possible. The glutaraldehyde-fixed specimens may be further processed for TEM. With a scanty pellet, the procedure can also be performed in a glass microhematocrit tube.

### B. Staining and Storage of Cytological Preparations

A quick stain for first cytological impression can be done with toluidine blue (30) or 5% aqueous methylene blue (own experience). A drop of methylene blue is applied on the air-dried smear, covered with a coverslip and immediately examined by light microscopy. Quick stain procedures enable an early decision on whether or not to proceed with the technical processing of the sample. When an abundance of (suspect) cells is present it can be decided to prepare cell blocks for routine paraffin embedding or for transmission electron microscopy.

Several smears of the cell pellet are always immediately fixed for Papanicolaou stain and cytochemistry, in addition to some that are air-dried for Giemsa stain. It is recommended that several spare slides be stored for immunocytochemistry at −20°C. Acetone-dehydrated smears should be wrapped in tinfoil to prevent deposition of condensate after their removal from the freezer (31).

Occasionally, the puncture fluids contain large numbers of tumor cells. In those cases the remainder of the cell pellets can be frozen and stored at −20°C in a suspension of 10% dimethyl sulfoxide (OMSO; 32). If necessary these suspensions can be processed for light microscopy and TEM at any time.

### C.  Immuno(cyto)chemistry

*Techniques of Immunostaining*

The most commonly applied staining techniques are the indirect-conjugated method, the indirect-unconjugated method, and those based on the high-affinity binding of avidin to biotin-linked macromolecules. These three methods can be combined with different enzymes, such as horseradish peroxidase or alkaline phosphatase. The methods may differ in sensitivity and signal/background ratio (33,34).

*Preparation of the Specimen*

Immunocytochemistry can be applied on acetone-fixed or alcohol-fixed cytological smears of sediments of pleural effusions or on slides of formalin-fixed, paraffin-embedded sediments. The advantage of the former method is the ease of obtaining smear preparations and the large number of cells available for examination. Moreover, formalin-sensitive epitopes are also available for testing. Additionally, some authors have reported good immunostaining results after fixation of smears at 4°C with buffered formol-acetone (35,36). In smears of effusions that are heavily contaminated with blood, there may be a high background. Ficoll–Isopaque density separation appears to be very helpful in eliminating this problem. An advantage to the use of formalin-fixed, paraffin-embedded sediments (cell blocks) is the possibility of making multiple sections and the low background in immunocytochemistry.

### Storage or Fixed Specimens

Air-dried cytological smears can be stored for approximately 1 week at room temperature before immunostaining with most antibodies. If storage for prolonged periods is envisaged, air-dried, acetone-fixed slides may be kept in a tightly closed box or enveloped in tinfoil at $-20°C$ until use. Condensate formation on the slides should be prevented when slides are removed from the freezer.

### Destaining of Archival Slides

For several antibodies [e.g., to epithelial membrane antigen (EMA) or carcinoembryonic antigen (CEA)], it is possible to destain Papanicolaou-stained and Giemsa-stained slides, by incubation in pure methanol and then to perform immunostaining (37). From our experience, Papanicolaou-stained slides stored for many years in the archives may be used for immunostaining.

### Blocking of Endogenous Peroxidase Activity

The presence of granulocytes (and erythrocytes) in a pleural effusion may lead to substantial endogenous peroxidase activity if a peroxidase conjugate is being used as secondary antibody. This background activity is blocked by incubation of the slides with methanol-containing hydrogen peroxide. By this procedure a simultaneous fixation of the cells is achieved; however, some epitopes are sensitive to this hydrogen peroxide treatment. Alternatively, conjugates of secondary antibody with alkaline phosphatase can be used, obviating the need for endogenous peroxidase blocking and resulting in lower background staining.

### General Remarks

Currently, more sensitive methods that are based on high-affinity streptavidin–biotin binding are being increasingly employed, using either horseradish peroxidase or alkaline phosphatase as the visualizing enzyme. In general, an indirect-conjugated immunocytochemical-staining method is sufficiently sensitive to visualize the presence of relevant markers. It should be realized that, occasionally, the method employed may influence the outcome of a staining reaction. It is recommended that, before the routine application of a monoclonal antibody, a reference set of smears or slides of cell blocks containing either benign or malignant mesothelial cells from a series of patients be examined. Once an immunocytochemical staining technique has become selected, it should not be replaced by another method before checking its specificity and sensitivity in diagnosis of malignant mesothelioma.

### D.  Transmission Electron Microscopy

For TEM, cells in the fluid must be fixed quickly. Usually, the effusion
obtained by puncture is collected in an anticoagulant, such as sodium ci-
trate, mixed with an equal volume of the fixative solution for 1 h, then
centrifuged (1500 rpm for 10 min), and the pellet fixed at 4°C for 2 h. The
fixative solution used is 2.5% glutaraldehyde in cacodylate buffer, 0.1 $M$
pH 7.4. The pellet is then washed, postfixed, dehydrated, and embedded in
Epon for TEM as usual. Cytochemistry and immunocytochemistry can be
performed at the ultrastructural level using pre- or postembedding methods
(38). The method described by Kaps (29) (see Sec. II.A.3) is particularly
useful if the pellet is scant. In fact, we often apply this procedure, even if a
large pellet is present.

## III.  Efficacy of Cytology for the Diagnosis of Malignant Mesothelioma

### A.  Comparison of Diagnostic Methods

The diagnosis of malignant mesothelioma can be based on histological or
cytological examination of tumor specimens obtained by several different
approaches. Large differences in sensitivity among the different methods
employed exist within and between institutions (Table 1). In autopsy-
proved malignant mesothelioma, previous thoracotomy and biopsy established the diagnosis in 90% of cases (42). However, thoracotomy can be
complicated by intractable pain along the incision line and metastatic lesions in the thoracotomy wound (3). Among the 327 patients reported by

**Table 1**  Sensitivity of Diagnostic Procedures for Malignant Mesothelioma

| | Diagnostic procedure | | | |
| Ref. | Effusion cytology | Closed-needle biopsy | Thoracoscopy biopsy | Open pleural biopsy |
|---|---|---|---|---|
| 3 | 3[a] (35)[b] | 36 (49) | 81  (89) | 93 (97) |
| 39 | 0  (0) | 79 (79) | 100 (100) | |
| 40 | 19  (42) | 56 (73) | | |
| 41 | 48 | 39 | | |
| 11 | 10  (32) | 10 (48) | | 77 (92) |
| 6 | (45) | (43) | | |

[a]Figures represent percentages of established diagnosis of malignant mesothelioma.
[b]Between parentheses is the percentage of cases in which malignancy could be determined.

Elmes and Simpson (43) only 35 developed a chest wall mass, 80% of these arising from the site of a previous pleural biopsy, thoracotomy, or chest tube drainage. Dorward and Stack (40) reported that a tumor in the chest wall developed in the 4 patients who underwent thoracotomy, whereas 5 of 23 patients with a percutaneous needle biopsy developed subcutaneous tumor growth in the needle tract. Although some authors implied that these iatrogenic complications are the cause of much discomfort to the patient, Ruffie et al. (3) reported that in his series of patients these lesions were rarely a cause of pain, and they did not contribute to death.

Comparison of the diagnostic value of different methods of tumor tissue retrieval demonstrates that both closed-needle biopsies and exfoliative cytology are associated with a low diagnostic sensitivity, whereas in 80–90% of cases a definite diagnosis of malignant mesothelioma can be established by thoracoscopy or open pleural biopsy (see Table 1). Similarly, the overall picture emerging from these comparative studies is that exfoliative cytology is of limited value for the diagnosis. Some authors put forward that combined assessment of a needle biopsy and cytological preparations would lead to an improved diagnostic accuracy. Histological examination of needle biopsies and cytological assessment of effusions can yield complementary information, leading to an increased number of correct diagnoses of malignant mesothelioma. Thus, features of malignancy evident in histopathological preparations may be linked to features of mesothelial differentiation of atypical cells in cytological smears, or vice versa. Whitaker and Shilkin (5) claimed that, in 39% of a series of 70 cases of confirmed malignant mesothelioma, a definite diagnosis could be made on a pleural biopsy and, in 50%, by cytological methods alone. Combining the two methods led to an 80% score of correct diagnoses.

Antman et al. (44) collected the data from five different studies for comparison of the diagnostic efficacy of effusion cytology, closed-needle biopsy, and thoracotomy (Table 2). On the basis of these data the authors

**Table 2** Sensitivity of Diagnostic Procedures for Malignant Mesothelioma

| Technique | Number | Percentage positive for mesothelioma |
|---|---|---|
| Effusion cytology | 270 | 9 |
| Needle biopsy | 115 | 24 |
| Thoracotomy | 242 | 60 |

*Source*: Ref. 44.

concluded that pleural fluid cytological analysis was the least sensitive technique for diagnosis of malignant mesothelioma (9% sensitivity), followed by needle biopsy (24%) and thoracotomy (60%). An objection to the approach by Antman is that results of different techniques within one institution or one study were not compared, but rather, data obtained with different techniques in different clinical settings were used.

### B. Sensitivity of Cytological Methods

In contrast with the poor diagnostic performance of cytology apparent from the aforementioned studies, data from several publications largely devoted to cytology of pleural effusions as the single diagnostic criterion revealed a more heterogeneous picture (Table 3). In these studies on confirmed cases of malignant mesothelioma, the percentage of a definite diag-

**Table 3**  Accuracy of a Cytological Diagnosis of Malignant Mesothelioma

| Author (Ref.) | Number of mesotheliomas | Sensitivity for mesothelioma (%) | Sensitivity for malignancy (%) |
|---|---|---|---|
| Klempman (45) | 27 | 63 | 70 |
| Naylor (46) | 7 | 57 | 86 |
| Roberts (47) | 14 | 57 | 71 |
| Elmes (43) | 172 | 4 | 15 |
| Jara (48) | 20 | 5 | 40 |
| Whitaker (49) | 12 | 60 | 83 |
| Edge (50) | 26 | 77 | 77 |
| Tao (16) | 22 | 77 | 77 |
| Antman (14) | 28 | 4 | 28 |
| Lewis (51) | 46 | 6 | 6 |
| Brenner (52) | 60 | 12 | 37 |
| Nauta (53) | 26 | 15 | 35 |
| Law (54) | 80 | 0 | 25 |
| Triol (55) | 75 | 56 | 67 |
| Martensson (12) | 31 | 3 | 35 |
| Matzel (56) | 51 | 41 | 76 |
| Adams (11) | 69 | 26 | 32 |
| Whitaker (57) | 103 | 72 | 81 |
| Strankinga (39) | 25 | 0 | 0 |
| Whitaker (17) | 30 | 80 | 90 |
| Ruffie (3) | 152 | 3 | 35 |
| Sherman (58) | 36 | 64 | 72 |
| Delahaye (in press) | 74 | 68 | 73 |

nosis of malignant mesothelioma and the percentage of a definite diagnosis of malignancy were reported. The sensitivity for correctly diagnosing malignant mesothelioma ranges from 0 to 80%. Particularly, the outcome of the large series of Elmes and Simpson (43) is often referred to as an example of low sensitivity of cytological methods for demonstration of malignant mesothelioma. As pointed out in the review by Whitaker and Shilkin (5), the alleged low sensitivity of cytology in diagnosis of this malignancy, apparent from the foregoing study, can partially be attributed to the composition of this large series. In fact, all cases were collected from a large number of hospitals and associated pathological laboratories, each with their own relative experience.

The data listed in Table 3 indicate that the sensitivity for establishing malignancy fluctuates in close relation to the sensitivity of the diagnosis of malignant mesothelioma. In the studies reporting a low frequency of definite cytological diagnosis of malignant mesothelioma, this seems to be partly due to the failure to recognize features of malignancy in the exfoliated cells.

## IV. Cytomorphological Features of Malignant Mesothelioma

The cytological diagnosis of malignant mesothelioma is based on the recognition of features suggestive of *malignancy* and *mesothelial differentiation*. Although a combination of these features will generally lead to a diagnosis, for clarity sake we will deal with the criteria separately.

### A. Criteria of Malignancy

#### Size and Shape of Cell Clusters

During low-power examination of a cytological preparation of an effusion, abnormal cell clusters may be the first feature noticed. If present, they point to possible malignancy. Papillary aggregates and morules are three-dimensional clusters of mesothelial cells in which the nuclei are located peripherally in the cytoplasm (Figs. 1 and 2). The presence of these structures in a smear are a strong argument in favor of malignancy. Morules may be seen occasionally in reactive mesothelial proliferations, but if present in larger numbers, they are a strong indication for malignancy. Kwee et al. (59) found morules in only 3.7% of reactive pleural effusions, but in 87.2% of effusions of patients with a malignant mesothelioma. In cytological smears of benign effusions, large groups of mesothelial cells may occasionally be present, but they generally have a two-dimensional sheet arrangement in which the mesothelial cells form a regular pattern, with tiny slits

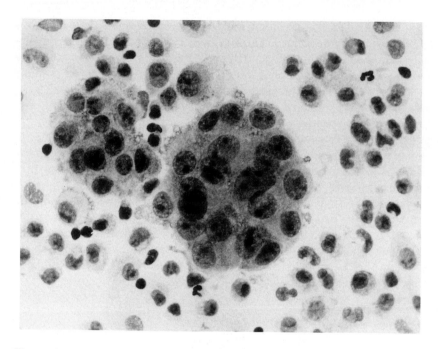

**Figure 1**  Aggregate of malignant mesothelioma cells forming a morula. Compact cell group with knobby edge. Giemsa stain.

between the cells. Stevens et al. (60) also quantitated several cytological features of malignant mesothelioma on a series of 44 histologically confirmed malignant mesotheliomas, 46 metastatic adenocarcinomas, and 30 benign mesothelial proliferations of patients with a negative clinical follow-up. These authors observed three-dimensional aggregates in about 65% of malignant mesotheliomas and in 40% of adenocarcinomas, but in only 6.7% of benign effusions.

### Nuclear Features

Although general cytological criteria of malignancy also apply to the assessment of effusions suggestive of malignant mesothelioma, some features suggestive of malignancy are rather exclusive for malignant mesothelioma. The general criteria of malignancy include increased nuclear size, nuclear indentations, hyperchromasia, and atypical or enlarged nucleoli. The morphometric study by Kwee et al. (59), on a series of 40 effusions with a previously diagnosed malignant mesothelioma and 20 reactive cases, clearly indicated that in most cases of pleural malignant mesothelioma it is possible to distinguish malignant from reactive mesothelial cells on the basis of nuclear size and cytoplasmic area. Both nuclear size and cytoplasmic area are increased in malignant mesothelioma cells, resulting in a somewhat increased nuclear/cytoplasmic ratio. A major drawback of the application of morphometry to cytological diagnosis is that the observer must select for the malignant cells in an effusion. It is well-known that in pleural effusions with a malignant mesothelioma a large proportion of reactive (nonmalignant) mesothelial cells may be present. As the efficacy of morphometry depends on the skill of the investigator, this approach seems to be a less objective diagnostic tool in cytodiagnosis of malignant mesothelioma than may be assumed. Nevertheless, morphometry is important to substantiate morphological differences claimed to exist between different pathological conditions.

In the study by Kwee et al. the nuclear shape, nuclear size, and chromatin pattern of reactive and malignant mesothelial cells were compared (59). A summary of the most relevant findings are listed in Table 4. It is apparent that differences in nuclear shape are hardly significant, but that

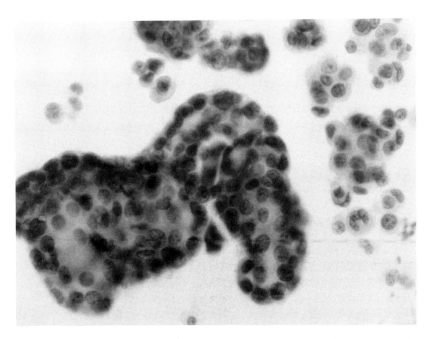

**Figure 2** Compact cell group of malignant mesothelioma cells with a papillary structure. Papanicolaou stain.

**Table 4**  Nuclear Parameters of Reactive and Malignant Mesothelial Cells in Pleural Effusion

| | Nuclear shape | | | | Chromatin pattern | | |
|---|---|---|---|---|---|---|---|
| Cells | Round | Poly-morph | Nuclear area | N/C ratio | Regular | Irregular | Coarse |
| Reactive | 72.0 | 8.4 | 91.4 ± 21.9 | 0.45 ± 0.97 | 81.6 | 18.4 | 19.6 |
| Malignant | 57.2 | 17.6 | 139.8 ± 39.2 | 0.39 ± 0.63 | 13.2 | 86.8 | 83.2 |

*Source*: Ref. 59.

more subjective characteristics, based on the assessment of chromatin pattern, may indeed contribute to the recognition of malignancy in the cytodiagnosis of malignant mesothelioma. Nevertheless, a great variability among the different cases exists. Stevens et al. (60) reported the presence of nuclear polymorphism in 70% of their cases of malignant mesothelioma, whereas this feature was lacking in benign effusions. The diagnostic value of macronucleoli was also substantiated by their quantitative study: macronucleoli, with diameters larger than 2 $\mu$m were seen in 72.7% of malignant mesotheliomas and in 13.3% of benign mesothelial proliferations.

### Other Cellular Features

Engulfment in which one large cell contains one or more smaller cells within its cytoplasm—also described as cannibalism or autophagocytosis—is another feature that is frequently present in malignant mesothelioma, but not in reactive effusions (46,47) (Fig. 3). In the series of Stevens et al., engulfment was present in 93.2% of malignant mesotheliomas and in 10% of benign mesothelial proliferations (60).

### Summary of Data

In Table 5, the significance of a number of cytological features of malignant mesothelioma in smear preparations is listed relative to their contribution to the establishment of malignancy. By stepwise, logistic regression analysis of the cytomorphological data scored on specimens from effusions with benign and malignant mesothelial proliferations, Stevens et al. identified papillary aggregates, nuclear polymorphism, the presence of macronucleoli, and engulfment as major features predictive of malignant mesothelioma (60) (Table 6).

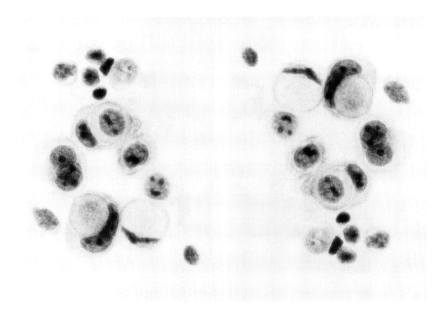

**Figure 3** Cell-in-cell engulfment of malignant mesothelioma cells. Giemsa stain.

**Table 5** Significance of Cytological Criteria for Malignancy

| Cytological feature | Significance |
|---|---|
| Nuclear shape | No |
| Nuclear position | No |
| Mitotic figures | No |
| Multinucleation | No |
| Presence of few morules (< 3/smear) | No |
| Increased nuclear/cytoplasm ratio | No |
| Peripheral cytoplasmic blebbing | No |
| Several morules (> 3/smear) | Yes |
| Nuclear hyperchromasia | Yes |
| Macronucleoli | Yes |
| Increased nuclear size | Yes |
| Increased cytoplasm | Yes |
| Engulfment | Yes |

**Table 6**  Diagnostic Cytological Features in Serous Effusions

| Feature | *p*-value |
|---|---|
| Distinction of malignant from benign mesothelial proliferation | |
|     Nuclear pleomorphism | 0.0001 |
|     Macronucleoli | 0.0495 |
|     Engulfment | 0.0001 |
| Distinction of adenocarcinoma from malignant mesothelioma | |
|     Papillary aggregates | 0.012 |
|     Multinucleation with atypia | 0.045 |
|     Apposition | 0.0001 |
|     Acinuslike structures | 0.0001 |
|     Balloonlike vacuolization | 0.0001 |

*Source*: Adapted from Ref. 60.

## B.  Criteria for Mesothelial Differentiation

### Staining Properties

Unfortunately, most of the features of mesothelial differentiation are not particularly specific as single characteristics, since malignancies of other origins may also share some of these features. In Giemsa-stained smears malignant mesothelioma cells have an amphophilic cytoplasm that is optically dense and very ample, whereas in Papanicolaou-stained smears a change in color can be seen from orange, in the direct vicinity of the nucleus, to green at the edge of the cell. This "two-tone" effect, although quite specific for malignant mesothelioma, is present only in a few cases (60). The presence of dense cytoplasm is not fully specific for mesothelial differentiation, as this feature may be present in a large proportion of adenocarcinomas, for example, in pulmonary adenocarcinoma cells (60).

### Cytomorphological Features

Cytoplasmic blebs and microvilli frequently can be seen in malignant mesothelial cells, but, again, this criterion is not sufficient on its own for diagnosis (59) (Fig. 4). The presence of peripheral vacuolization of the cytoplasm of tumor cells is considered to suggest mesothelial, rather than adenocarcinomal, differentiation (Fig. 5).

### Cell-to-Cell Apposition

In small clusters of (malignant) mesothelial cells the adjacent cells may be attached on the edges, leaving a gap in the center (apposition). These windows between cells are quite characteristic of mesothelial differentiation

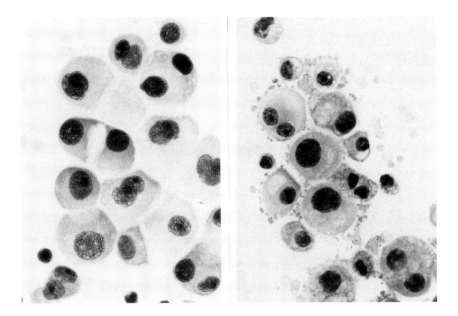

**Figure 4** Doublet of tumor cells with cell-to-cell apposition (window formation) (left). Malignant mesothelioma cells with cytoplasmic blebs (right). Giemsa stain.

(see Fig. 4). Multinucleation is a common feature of malignant and mesothelial cells.

### Morules

Three-dimensional clusters of tumor cells may assume the shape of a morule, with the nuclei somewhat bulging out (see Fig. 1). The latter feature is particularly characteristic of mesothelial differentiation.

### Collagenous Cores

Malignant mesothelial cells in effusions are frequently arranged in larger three-dimensional clusters that may have the appearance of a morule or a papillary structure (see later discussion). A somewhat underestimated feature of mesothelial differentiation is the presence of amorphous acellular material within clusters of (mesothelial) cells. These collagenous cores are sharply demarcated and should be distinguished from stromal fragments, which may also be present in tumor clusters. The collagenous cores can be identified easily in Giemsa-stained smear preparations. However, it should be stressed that, in Papanicolaou-stained preparations, these collagenous

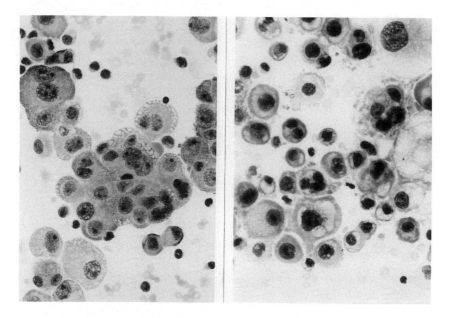

**Figure 5**  Peripheral cytoplasmic vacuolization resulting in brush border (left). Tumor cell with large cytoplasmic vacuoles (right). Giemsa stain.

cores are often hardly stained (Fig. 6). In earlier publications, the presence of collagenous cores in malignant mesothelioma was evaluated in Van Gieson-stained sections of paraffin-embedded sediments of effusions (55,61). This approach led to an underestimation of their diagnostic significance.

More recently, Delahaye et al. found collagenous cores in 51% of Giemsa-stained and in 64% of Azan-stained smears of effusions from malignant mesothelioma (62). In effusions from metastatic adenocarcinomas of the ovary and breast, collagenous cores may occasionally be found. The use of smears allows the examination of larger cell numbers and of cell groups. The need to examine numerous cells and cell groups was underscored by the observation by Delahaye et al. that, in 25% of their cases, only a few collagenous cores could be found, requiring a careful search for their presence (62). It is important to realize that collagenous cores also occur in clusters of reactive mesothelial cells that may be contaminating effusions with adenocarcinoma. The presence of collagenous cores in reactive mesothelial proliferations complicates use of this characteristic as an argument for malignancy.

### Papillary Formations

The presence of papillary groups (lacking collagenous cores) of tumor cells does not serve as a criterion for the mesothelial differentiation of tumor cells (see Table 6), as well-differentiated adenocarcinomas and bronchoalveolar carcinomas of the lung, and papillary thyroid carcinomas may also exfoliate these structures (see Fig. 2). Stevens et al. distinguished true papillary aggregates as an important morphological feature for mesothelial differentiation (60). They occurred in 61% of malignant mesotheliomas and in 28% of metastatic adenocarcinomas. These true papillary aggregates are defined as papillary frondlike structures or rosettes of cells arranged around a central amorphous or fibrovascular core. This definition implies that these "true papillary aggregates" also include the more narrowly defined collagenous cores.

Papillary groups from different localizations may additionally show psammoma bodies, including those originating from reactive mesothelial proliferations and malignant mesothelioma. Table 7 lists the validity of the

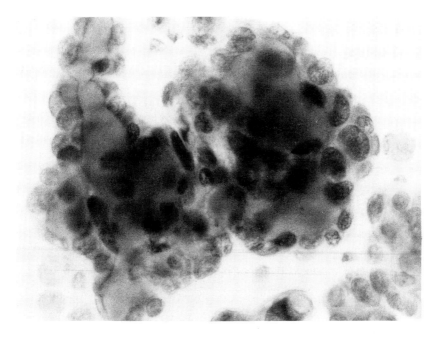

**Figure 6** Cell group of malignant mesothelioma cells with amorphous, faintly visible collagen cores. Papanicolaou stain.

**Table 7**  Cytological Criteria of the
Mesothelial Nature of a Malignancy

| Feature | Verification |
|---|---|
| Morules | Strong |
| Collagen core | Strong |
| Abundant glycogen | Strong |
| Windows | Strong |
| Presence of hyaluronic acid | Intermediate |
| Brush border | Intermediate |
| Multinucleation | Intermediate |
| Dense cytoplasm | Intermediate |
| Cytoplasmic blebs | Intermediate |
| Engulfment | Poor |
| Two-tone effect | Poor |
| Presence of fat droplets | Poor |
| Vacuolization pattern | Poor |
| Psammoma bodies | Poor |
| Papillary groups | Poor |

cytological criteria that can be used for establishing the mesothelial nature of malignant cells in cytological smears.

### Glandular Formations

Some authors have claimed that examination of slides of paraffin-embedded sediments from effusions can be very helpful in distinguishing adenocarcinoma from malignant mesothelioma (5). With this technique, the presence of glandlike structures composed of columnar cells in adenocarcinoma can easily be recognized. In contrast, in malignant mesothelioma the tumor cells are more rounded and contain peripherally located nuclei.

### Variants of Malignant Mesotheliomas

Rare forms of malignant mesothelioma, such as small-cell malignant mesothelioma, adenosquamous mesothelioma, carcinosarcoma, and signet-ring type of malignant mesothelioma, may not pose a problem in establishing the malignant nature of the process, but a precise cytological diagnosis is very difficult (5).

## V. The Role of Cytochemistry and Immunocytochemistry

### A. Cytochemical Staining

The presence of mucins in secretory vacuoles is an important distinctive feature of adenocarcinomas, as mucin-containing secretory vacuoles are lacking in malignant mesotheliomas. To demonstrate their presence, cytochemical examinations can be performed on cytological smears using alcian blue, mucicarmine or periodic acid-Schiff (PAS)-staining after enzymatic digestion of glycogen with diastase. Unfortunately, mucin-containing secretory vacuoles are present in only 40–60% of adenocarcinomas (63,64). Therefore, the lack of staining of tumor cells for neutral mucins is not considered a reliable positive criterion for mesothelial differentiation. Moreover, not all PAS-positive, diastase-resistant material is mucin, and one should be cautious about assigning the diagnosis "adenocarcinoma" based on the presence of globules of this kind in tumor cell cytoplasm. This latter point is reinforced by the observation that mucicarmine-positive cytoplasmic vacuoles can be present in malignant mesothelioma cells (65). More recently, Triol et al. observed that the presence of mucicarmine-, alcian blue-, or colloidal iron-positive cytoplasmic vacuoles is due to the presence of hyaluronic acid in these vacuoles, as pretreatment with hyaluronidase abolishes these staining reactions (66).

In mesothelial (tumor) cells, substantial amounts of glycogen may be present that may be revealed by PAS stain: characteristic speckled cytoplasmic staining arises. However, glycogen may also be present in adenocarcinomas, most notably in renal cell carcinomas and other clear cell carcinomas.

It has been generally appreciated that the production of hyaluronic acid by malignant mesothelioma cells may serve as an aid in the differential diagnosis with adenocarcinoma. In pleural effusions, a high hyaluronic acid content, determined in a biochemical assay, is consistent with malignant mesothelioma. Similarly, cytochemical demonstration of hyaluronic acid in cytoplasmic vacuoles or at the peripheral rim of a tumor cell makes a diagnosis of malignant mesothelioma more likely. Cytochemical demonstration of hyaluronic acid in tumor cells present in a cell smear depends on the demonstration that hyaluronidase pretreatment is able to abolish the cytochemical staining with alcian blue (optimal at pH 2.5). Failure to identify hyaluronic acid is not uncommon in smears containing malignant mesothelioma cells.

The presence of cytoplasmic fat droplets by an oil Red O staining on fixed smears is also considered as a criterion for malignant mesothelioma. The absence of lipid droplets in tumor cells does not exclude a diagnosis of malignant mesothelioma. Their presence is not fully specific for malignant mesothelioma.

## B.  Immunocytochemistry

Immunocytochemistry is increasingly applied as an adjunct to morphological diagnosis of malignant mesothelioma in cytological laboratories. It is apparent from Section IV that the availability of objective features to help identify malignant cells among the benign cells is of utmost importance in cytodiagnostics of effusions. The efficacy of diagnosis of malignant mesothelioma is largely determined by the cytologist's ability to establish the malignant nature of the suspect cells.

Immunohistochemical studies on histological, pleural-derived, tissue specimen largely focus on the differential diagnosis of adenocarcinoma versus malignant mesothelioma. In those studies there is less emphasis on markers distinguishing reactive mesothelial cells from malignant cells (67).

### General Aspects

To some extent, the immunocytochemical detection of malignant cells in (pleural) effusions relies on the restricted number of cell types normally present in this body compartment. These cell types include (reactive) mesothelial cells, macrophages, lymphoid cells, and granulocytes. Many markers for epithelial differentiation are also present in reactive and malignant mesothelial cells. Thus, several types of cytokeratins are expressed by both malignant and reactive mesothelial cells as well as adenocarcinoma cells. Blobel et al. demonstrated, with gel electrophoresis on tissue homogenates, that adenocarcinomas and malignant mesotheliomas both express cytokeratins 7, 8, 18, and 19 (68). Additionally, epithelial and biphasic malignant mesotheliomas contain cytokeratins 4, 5, 6, 14, and 17. Although the expression of these cytokeratins could be useful for the distinction of adenocarcinomas from malignant mesotheliomas, no immunocytochemical studies using them on serous effusions have yet been published. Initially, it was thought that coexpression of cytokeratins and vimentin would be of value to separate adenocarcinomas from malignant mesotheliomas, but now it has become apparent that this coexpression is frequently observed in both malignancies. In particular, reactive mesothelial cells strongly express vimentin, whereas adenocarcinomas tend to have a lower expression (69).

Most antibodies now applied for immunocytochemical demonstration of malignancy in an effusion are reactive with (adeno)carcinomas, but not with reactive or malignant mesothelial cells (Table 8). The expression of these markers is used to confirm malignancy, on the one hand, and to exclude a diagnosis of malignant mesothelioma, on the other. As not all adeno-

**Table 8** Markers of Malignancy Employed in Effusion Cytology

| Marker | Reactive mesothelium | Malignant mesothelioma | Adenocarcinoma |
|---|---|---|---|
| CEA | − | − | + |
| TAG-72.3 | − | − | + |
| Leu-M1 (CD-15) | − | − | + |
| GICA | − | − | + |
| Ber-EP4 | − | − | + |
| MOC31 | − | − | + |
| 44-3A6 | − | − | + |
| AUA1 | − | − | + |
| Secretory component | − | − | + |
| EMA (E29)/HMFG2 | − | + | + |

carcinomas express these markers and within a carcinoma a considerable heterogeneity for a particular marker exists, this approach is likely to lead to misdiagnosis of malignant mesothelioma in a number of cases. This can be prevented, to some extent, if multiple markers for adenocarcinoma are applied, reducing the chance of false-negative results. Antibodies directed against mesothelioma-specific markers would be more suitable, as they would permit the positive identification of malignant mesothelioma cells.

Because of the heterogeneity of tumor cells in their expression of immunocytochemically detectable markers, occasionally very low percentages of the tumor cells may express a particular antigen. Moreover, some malignancy-associated antigens (most notably anti–epithelial membrane antigen) may be expressed—although faintly—by a small fraction of benign (mesothelial) cells. This raises the important question of what is the minimum number or minimum frequency of immunostained cells required for a positive diagnosis of malignancy. A general rule is not to make a strong statement about malignancy if it is based only on the presence of sporadic immunostained cells lacking nuclear features of malignancy. Most authors feel more confident about a definite diagnosis of malignancy in a suspect effusion if this is supported by more than one marker.

### Episialins

One of the earliest immunocytochemical markers for improving the accuracy of the cytological diagnosis from effusions is epithelial membrane antigen (EMA), also known as human milk fat globule (HMFG) membrane glycoproteins (70). These high relative molecular mass ($M_r$) glycoproteins, expressed by most normal epithelia and most carcinomas, are now characterized as episialins (71). Currently, the two most frequently used monoclonal antibodies for demonstration of episialins are anti-EMA (designation E29) raised by Gatter et al. (72) and antibody HMFG2 raised by Burchell et al. (73). Comparison of data from the literature does not reveal significant differences between these antibodies in staining results. In most studies on serous effusions with metastatic adenocarcinoma, a high sensitivity and specificity of anti-EMA/HMFG2 for adenocarcinoma was noted (Table 9). Although some early immunohistochemical studies on tissue sections of paraffin-embedded material denied expression of EMA in malignant mesothelioma, subsequent studies on larger series of tumors unequivocally demonstrated its presence. Similarly, the collected data of several immunocytochemical studies on serous effusions with malignant mesothelioma indicate that approximately 80% of malignant mesotheliomas contain significant numbers of EMA/HMFG2-positive cells. The dectection of EMA-positive cells in a pleural effusion does not serve to distinguish adenocarcinoma from malignant mesothelioma.

In several studies (a generally faint) immunostaining of mesothelial cells in cytologically negative effusions by antibodies to EMA or HMFG was observed (31,74,85).

Hilkens et al. showed that the epitope specificity of monoclonal antibodies to episialins determines their reactivity with benign mesothelial cells (89). Thus, the specificity of anti-EMA or anti-HMFG antibody for malignant mesothelioma is dependent on the epitope specificity (89,90). Furthermore, it is conceivable that the sensitivity of the detection technique may influence the reactivity of these antibodies with benign mesothelial cells if the amount of episialins present on a particular mesothelial cell is below detection level by one technique and just detectable by another technique. In fact, one immunoelectron microscopic study with anti-EMA antibody revealed the presence of small amounts of EMA on the cell membranes of reactive mesothelial cells (80). In our experience the presence of several cells with an intense membranous staining for EMA or HMFG2 indicates malignancy. In contrast, sporadic or faintly cytoplasmic EMA/HMFG2-positive cells do also occur in reactive effusions without malignancy.

### Antibodies to Carcinoembryonic Antigen

To address the differential diagnostic problem of separating adenocarcinoma from malignant mesothelioma, the earliest and most frequently used marker is carcinoembryonic antigen (CEA). Both polyclonal and various monoclonal antibodies are in use for the immunocytochemical detection of CEA. A review of literature data shows the supreme reliability of anti-CEA antibodies in distinguishing adenocarcinomas from malignant mesotheliomas. The latter tumor type rarely expresses substantial amounts of CEA

**Table 9** Immunocytochemistry of Effusions

| Authors (Ref.) | Reactive mesothelium | | | | Malignant mesothelioma | | | | Adenocarcinoma | | | |
|---|---|---|---|---|---|---|---|---|---|---|---|---|
| | EMA/HMFG2 | CEA | CD15 | TAG 72 | EMA/HMFG2 | CEA | CD15 | TAG 72 | EMA/HMFG2 | CEA | CD15 | TAG 72 |
| Ghosh et al. (74) | 14/22 | 0/22 | | | 1/1 | 1/1 | | | 39/40 | 30/36 | | |
| Schested et al. (75) | | 0/34 | | | | 0/1 | | | | 22/32 | | |
| Johnston et al. (28) | | | | 0/24 | | | | | | | | 60/61 |
| Ernst et al. (76) | | | | | 4/4 | 0/6 | | | | | | |
| Martin et al. (34) | | | | 0/10 | | | | | | | | 26/26 |
| Ghosh and Butler (77) | 0/5 | 0/5 | | | 10/12 | 1/12 | | | | | | |
| Mason et al. (78) | 1/9 | 0/9 | | | 0/4 | 0/4 | | | 34/37 | 32/37 | | |
| Duggan et al. (79) | | 0/5 | | | | 0/5 | | | | 4/5 | | |
| Walts et al. (80) | 4/12 | | | | 2/2 | | | | 27/27 | | | |
| Croonen et al. (81) | 1/43 | 0/43 | | | 6/6 | 0/6 | | | 29/29 | 21/29 | | |
| van der Kwast et al. (38) | 2/52 | | | | 23/25 | | | | 38/39 | | | |
| Lauritzen (82) | | 0/9 | 0/9 | 0/9 | | 0/3 | 0/3 | 0/3 | | 21/29 | 15/29 | 20/29 |
| Guzman (83) | | 0/31 | | | 12/12 | 0/12 | | | 57/57 | 36/57 | | |
| Shield (84) | | | | | | 0/1 | | | | 24/46 | | |
| Esteban et al. (85) | 7/18 | 0/18 | | 2/18 | 2/2 | 1/2 | 0/2 | 0/2 | 18/18 | 11/18 | | 17/18 |
| Tickman et al. (86) | 1/19 | 1/19 | 1/19 | 0/19 | 0/1 | 0/1 | 0/1 | 0/1 | 63/69 | 18/69 | 30/69 | 45/69 |
| Nance and Silverman (87) | 0/28 | 0/28 | 0/28 | 0/28 | 9/12 | 0/12 | | 1/12 | 25/26 | 20/26 | 11/26 | |
| Daste et al. (36) | 7/20 | 0/20 | | | | | | | 42/42 | 31/42 | | 14/16 |
| Donna et al. (88) | | | | | | | | | | | | |
| Total | 37/228 | 1/263 | 1/56 | 2/108 | 69/81 | 3/66 | 0/6 | 1/18 | 372/388 | 270/426 | 56/124 | 182/219 |
| % positive | 16.2 | 0.4 | 1.8 | 1.9 | 85.2 | 4.5 | | 5.6 | 95.9 | 63.4 | 39.4 | 83.1 |

(4.5% of cases), whereas variable proportions of adenocarcinomas do express it (see Table 9). Moreover, reactive mesothelial cells rarely, if ever, are labeled with anti-CEA antibodies.

It is clear from Table 9 that the sensitivity of anti-CEA as a marker in detecting malignancy varies strongly. This variation can be attributed to the tumor type-specificity of CEA expression. More than 80% of gastrointestinal and pulmonary adenocarcinomas are CEA-positive, whereas breast and ovarian cancers have a much lower frequency of CEA expression.

### Antibody B72.3

To increase the sensitivity of immunocytochemical diagnosis of metastatic adenocarcinoma, several additional markers have been added to the diagnostic repertoire. B72.3 is a monoclonal antibody raised against a human breast carcinoma membrane preparation (28), but this antibody also reacts with adenocarcinomas of other origins, including pulmonary, colon, and ovarian adenocarcinoma. TAG-72, the high $M_r$ glycoprotein against which B72.3 is directed (91), is detectable only rarely in reactive or malignant mesothelial cells. Combining the data from various investigators (see Table 9), it appears that, in serous effusions, B72.3 has a higher sensitivity for detection of metastatic adenocarcinoma than CEA (83.1 vs 63.4%). It should be kept in mind that these figures are influenced by the frequency of adenocarcinomas of different primary origin, similar to the aforementioned.

### Antibody Leu-M1

Another marker examined for its diagnostic value in cytological smears of serous effusions is Leu-M1, a monoclonal antibody directed against the X-hapten, which is a carbohydrate antigen also referred to as lacto-*N*-fucose-pentosyl III. The antibody 624A12 is also reactive with this carbohydrate epitope (92). Leu-M1 and other antibodies directed to this carbohydrate antigen have now been designated CD15. The antigen probably is similar to stage-specific embryonic antigen, and antibodies raised against the latter antigen have also been used to discriminate malignancy in serous effusions (76). Leu-M1 is expressed in a variety of myeloproliferative disorders and in various carcinomas (93), but is rarely detectable in reactive or malignant mesothelial cells. In serous effusions Leu-M1 is highly specific for malignancy, but has a rather limited sensitivity of about 40% for adenocarcinoma (see Table 9). This low figure is in contrast with a previously published percentage (94%) determined on histological material of adenocarcinomas (94). The number of effusions with malignant mesothelioma investigated so far is very limited, but, from comparative studies on histological material, it is clear that CD15 is present only rarely in malignant mesotheliomas (92,94–96).

### Antibody BER-EP4

Latza et al. recently described a monoclonal antibody designated BER-EP4 that was able to distinguish epithelial cells from mesothelial cells (97). BER-EP4 was raised against the human mammary carcinoma cell line MCF-7 and recognizes a partially formol-resistant epitope on a glycoprotein composed of two 34-kDa and one 39-kDa polypeptides. It was claimed from studies on formalin-fixed, paraffin-embedded tissues that BER-EP4 reacts with virtually all carcinomas, but with only 1–20% of malignant mesotheliomas (98,99). In the study by Latza et al. (97), the 11 examined serous effusions that contained carcinoma cells also contained BER-EP4-positive tumor cells, whereas immunostained cells were not detectable in any of 25 reactive effusions. More studies on serous effusions, including those with malignant mesothelioma cells, are required to define the use of this antibody in the differential diagnosis of adenocarcinoma from malignant mesothelioma.

### Other Monoclonal Antibodies Selectively Reactive with Adenocarcinomas

Several additional monoclonal antibodies have been reported with a potential use in the differential diagnosis of adenocarcinoma from malignant mesothelioma in serous effusions (Table 10). Monoclonal antibody 44-3A6 is directed against a membrane-associated protein with an $M_r$ of 40 kDa (100). A major drawback of this antibody seems to be that reactive mesothelial cells and some histiocytes are occasionally stained. Spagnolo et al. give no information about the frequency of this observation (100). MOC31 is a monoclonal antibody reactive with a large proportion of squamous cell carcinomas, adenocarcinomas, and small-cell carcinomas of the lung (101). Delahaye et al. (102) demonstrated, on cytological smears of serous effu-

**Table 10**  Additional Adenocarcinoma-Specific Monoclonal Antibodies

| Designation | Ref. | % positive adenocarcinoma | % positive mal mesothelioma |
|---|---|---|---|
| 44-3A6 | 100 | 90 | 9 |
| MOC31 | 102 | 58 | 9 |
| GICA | 76 | 38 | 0 |

sions, that this antibody reacted with 2 of 24 malignant mesotheliomas and with 18 of 31 adenocarcinomas. As no MOC31-positive cells were observed in cytological smears of reactive effusions, this marker may have some value as a marker of malignancy. The low sensitivity of the antibody to gastrointestinal carcinoma antigen (GICA) seems to limit its use for distinguishing adenocarcinoma from malignant mesothelioma (76).

### Mesothelioma-Specific Antibodies

A marker specifically reactive with malignant mesothelioma cells, but not with adenocarcinoma cells, would have great diagnostic import, as such a marker could lead to the positive identification of malignant mesothelioma. Since most serous effusions of malignant mesothelioma also contain variable numbers of benign or reactive mesothelial cells, such an antibody would be most useful if it lacked reactivity with the latter cells.

Two polyclonal mesothelioma-specific antibodies have been described (88,103,104), but neither is commercially available. The antimesothelial cell antiserum was reported by Donna et al. to stain malignant mesothelial cells intensely, whereas it yields weak immunoreactivity in benign mesothelial cells in paraffin sections of cell blocks. The antigen with which this antibody reacts has not yet been identified with full certainty. The antiserum probably recognizes a mesothelium-specific autocrine growth factor (105).

Four promising monoclonal antibodies capable of discriminating malignant mesotheliomas from pulmonary adenocarcinomas by their selective reactivity with malignant mesothelioma cells have been recently described (Table 11). Monoclonal antibodies ME1 (106,107) and K1 (108), and a monoclonal antibody specific for thrombomodulin (109) were reported to distinguish malignant mesothelioma cells from adenocarcinoma cells on tissue sections. Unfortunately, the three monoclonal antibodies also react with benign mesothelial cells. Double-labeling with one of these antibodies and monoclonal anti-EMA antibody may lead to the selective identification of malignant cells expressing markers characteristic of mesothelial differen-

**Table 11**   Mesothelioma-Specific Monoclonal Antibodies

| Designation | Antigen | Formalin resistance | Benign mesothelium | Ref. |
|-------------|---------|---------------------|--------------------|------|
| ME1 | 200-kDa glycoprotein | − | + | 106,107 |
| K1 | 40-kDa membrane protein | + | + | 108 |
| TM | Thrombomodulin | + | + | 109 |
| OV632 | Unknown | − | − | 102 |

tiation. No studies on the application of K1 or thrombomodulin on cytological smears or cell blocks of serous effusions have yet been reported.

Another recently described marker is OV632, originally raised against human ovarian carcinoma cells. The OV632-reactive antigen has not yet been identified. The epitope is formalin-sensitive. The selective reactivity of OV632 with ovarian carcinomas was reported in previous studies (110,111). In the latter study, it was noted that OV632 did not react with benign mesothelial cells. Delahaye et al. reported that over 80% of serous effusions with malignant mesothelioma contained OV632-positive tumor cells, whereas it was also noted that reactive mesothelial cells did not label with this antibody (102). Although about 20% of pulmonary adenocarcinomas showed reactivity with OV632, this antibody seems to be highly useful in improving the cytodiagnosis of malignant mesothelioma, as it distinguishes malignant from reactive mesothelial cells. If the foregoing data can be confirmed by other investigators, the specificity of OV632 for malignant mesotheliomas in male patients can be used as a rather specific criterion in the differential diagnosis of malignant mesothelioma and adenocarcinoma. The suggested common histogenesis of malignant mesothelioma and ovarian carcinoma is in line with the reactivity pattern of OV632.

### Effect of Immunocytochemistry

A few retrospective studies have attempted to evaluate the influence of immunocytochemistry on cytologically problematic cases (112–114). In each of these three studies small panels of antibodies were used, which led to an improvement in accuracy of the cytological diagnosis. For a differential diagnosis of adenocarcinoma from malignant mesothelioma, a definite and correct diagnosis of malignant mesotheliomas was obtained in 21 of 22 cases. Similar studies focused on the use of panels of monoclonal antibodies for the cytological diagnosis of malignant mesotheliomas in effusions still need to be performed. It is recommended that, for evaluation of cost-effectiveness, the relative effect of each marker should be examined to compose a minimum package of markers with optimal influence on the cytological diagnosis.

## VI. The Role of Transmission Electron Microscopy

Despite the increasing importance of immunocytochemistry with monoclonal antibodies, ultrastructural analysis is still a useful tool in the diagnosis of pleural malignant mesothelioma. The first complete description of ultrastructural characteristics of this tumor was performed on biopsies from four pleural mesotheliomas by Wang (115). Thereafter, TEM was used as the ultimate criterion in the diagnosis of malignant mesothelioma (116,117), especially in biopsy specimens. Only a few reports focused on the ultrastructural characteristics from pleural fluid (118–121). However, the phenotype of cells is not always characteristic and specific, and TEM analysis alone does not resolve the differential diagnostic problems, so combination with light microscopy and immunocytochemistry is necessary to confirm the positive diagnosis of malignant mesothelioma.

### A. Ultrastructural Characteristics

Epithelial and sarcomatous mesotheliomas show different cellular patterns on biopsy samples (122,123); however, as described earlier, only the epithelial cells from malignant pleural mesothelioma can be observed in effusions (124). The ultrastructural pattern of mesothelioma is characterized first by epithelial effusion; that is, cells organized in clusters, sometimes circumscribed by basal lamina, and joined by adherent junctions (spot or belt desmosomes), with or without tight junctions (115,125). The mesothelial differentiation of this epithelial tumor is characterized by three major criteria: (1) the specific features of the microvilli, (2) the abundant intermediate filaments, and (3) the absence of secretory granules.

#### Microvilli

The microvilli are usually abundant, elongated, and slender (up to 3 $\mu$m in length), sometimes with a branching pattern. A length:diameter ratio (LDR) greater than 10:1 is very suggestive (126,127) for mesothelioma, and in Warhol's study, a LDR greater than 15 was observed only in malignant mesotheliomas (Fig. 7). The microvilli often have a circumferential cell distribution and projections through deficiencies in the basal lamina (121) (Fig. 8). Interdigitations of microvilli with stromal collagen fibers is, for some authors, also characteristic of mesothelial differentiation (120,125). The microvilli of malignant mesothelioma may have filamentous cores, but no glycocalyceal bodies and rootlets are present (123,125).

Studies performed using immunocytochemistry with anti-EMA antibodies (38) have demonstrated the presence of EMA on the outer cytoplasmic membranes of the long villi of cells with ultrastructural features of mesothelium (Fig. 9). Intracellular lacunae, when observed, are often surrounded by long microvilli.

#### Intermediate Filaments

Intermediate filaments are abundant and are particularly concentrated in a ringlike fashion immediately adjacent to the nuclear envelope (Fig. 10). Studies using immunocytochemical methods applied to TEM (126) have

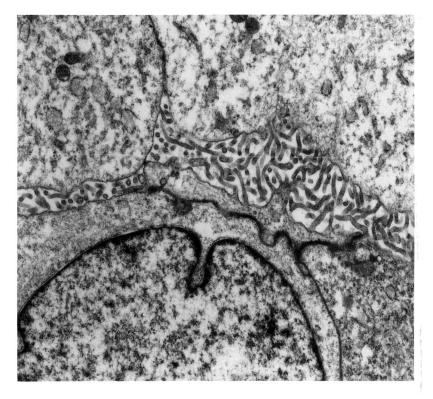

**Figure 7** TEM of malignant pleural mesothelial cells in pleural effusion. Note the typical long and slender microvilli with microfilamentous cores and absence of rootlets (magnification × 12,500).

demonstrated that the intermediate filaments observed were composed of cytokeratin, as they inserted into desmosomes that define a network of tonofilaments immediately under the terminal web of the microvilli.

### Secretory Granules

The absence of any secretory granules is a constant feature (123). Their presence unequivocally excludes the diagnosis of malignant mesothelioma.

### Other Ultrastructual Features

Other ultrastructural features observed are less specific for mesotheliomas; that is, intracellular lumina, pools of glycogen granules, lipids, Golgi complexes, and rough-surfaced endoplasmic reticulum. These characteristics

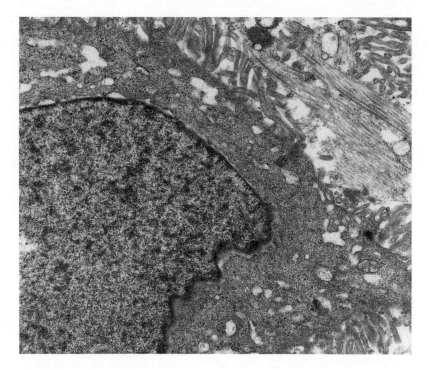

**Figure 8**  TEM of malignant mesothelioma from biopsy sample showing interdigitations of microvilli (arrow) with collagen fibers (arrowhead) (magnification ×13,000).

are not present in all mesotheliomas. Those lacking microvilli or with low LDR have been observed (128), as well as those in which the cytoplasmic intermediate filaments were not abundant or typical in distribution.

### B.  Differential Diagnosis

The aim of TEM analysis is to determine the differentiation of the tumor cells. The differential diagnosis of malignant mesothelioma, as stated earlier, involves two questions: First, are the mesothelial cells malignant or reactive? Second, is it indeed a malignant mesothelioma, or is it a pleural metastasis of an adenocarcinoma? It has been generally accepted that there are no ultrastructural features that distinguish between malignant and benign mesothelioma cells. However, some authors have described features they consider specific for malignancy. Wueker et al. reported that benign mesothelial cells do not show the long, complex, and branching microvilli characteristic of malignant mesothelioma (121); instead, they display short

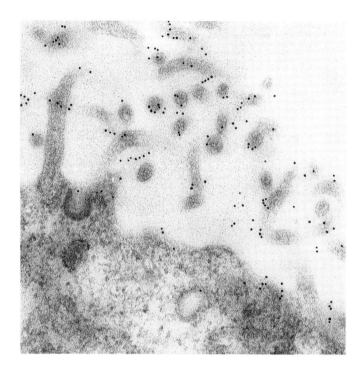

**Figure 9** TEM demonstrating immunogold labeling of malignant mesothelioma cells for EMA. Gold particles are situated along the surface of the slender villi.

surface microvilli. Dewar et al. reported (125) that interdigitation of microvilli with collagen fibers through the basal lamina defects was observed only in malignant cells and not in their benign counterparts, in which microvilli projected into lumens. More recently, Leong et al. observed apparent incorporation of collagen fibers in the cytoplasm of malignant mesothelial cells, resulting from cross-cutting of interdigitating microvilli and extracellular collagen fibers (120). For these authors, this feature is diagnostic for malignant mesothelioma. In a study using immunoelectron microscopy, van der Kwast et al. demonstrated that labeling by anti-EMA occurred selectively on the villi of malignant mesothelial cells (38). However, these reports are sparse, and TEM alone is not sufficient to make a diagnosis of malignancy.

In TEM analysis, the main differential diagnosis concerns metastasis of carcinoma and, especially, of poorly differentiated adenocarcinoma.

Usually adenocarcinomas are characterized ultrastructurally by the inconsistent presence of microvilli; when present, they are short or of medium length (LDR < 5) and associated with glycocalyceal bodies or root-

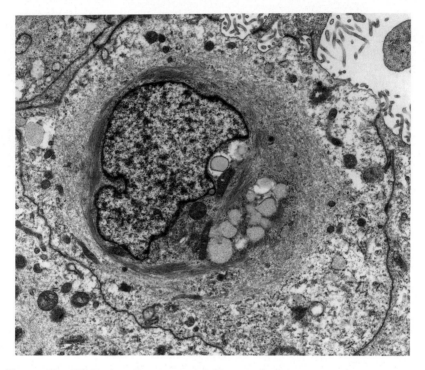

**Figure 10** TEM of malignant mesothelioma cells from pleural fluid, showing typical perinuclear arrangement of intermediate filaments (magnification × 7700).

lets and terminal bars (Fig. 11). Moreover, microvilli are generally confined to the apical pole of the carcinoma cells. It has been generally considered that, in metastasis of adenocarcinoma, microvilli show no contact with connective tissue elements (125).

Secretory granules are often observed in adenocarcinoma as mucous granules or granules from Clara cells, or as alveolar cells in bronchioloalveolar carcinomas; but they are not present in every kind of adenocarcinoma.

Cytoplasmic filaments are often observed joined to desmosomes; perinuclear arrangements are usually not observed.

However, the distinction between mesothelioma and pleural metastasis of adenocarcinoma is not always so clear-cut. Warhol and Corson reported that of 30 adenocarcinomas, 2 cases had long microvilli (126). Dewar et al. reported the same observation in 2 of 20 adenocarcinomas (125). However, in these cases, other features of adenocarcinoma, such as

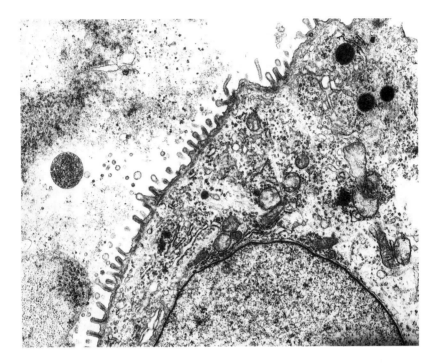

**Figure 11**   TEM of metastasis of adenocarcinoma in pleural fluid. Note the typical short microvilli with filamentous cores and rootlets (magnification × 10,000).

secretory granules or glycocalyceal bodies or rootlets, were present. The presence of abluminal microvilli making contact with collagen fibrils through discontinuities in the basal lamina has been suggested, by some authors, to be highly characteristic for mesothelial differentiation. But these features have been recently demonstrated in some cases of pleural metastases of adenocarcinoma (129). The perinuclear organization of tonofilaments can be observed in adenocarcinoma, and it has been well described in breast carcinoma (126). In these cases, other characteristics, such as length of microvilli, are helpful to distinguish the two tumors. Conversely, true malignant mesothelioma can present short or few microvilli, but without glycocalyceal bodies or rootlets.

   In conclusion, TEM remains a well-accepted method to establish diagnosis of pleural malignant mesothelioma in pleural fluid. The main ultrastructural features — slender and elongated microvilli, abundant perinuclear intermediate filaments, and lack of secretory granules, when present — are highly suggestive of malignant mesothelioma and remain an important complement to standard methods as well as to immunocytochemistry in the diagnosis of malignant mesothelioma. When these features, as well as those typical of adenocarcinoma, are absent a diagnosis of mesothelial malignancy cannot be made.

## VII.  Perspectives in the Cytological Diagnosis of Malignant Mesothelioma

### A.  DNA Ploidy Measurements and In Situ Hybridization

*DNA Flow Cytometry*

The use of DNA flow cytometry of cells in serous effusions has the great advantage of rapid and objective analysis of large numbers of cells. An objection to the method is that no morphological analysis can be performed on the same cells. The applicability of DNA flow cytometry is based on the observation that most malignancies are DNA aneuploid. Studies on paraffin-embedded tumor tissue specimens of malignant mesotheliomas have shown that 35–61% of cases are DNA diploid (130–132). In contrast, a much larger proportion of pulmonary adenocarcinomas were reported to be DNA aneuploid.

The sensitivity of DNA flow cytometry in detection of epithelial malignancy in serous effusions is rather low (average 60%) and tends to vary strongly among the different studies (133). The generally low sensitivity of this method has been attributed to heavy contamination with nucleated blood cells and other reactive cells. In spite of incorporation of additional parameters, such as S-phase fraction determination, DNA flow cytometry is of additional value in cytological analysis of only a small percentage of pleural effusions (134).

Another approach to improve the sensitivity of DNA flow cytometry has been adopted by Croonen et al. (81). They performed a double-labeling of the cells in serous effusions that uses propidium iodide for DNA staining and keratin for selective identification of epithelial cells. However, in 5 of 26 benign effusions, an aneuploid pattern was found, whereas 18 of 24 adenocarcinomas were clearly DNA aneuploid. All samples of malignant mesothelioma, but one, were DNA diploid or near diploid. Currently, the application of DNA flow cytometry as a routine technique to make a diagnosis of malignant mesothelioma is obviated because (1) a large proportion of malignant mesotheliomas yields a DNA diploid pattern in flow cytometry; (2) in malignant mesotheliomas, a heavy contamination of reactive mesothelial cells is frequently present that may show multinucleation as a compounding factor; and (3) if DNA aneuploid tumor cells represent fewer than 5% of the total number of nucleated cell population, they may not be detectable.

### In Situ Hybridization

In situ hybridization with chromosome-specific probes on cytological smears now belongs to the diagnostic possibilities (135). Nevertheless, its practical use seems to be limited, since cytogenetic studies have not indicated specific chromosomal changes in malignant mesotheliomas that distinguish them from adenocarcinomas (136). Admittedly, some chromosomes (e.g., chromosome 22) are more often involved in malignant mesothelioma, and their specific loss or increase may be used to distinguish malignant from reactive mesothelial cells.

### B. Oncogenes

Oncogenes may be activated or inactivated by mutations or other genetic alterations. Among the oncogenes most frequently involved in carcinogenesis are the *ras* genes and the *p53* suppressor gene. In addition, overexpression of genes coding for growth factors or growth factor receptors can be observed in several tumor types.

### Mutations of the ras Gene

Activating *ras* gene mutations preferentially occur in codons 12, 13, and 61 of the first exon of the Ki(rsten)-, Ha(rvey)-, or N-*ras* gene. Although, in pulmonary adenocarcinomas, a high prevalence of mutations in the Ki-*ras* gene has been observed (137), in none of 20 human malignant mesothelioma cell lines has a Ki-*ras* mutation been observed. Similarly, in a series of seven mesothelioma cell lines, we were not able to detect mutations in the Ki-*ras* gene. Neither did Sheibani et al. (138) find an Ha-*ras* mutation in tumor tissue of three malignant mesothelioma patients. The data indicate that determination of mutations in the Ha- or Ki-*ras* gene is not contributory to the diagnostics of malignant mesothelioma.

### Mutation of the p53 Gene

A 53-kDa nuclear phosphoprotein, p53, is normally involved in the negative regulation of cell proliferation (139). Mutation of the *p53* gene is often associated with a stabilization of the p53 protein, causing an intranuclear accumulation that is detectable by immunohistochemistry. Preliminary experiments showed that proper fixation of the smears is required to prevent leakage of the p53 protein from the nuclei. The wild-type p53 is generally present in small amounts, below the detection level, but exceptions are noted in which immunohistochemically detected p53 occurs without accompanying mutation of the *p53* gene (140). In a few human malignant mesothelioma cell lines, a point mutation in the *p53* gene was found by direct sequencing (141,142). In the one study, *p53* alterations were found in two of four examined cell lines (141), whereas, in the other study, these mutations were detected in cell lines of only 2 of 17 patients (142). Although particularly the latter data suggest a rather low frequency of p53 abnormalities in human malignant mesothelioma, immunohistochemical studies on paraffin-embedded malignant mesothelioma tissue revealed overexpression of *p53* in most malignant mesotheliomas (143–145). Unfortunately, these authors did not examine the presence of *p53* gene mutations in the patients' tumor tissue. Until now reactive mesothelium proved to be nonimmunoreactive with the employed anti-p53 antibodies (143,144). Although p53 overexpression may be a useful marker to distinguish malignant from reactive mesothelial cells in pleural effusions, p53 cannot be used to differentiate malignant mesothelioma from adenocarcinoma, owing to the high frequency of *p53* mutations in the latter population of tumors. Further data are required to substantiate the potential diagnostic usefulness of p53 immunocytochemistry. The possibility of wild-type p53 overexpression in (proliferating) reactive mesothelial cells should particularly be taken into account.

### Overexpression of the sis Oncogene

In human malignant mesothelioma cell lines, high levels of platelet-derived growth factor (PDGF) A- and B-chain may be present (146,147). Strikingly, expression of PDGF-B (coded by the *sis* oncogene on chromosome 22) was much increased, both at the mRNA and the protein level in malignant mesothelioma cell lines, compared with cell lines of nonmalignant human mesothelial cells. No structural changes in the *sis* gene of malignant mesotheliomas have been observed, although chromosome 22 is often involved in chromosomal aberrations in malignant mesothelioma (147). Immunocytochemistry with specific monoclonal antibodies for PDGF-B chain molecules could be a potential approach for distinction of malignant mesothelioma from reactive mesothelial proliferations. A drawback of this approach is the presence of PDGF-B in macrophages, requiring the employment of a double–immunohistochemical-staining technique to distinguish them from the putative malignant cells.

### References

1. Senger DR, Perruzzi CA, Feder J, Dvorak HF. A highly conserved vascular permeability factor secreted by a variety of human and rodent tumor cell lines. Cancer Res 1986; 46:5629–5632.

2. Pisani RJ, Colby TV, Williams DE. Subject review. Malignant mesothelioma of the pleura. Mayo Clin Proc 1988; 63:1234–1244.

3. Ruffie P, Feld R, Minkin S, Cormier Y, Boutan-Laroze A, Ginsberg R, Ayoub J, Sheperd FA, Evans WK, Figueredo A, Pater JL, Pringle JF, Kreisman H. Diffuse malignant mesothelioma of the pleura in Ontario and Quebec: a retrospective study of 332 patients. J Clin Oncol 1989; 7:1157–1168.

4. Chahinian AP, Pajak TF, Holland JF, Norton L, Ambinder RM, Mandell EM. Diffuse malignant mesothelioma. Prospective evaluation of 69 patients. Ann Intern Med 1982; 96:746–755.

5. Whitaker D, Shilkin K. Diagnosis of pleural malignant mesothelioma in life. A practical approach. J Pathol 1984; 143:147–175.

6. Achatzy R, Beba W, Ritschler R, Wörn H, Wahlers B, Macha, HN, Morgan JA. The diagnosis, therapy and prognosis of diffuse malignant mesothelioma. Eur J. Cardiothorac Surg 1989; 3:445–448.

7. Tao L-C. Aspiration biopsy cytology of mesothelioma. Diagn Cytopathol 1989; 5:14–21.

8. Wada H, Chihara K, Ito M, Inukai K, Shindou T, Reshad K, Terada Y, Matunobe S. Pleural mesothelioma in Japan: a review of 37 cases in Japan. Jpn J Chest Dis 1983; 42:1020–1030 [in Japanese].

9. Nakajima M, Manabe S, Yagi S. Appearance of mesothelioma cells in sputum. A case report. Acta Cytol 1992; 36:731–736.

10. Van Gelder T, Hoogsteden HC, Vandenbroucke JP, van der Kwast TH, Planteydt HT. The influence of the diagnostic technique on the histopathological diagnosis in malignant mesothelioma. Virchows Archiv [A] 1991; 418: 315–317.

11. Adams VI, Unni KK, Muhm JR, Jett JR, Ilstrup DM, Bernatz PE. Diffuse malignant mesothelioma of pleura. Diagnosis and survival in 92 cases. Cancer 1986; 58:1540–1551.

12. Martensson G, Hagmar B, Zettergren L. Diagnosis and prognosis in malignant pleural mesothelioma: a prospective study. Eur J Respir Dis 1984; 65: 169–178.

13. Huncharek M, Muscat J. Metastases in diffuse pleural mesothelioma: influence of histological type. Thorax 1987; 42:897–898.

14. Antman KH, Blum RH, Greenberger JS, Flowerdew G, Skarin AT, Canellos GP. Multimodality therapy for malignant mesothelioma based on a study of natural history. Am J Med 1980; 68:356–362.

15. Chailleux E, Dabouis G, Pioche D, De Lajartre M, De Lajartre AY, Rembeaux A, Germaud P. Prognostic factors in diffuse malignant pleural mesothelioma. Chest 1988; 93:1–162.

16. Tao L-C. The cytopathology of mesothelioma. Acta Cytol 1979; 23:209–213.

17. Whitaker D, Sterrett G, Shilkin K. Early diagnosis of malignant mesothelioma: the contribution of effusion and fine needle aspiration cytology and ancillary techniques. In: Source book on asbestos diseases. New York: Garland Law Publishing, 1989:71–115.

18. Gupta PK, Frost JK. Cytologic changes associated with asbestos exposure. Semin Oncol 1981; 8:283–289.

19. Spriggs AI, Boddington MM. Atlas of serous fluid cytopathology. London: Kluwer Academic Publishers, 1989:127.

20. Boon ME, Drijver JS. Routine cytological staining techniques. Theoretical background and practice. London: MacMillan Education, 1986:106.

21. Keebler CM. Cytopreparatory techniques. In: Bibbo M. Comprehensive cytopathology. Philadelphia: WB Saunders, 1991:881.

22. Pool EH, Dunlop GR. Cancer cells in the blood stream. Am J Cancer 1934; 21:99–102.

23. Malgren RA. Problems in techniques used in blood specimen preparation. Acta Cytol 1965; 9:97–99.

24. Yam LT, Janickla AJ. A simple method of preparing smears from bloody effusions for cytodiagnosis. Acta Cytol 1983; 27:114–118.

25. Boyum A. Separation of leucocytes from blood and bone marrow. Scand J Clin Lab Invest [Suppl] 1968; 21:97.

26. Nagasawe T, Nagasawa S. Enrichment of malignant cells from pleural effusions by Percoll density gradients. Acta Cytol 1983; 27:119–123.

27. Sayk J. Ergebnisse neuer liquorcytoloische Untersuchungen mit den Sedimentkammerverfahren. Arts Wochenschr 1954; 9:1042–1046.

28. Johnston WW, Szpak CA, Lottich SC, Thor A, Schlom J. Use of a monoclonal antibody (B72.3) as an immunocytochemical adjunct to the diagnosis of adenocarcinoma in human effusions. Cancer Res 1985; 45:1894–1900.

29. Kaps M, Burkhardt E. An improved method for electron microscopic observation of cerebrospinal fluid cells. Acta Cytol 1985; 29:484–486.

30. McCormack LJ, Hazard JB, Belovich D, Gardner WJ. Identification of neoplastic cells in cerebrospinal fluids by wet-film method. Cancer 1957; 10: 1293–1299.

31. Daste G, Serre G, Mauduyt M-A, Vincent C, Caveriviere P, Soleilhavoup J-P. Immunophenotyping of mesothelial cells with monoclonal antibodies to cytokeratins, vimentin, CEA and EMA improves the cytodiagnosis of serous effusions. Cytopathology 1991; 2:19–28.

32. Freshney RT. Culture of animal cells. A manual of basic techniques, 2nd ed. New York: Alan R Liss, 1987.

33. Hsu SM, Raine L, Fanger H. The use of avidin–biotin–peroxidase complex (ABC) in immunoperoxidase techniques: a comparison between ABC and unlabelled (PAP) procedures. J Histochem Cytochem 1981; 29:577–581.

34. Mason DY, Sammons R. Alkaline phosphatase and peroxidase for double immunoenzymatic labeling of cellular constituents. J Clin Pathol 1978; 31: 454–459.

35. Martin SE, Moshiri S, Thor A, Vilasi V, Chu EW, Schlom J. Identification of adenocarcinoma in cytospin preparations of effusions using monoclonal antibody B72.3. Am J Clin Pathol 1986; 86:10–18.

36. Li Cy, Laczano-Villareal O, Pierre RV, Yam LT. Immunocytochemical identification of cells in serous effusion. Technical consideration. Am J Clin Pathol 1987; 88:696–706.

37. DiBonito L, Falconieri G, Colautti I, Bonifacio Gori D, Dudine S, Giarelli

L. Cytopathology of malignant mesothelioma: a study of its patterns and histological bases. Diagn Cytopathol 1993; 9:25–31.

38. van der Kwast TH, Versnel MA, Delahaye M, De Jong AAW, Zondervan PE, Hoogsteden H. Expression of epithelial membrane antigen on malignant mesothelioma cells. An immunocytochemical and immunoelectron microscopic study. Acta Cytol 1988; 32:169–174.

39. Strankinga WFM, Sperber M, Kaiser MC, Stam J. Accuracy of diagnostic procedures in the initial evaluation and follow-up of mesothelioma patients. Respiration 1987; 51:179–187.

40. Dorward AJ, Stack BHR. Diffuse malignant pleural mesothelioma in Glasgow. Br J Dis Chest 1981; 75:397–402.

41. Prakash UBS. Comparison of needle biopsy with cytologic analysis for the evaluation of pleural effusion: analysis of 414 cases. Mayo Clin Proc 1985; 60:158–164.

42. Ryan CJ, Rodgers RF, Unni KK, Hepper NGG. The outcome of patients with pleural effusion of indeterminate cause at thoracotomy. Mayo Clin Proc 1981; 56:145–149.

43. Elmes PC, Simpson MJC. The clinical aspects of mesothelioma. Q J Med 1976; 45:427–429.

44. Antman KH. Clinical presentation and natural history of benign and malignant mesothelioma. Semin Oncol 1981; 8:313–320.

45. Klempman, S. The exfoliative cytology of diffuse pleural mesothelioma. Cancer 1962; 15:691–704.

46. Naylor B. The exfoliative cytology of diffuse malignant mesothelioma. J Pathol Bacteriol 1963; 86:293–298.

47. Roberts GH, Campbell GM. Exfoliative cytology of diffuse mesothelioma. J Clin Pathol 1972; 25:577–582.

48. Jara F, Hiroshi T, Uma NMR. Malignant mesothelioma of pleura. NY State J Med 1977; 77:1885–1888.

49. Whitaker D, Shilkin KB. The cytology of malignant mesothelioma in western Australia. Acta Cytol 1978; 22:67–70.

50. Edge JR, Choudhury SL. Malignant mesothelioma of the pleura in Barrow-in Furness. Thorax 1987; 33:26–30.

51. Lewis RJ, Sisler GE, MacKenzie JW. Diffuse, mixed malignant pleural mesothelioma. Ann Thorac Surg 1981; 31:53–60.

52. Brenner J, Sordillo PP, Magill GB, Golbey RB. Malignant mesothelioma of the pleura: review of 123 patients. Cancer 1982; 49:2431–2435.

53. Nauta RJ, Osteen RT, Antman KH, Koster JK. Clinical staging and the tendency of malignant pleural mesotheliomas to remain localized. Ann Thorac Surg 1982; 34:66–70.

54. Law MR, Hodson ME, Turner-Warwick M. Malignant mesothelioma of the pleura. Clinical aspects and symptomatic treatment. Eur J Respir Dis 1984; 65:162–168.

55. Triol JH, Conston AS, Chandler SV. Malignant mesothelioma, cytopathlogy of 75 cases seen in a New Jersey community hospital. Acta Cytol 1984; 28:37–45.

56. Matzel W. Biochemical and cytological features of diffuse mesotheliomas of the pleura. Arch Geschwulstforsch 1985; 55:2-264.
57. Whitaker D. The validity of a cytological diagnosis of mesothelioma. Aust NZ J Med 1987; 17:519.
58. Sherman ME, Mark EJ. Effusion cytology in the diagnosis of malignant epithelioid and biphasic pleural mesothelioma. Arch Pathol Lab Med 1990; 114:845-851.
59. Kwee WS, Veldhuizen RW, Alons CL, Morawetz F, Boon ME. Quantitative and qualitative differences between benign and malignant mesothelial cells in pleural fluid. Acta Cytol 1982; 26:401-406.
60. Stevens MW, Leong AS-Y, Fazzalari NL, Dowling KD, Henderson DW. Cytopathology of malignant mesothelioma: a stepwise logistic regression analysis. Diagn Cytopathol 1992; 8:333-341.
61. Whitaker D. Cell aggregates in malignant mesothelioma. Acta Cytol 1977; 21:236-239.
62. Delahaye M, De Jong AAW, Versnel MA, Hoogsteden HC, Teeling P, van der Kwast TH. Cytopathology of malignant mesothelioma. Reappraisal of the diagnostic value of collagen cores. Cytopathology 1990; 1:137-145.
63. Silverman JF, Nance K, Phillips B, Norris HT. The use of immunoperoxidase panels for the cytologic diagnosis of malignancy in serous effusions. Diagn Cytopathol 1987; 3:134-140.
64. Cibas ES, Corson JM, Pinkus GS. The distinction of adenocarcinoma from malignant mesothelioma in cell blocks of effusions. Hum Pathol 1987; 18:67-74.
65. Ernst CS, Atkinson BF. Mucicarmine positivity in malignant mesothelioma. Lab Invest 1980; 42:113-114.
66. Triol JH, Conston AS, Van D. Distinguishing adenocarcinoma from mesothelioma in effusions [letter]. Hum Pathol 1987; 18:969.
67. Sheibani K, Esteban JM, Bailey A, Battifora H, Weiss LM. Immunopathologic and molecular studies as an aid to the diagnosis of malignant mesothelioma. Hum Pathol 1992; 23:107-116.
68. Blobel GA, Moll R, Franke WW, Kayser KW, Gould VE. The intermediate filament cytoskeleton of malignant mesotheliomas and its diagnostic significance. Am J Pathol 1985; 121:235-247.
69. Tickman RJ, Cohen C, Varma VA, Fekete PS, DeRose PB. Distinction between carcinoma cells and mesothelial cells in serous effusions. Usefulness of immunohistochemistry. Acta Cytol 1990; 34:491-496.
70. To A, Coleman DV, Dearnaley DP, Ormerod MG, Stelle K, Neville AM. Use of antisera to epithelial membrane antigen for the cytodiagnosis of malignancy in serous effusions. J Clin Pathol 1981; 34:1326-1332.
71. Ligtenberg MJ, Vos HL, Gennissen AM, Hilkens J. Episialin, a carcinoma-associated mucin, is generated by a polymorphic gene encoding splice variants with alternative amino termini. J Biol Chem 1990; 265:5573-5578.
72. Gatter KC, Alcock C, Herget A, Pulford KA, Heyderman E, Taylor-Papadimitriou J, Stein H, Mason DY. The differential diagnosis of routinely

processed anaplastic tumors using monoclonal antibodies. Am J Clin Pathol 1984; 82:33–43.

73. Burchell J, Durbin H, Taylor-Papadimitriou J. Complexity of expression of antigenic determinants, recognized by monoclonal antibodies HMFG-1 and HMFG-2, in normal and malignant human mammary epithelial cells. J Immunol 1983; 131:508–513.

74. Ghosh AK, Mason DY, Spriggs AI. Immunocytochemical staining with monoclonal antibodies in cytologically "negative" serous effusions from patients with malignant disease. J Clin Pathol 1983; 36:1150–1152.

75. Sehested M, Ralfkjaer E, Rasmussen J. Immunoperoxidase demonstration of carcinoembryonic antigen in pleural and peritoneal effusions. Acta Cytol 1983; 27:124–127.

76. Ernst CS, Atkinson B, Chianese D, Peters J, Perry M, Herlyn M, Koprowski H. Differential diagnosis between mesotheliomas and metastatic adenocarcinomas using monoclonal antibodies against gastrointestinal carcinoma antigen and stage-specific embryonic antigen. Appl Pathol 1986; 4:115–124.

77. Ghosh AK, Butler EB. Immunocytochemical staining reactions of anticarcinoembryonic antigen, Ca, and anti-human milk fat globule monoclonal antibodies on benign and malignant exfoliated cells. J Clin Pathol 1987; 40: 1424–1427.

78. Mason MR, Bedrossian WM, Fahey CA. Value of immunocytochemistry in the study of malignant effusions. Diagn Cytopathol 1987; 3:215–221.

79. Duggan MA, Masters CB, Alexander F. Immunohistochemical differentiation of malignant mesothelioma, mesothelial hyperplasia and metastatic adenocarcinoma in serous effusions, utilizing staining for carcinoembryonic antigen, keratin and vimentin. Acta Cytol 1987; 31:807–814.

80. Walts AE, Said JW, Shintaku IP. Epithelial membrane antigen in the cytodiagnosis of effusions and aspirates: immunocytochemical and ultrastructural localization in benign and malignant cells. Diagn Cytopathol 1987; 3: 41–49.

81. Croonen AM, Van der Valk P, Herman C, Lindeman J. Cytology, immunopathology and flow cytometry in the diagnosis of pleural and peritoneal effusions. Lab Invest 1988; 58:725–732.

82. Lauritzen AF. Diagnostic value of monoclonal antibody B72.3 in detecting adenocarcinoma cells in serous effusions. Acta Pathol Microbiol Immunol Scand 1989; 97:761–766.

83. Gutzman J, Bross KJ, Würtemberger G, Costabel U. Immunocytology in malignant pleural mesothelioma. Expression of tumor markers and distribution of lymphocyte subsets. Chest 1989; 95:590–595.

84. Shield PW. Lectin binding properties of cells from serous effusion and peritoneal washing specimens. J Clin Pathol 1989; 42:1178–1183.

85. Esteban JM, Yokota S, Husain S, Battifora H. Immunocytochemical profile of benign and carcinomatous effusions. A practical approach to difficult diagnosis. Am J Clin Pathol 1990; 94:698–705.

86. Tickman RJ, Cohen C, Varma VA, Fekete PS, DeRose PB. Distinction

between carcinoma cells and mesothelial cells in serous effusions. Usefulness of immunohistochemistry. Acta Cytol 1990; 34:491–496.

87. Nance KV, Silverman JF. Immunocytochemical panel for the identification of malignant cells in serous effusions. Am J Clin Pathol 1991; 95:867–874.

88. Donna A, Betta P-G, Bellingeri D, Tallarida F, Pavesi M, Pastormerlo M. Cytologic diagnosis of malignant mesothelioma in serous effusions using an antimesothelial-cell antibody. Diagn Cytopathol 1992; 8:361–365.

89. Hilkens J, Buijs F, Hilgers J, Hageman P, Calafat J, Sonnenberg A, Van der Valk M. Monoclonal antibodies against human milk-fat globule membranes detecting differentiation antigens of the mammary gland and its tumors. Int J Cancer 1984; 34:197–206.

90. Heyderman E, Strudley I, Powell G, Richardson TC, Cordell JL, Mason DY. A new monoclonal antibody to epithelial membrane antigen (EMA)-E29. A comparison of its immunocytochemical reactivity with polyclonal anti-EMA antibodies and with another monoclonal antibody. Br J Cancer 1985; 52: 355–361.

91. Johnson VG, Schlom J, Paterson AJ, Bennett J, Magnani JL, Colcher D. Analysis of a human tumor-associated glycoprotein (TAG-72) identified by monoclonal antibody B72.3. Cancer Res 1986; 46:850–857.

92. Lee I, Radosevich JA, Chejvec G, Yixing M, Warren WH, Rosen ST, Gould VE. Malignant mesothelioma. Improved differential diagnosis from lung adenocarcinomas using monoclonal antibodies 44-3A6 and 624A12. Am J Pathol 1986; 123:497–507.

93. Pinkus GS, Said JW. Leu-M1 immunoreactivity in non-hematopoietic neoplasms and myeloproliferative disorders: an immunoperoxidase study of paraffin sections. Am J Clin Pathol 1986; 85:278–282.

94. Sheibani K, Battifora H, Burke JS. Antigenic phenotype of malignant mesotheliomas and pulmonary adenocarcinomas. An immunohistologic analysis demonstrating the value of Leu M1 antigen. Am J Pathol 1986; 123:212–219.

95. Ordonez NG. The immunohistochemical diagnosis of mesothelioma. Differentiation of mesothelioma and lung adenocarcinoma. Am J Surg Pathol 1989; 13:276–291.

96. Warnock ML, Stoloff A, Thor A. Differentiation of adenocarcinoma of the lung from mesothelioma. Periodic acid–Schiff, monoclonal antibodies B72.3, and Leu M1. Am J Pathol 1988; 133:30–38.

97. Latza U, Niedobitek G, Schwarting R, Nekarda H, Stein H. Ber-EP4: new monoclonal antibody which distinguishes epithelia from mesothelia. J Clin Pathol 1990; 43:213–219.

98. Sheibani K, Shin SS, Kezirian J, Weiss L. Ber-EP4 antibody as a discriminant in the differential diagnosis of malignant mesothelioma versus adenocarcinoma. Am J Surg Pathol 1991; 15:779–784.

99. Gaffey MJ, Mills SE, Swanson PE, Zarbo RJ, Shah AR, Wick M. Immunoreactivity for BER-EP4 in adenocarcinomas, adenomatoid tumors, and malignant mesotheliomas. Am J Surg Pathol 1992; 16:3–9.

100. Spagnolo DV, Whitaker D, Carrello S, Radosevich JA, Rosen ST, Gould

VE. The use of monoclonal antibody 44-3A6 in cell blocks in the diagnosis of lung carcinoma, carcinomas metastatic to lung and pleura, and pleural malignant mesothelioma. Am J Clin Pathol 1991; 95:322-329.

101. De Leij L, Postmus PE, Poppema S, Elema JD, The TH. The use of monoclonal antibodies for the pathological diagnosis of lung cancer. In: Hansen HH, ed. Lung cancer: basic and clinical aspects. Boston: Martinus Nijhoff, 1986:31-48.

102. Delahaye M, Hoogsteden HC, van der Kwast TH. Immunocytochemistry of malignant mesothelioma: OV632 as a marker of malignant mesothelioma. J Pathol 1991; 165:137-143.

103. Singh G, Whiteside TL, Dekker A. Immunodiagnosis of mesothelioma. Use of antimesothelial cell serum in an indirect immunofluorescence assay. Cancer 1979; 43:2288-2296.

104. Donna A, Betta PG, Bellingeri D, Marchesini A. New marker for mesothelioma. An immunoperoxidase study. J Clin Pathol 1986; 39:961-968.

105. Donna A, Betta PG, Cosimi MF, Robutti F, Bellingeri D, Marchesini A. Putative mesothelial cell growth-promoting activity of a cytoplasmic protein expressed by the mesothelial cell. Exp Cell Biol 1989; 57:193-197.

106. Stahel RA, O'Hara CJ, Waibel R, Martin A. Monoclonal antibodies against mesothelial membrane antigen discriminate between malignant mesothelioma and lung adenocarcinoma. Int J Cancer 1988; 41:218-223.

107. O'Hara CJ, Corson JM, Pinkus GS, Stahel RA. ME1: a monoclonal antibody that distinguishes epithelial-type malignant mesothelioma from pulmonary adenocarcinoma and extrapulmonary malignancies. Am J Pathol 1990; 136:421-428.

108. Chang K, Pai LH, Pass H, Pogrebniak HW, Tsao M-S, Pastan I, Willingham MC. Monoclonal antibody K1 reacts with epithelial mesothelioma but not with lung adenocarcinoma. Am J Surg Pathol 1992; 16:259-268.

109. Collins CL, Ordonez NG, Schaefer R, Cook CD, Xie S-S, Granger J, Hsu P-L, Fink L, Hsu S-M. Thrombomodulin expression in malignant pleural mesothelioma and pulmonary adenocarcinoma. Am J Pathol 1992; 141:827-833.

110. Fleuren GJ, Coerkamp EG, Nap M, Van den Broek LJCM, Warnaar SO. Immunohistological characterization of a monoclonal antibody (OV632) against epithelial ovarian carcinomas. Virchows Arch [A] 1987; 410:481-486.

111. Koelma IA, Nap M, Van Steenis FJ, Fleuren GJ. Tumor markers for ovarian cancer. A comparative immunohistochemical and immunocytochemical study of two commercial monoclonal antibodies (OV632 and OC125). Am J Clin Pathol 1988; 90:391-396.

112. Linari A, Bussolati G. Evaluation of impact of immunocytochemical techniques in cytological diagnosis of neoplastic effusions. J Clin Pathol 1989; 42:1184-1189.

113. Flens MJ, Van der Valk P, Tadema TM, Huysmans ACLM, Risse EKJ, Van Tol GA, Meijer CJLM. The contribution of immunocytochemistry in diagnostic cytology. Comparison and evaluation with immunohistology. Cancer 1990; 65:2704-2711.

114. Wazir JF, Martin-Bates E, Woodward G, Coleman DV. Evaluation of immunocytochemical staining as a method of improving diagnostic accuracy in a routine cytopathologic laboratory. Cytopathology 1991; 2:75–82.

115. Wang NS. Electron-microscopy in the diagnosis of pleural mesotheliomas. Cancer 1973; 31:1046–1054.

116. Stoebner P, Brambilla E. Ultrastructural diagnosis of pleural tumors. Pathol Res Pract 1982; 173:402–416.

117. Warhol MJ, Hickey WF, Corson JM. Malignant mesothelioma: ultrastructural distinction from adenocarcinoma. Am J Surg Pathol 1982; 6:307–314.

118. Bewtra C, Greer KP. Ultrastructural studies of cells in body cavity effusions. Acta Cytol 1985; 29:226–238.

119. Kobzik L, Antman KH, Warhol MJ. The distinction of mesothelioma from adenocarcinoma in malignant effusions by electron microscopy. Acta Cytol 1985; 29:219–225.

120. Leong AS, Stevens MW, Murkherjee TM. Malignant mesothelioma: cytologic diagnosis with histologic, immunohistochemical, and ultrastructural correlation. Semin Diagn Pathol 1992; 9:141–150.

121. Wueker RB, Guglietti LC, Nations ED. Comparison of light and transmission electron microscopy for the evaluation of body cavity effusions. Acta Cytol 1983; 27:614–624.

122. Bolen JW, Hammar SP, McNutt MA. Reactive and neoplastic tissue. A light-microscopic, ultrastructural, and immunocytochemical study. Am J Surg Pathol 1986; 10:34–47.

123. Bedrossion CW, Bonsib S, Moran C. Differential diagnosis between mesothelioma and adenocarcinoma: a multimodal approach based on ultrastructure and immunocytochemistry. Semin Diagn Pathol 1992; 9: 124–140.

124. Pedio G, Landolt-Weber U. Cytologic presentation of malignant mesothelioma in pleural effusions. Exp Cell Biol 1988; 56:211–216.

125. Dewar A, Valente M, Ring NP, Corrin B. Pleural mesothelioma of epithelial type and pulmonary adenocarcinoma: an ultrastructural and cytochemical comparison. J Pathol 1987; 152:309–316.

126. Warhol MJ, Corson JM. An ultrastructural comparison of mesotheliomas with adenocarcinomas of the lung and breast. Hum Pathol 1985; 16:50–55.

127. Wick MR, Loy T, Mills SE, Legier JF, Manivel JC. Malignant epitheloid pleural mesothelioma versus peripheral pulmonary adenocarcinoma. A histochemical, ultrastructural and immunohistologic study of 103 cases. Hum Pathol 1990; 21:759–766.

128. Dardick I, Al-Jabi M, McCaughey WTE. Diffuse epithelial mesothelioma: a revue of the ultrastructural spectrum. Ultrastruct Pathol 1987; 11:503–533.

129. Carstens HB. Contact between abluminal microvilli and collagen fibrils in metastatic adenocarcinoma and mesothelioma. J Pathol 1992; 166:179–182.

130. Burmer GC, Rabinovitch PS, Kulander BG, et al. Flow cytometric analysis of malignant pleural mesotheliomas. Hum Pathol 1989; 20:777–783.

131. Frierson F, Mills SE, Legier JF. Flow cytometric analysis of ploidy in immunohistochemically confirmed examples of malignant epithelial mesothelioma. Am J Clin Pathol 1988; 90:240–243.

132. Dazzi H, Thatcher N, Hasleton PS. DNA analysis by flow cytometry in malignant pleural mesothelioma: relationship to histology and survival. J Pathol 1990; 162:51–55.
133. Zarbo RJ. Flow cytometric DNA analysis of effusions. A new test seeking validation. Am J Clin Pathol 1991; 95:2–4.
134. Fuhr JE, Kattine AA, Sullivan TA, Nelson HS. Flow cytometric analysis of pulmonary fluids and cells for the detection of malignancies. Am J Pathol 1992; 141:211–215.
135. Giwercman A, Hopman AHN, Ramaekers FCS, Skakkebæk NE. Carcinoma in situ of the testis. Detection of malignant germ cells in seminal fluid by means of in situ hybridization. Am J Pathol 1990; 136:497–502.
136. Hagemeijer A, Versnel MA, Van Drunen E, Moret M, Bouts MJ, van der Kwast TH, Hoogsteden H. Cytogenetic analysis of malignant mesothelioma. Cancer Genet Cytogenet 1990; 47:1–28.
137. Rodenhuis S, Van de Wetering ML, Mooi WJ, Evers SG, Van Zandwijk N, Bos JL. Mutational activation of the K-*ras* oncogene: a possible pathogenetic factor in adenocarcinoma of the lung. N Engl J Med 1987; 317:929–935.
138. Sheibani K, Wu A, Ben-Ezra J, et al. Analysis of Ha-*ras* sequence in DNAs of malignant mesothelioma and pulmonary adenocarcinoma by a sensitive polymerase chain reaction (PCR) method [abstr]. Lab Invest 1989; 60:87.
139. Martinez M, Georgoff I, Levine A. Cellular localization and cell cycle regulation by a temperature-sensitive p53 protein. Genes Dev 1991; 5:151–159.
140. Wynford-Thomas D. p53 in tumour pathology: can we trust immunocytochemistry? J Pathol 1992; 166:329–330.
141. Cote RJ, Jhanwar SC, Novick S, Pellicer A. Genetic alterations of the p53 gene are a feature of malignant mesothelioma. Cancer Res 1991; 51:5410–5416.
142. Metcalf RA, Welsh JA, Bennett WP, Seddon MB, Lehman TA, Pelin K, Linnainmaa K, Tamimilehto L, Mattson K, Gerwin BI, Harris CC. p53 and Kirsten-*ras* mutations in human mesothelioma cell lines. Cancer Res 1992; 52:2610–2615.
143. Mayall FG, Goddard H, Gibbs AR. p53 immunostaining in the distinction between benign and malignant mesothelial proliferations using formalin-fixed paraffin sections. J Pathol 1992; 168:377–381.
144. Ramael M, Lemmens G, Eerdekens C, Buysse C, Jacobs W, Van Marck E. Immunoreactivity for p53 protein in malignant mesothelioma and non-neoplastic mesothelium. J Pathol 1992; 168:371–375.
145. Kafiri G, Thomas DM, Shepherd NA, Krausz T, Lane DP, Hall PA. p53 expression is common in malignant mesothelioma. Histopathology 1992; 21:331–334.
146. Gerwin BI, Lechner JF, Reddel RR, Roberts AB, Robbins KC, Gabrielson EW, Harris CC. Cancer Res 1987; 47:6180–6184.
147. Versnel MA, Claesson-Welsh L, Hammacher A, Bouts MJ, van der Kwast TH, Eriksson A, Willemsen R, Weima SM, Hoogsteden HC, Hagemeijer A, Heldin C-H. Human malignant mesothelioma cell lines express PDGF β-receptors whereas cultured normal mesothelial cells express predominantly PDGF α-receptors. Oncogene 1991; 6:2005–2011.

# 9

## Establishment and Characterization of Human Normal and Malignant Mesothelial Cell Lines

**MARJAN A. VERSNEL,**
**THEODORUS H. VAN DER KWAST,**
**and ANNE HAGEMEIJER**

Erasmus University Rotterdam
Rotterdam, The Netherlands

**HENK C. HOOGSTEDEN**

University Hospital Dijkzigt
Rotterdam, The Netherlands

## I. Introduction

For the study of the biological properties of malignant mesothelioma and the process of malignant transformation of mesothelial cells, a continuous source of viable tumor material is essential. Viable tumor tissue of malignant mesothelioma patients is difficult to obtain. The material that is available for research usually consists of pleural effusion cells and sometimes biopsy material. In pleural effusions of malignant mesothelioma patients, the frequency of malignant mesothelioma cells is usually low, and several other cell types, such as lymphocytes, macrophages, and reactive mesothelial cells, can be found.

In vitro-growing tumor cell lines are useful as a continuous source of tumor material of a constant quality. Cell lines have been established from many different tumor types, and these cell lines have contributed considerably to our knowledge about these tumors. However, until recently, only a few malignant mesothelioma cell lines were established and not much was known on the isolation procedure used and the characteristics of the cell lines. Furthermore, it is essential for the study of the biological properties of malignant cells to have the normal counterpart of this cell type also available for comparison. In general, normal cells are not available in large quantities, they are difficult to culture, and they have a limited life span.

In this review, we shall summarize the data available on the establishment and characterization of in vitro-growing normal and malignant mesothelial cells from the literature and describe our own experience. Furthermore, recently described characteristics of normal and malignant mesothelial cells will be considered as markers for characterization of newly established cell lines.

## II. Confirmation of Diagnosis of Malignant Mesothelioma

Patient material to be used for the establishment of cell lines has to be diagnosed with as much certainty as possible. As the diagnosis of malignant mesothelioma is difficult owing to lack of criteria for the differentiation between malignant mesothelioma cells, adenocarcinoma, and reactive mesothelial cells, we require the use of at least two different techniques to establish the diagnosis of malignant mesothelioma. Malignant mesothelioma was never diagnosed on cytological analysis only, but always confirmed by at least electron microscopy or histological techniques. We have collected material from untreated patients suspected of a malignant mesothelioma for the establishment of malignant mesothelioma cell lines. From approximately half of the patients suspected of malignant mesothelioma, the diagnosis could be confirmed by at least two different techniques, and only those cases were retained (1). Although treatment of malignant mesothelioma is generally palliative, one has to be cautious with the use of material derived from treated patients. Treatment, and especially radiation therapy, can induce chromosomal aberrations, and the influence of treatment on the biological properties of the material is unknown.

## III. Isolation of Human Malignant Mesothelioma Cell Lines

The material that is most frequently available to us for the establishment of malignant mesothelioma cell lines is pleural effusion cells. Solid tumor tissue is sometimes obtained from thoracoscopic investigations or open surgery. However, it is never certain that each biopsy indeed contains tumor tissue. Autopsy material is another useful source of tumor tissue, provided that autopsy is performed within 4 h of death. As many malignant mesothelioma patients die at home, this is only occasionally possible. To get sterile tumor tissue from an autopsy, different sets of instruments should be used for incision of the skin and removal of tumor tissue. In Table 1, data

**Table 1** Derivation of Human Malignant Mesothelioma Cell Lines Described in the Literature[a]

| Author (Ref.) | Total number of isolated malignant mesothelioma cell lines | Patient material | | |
|---|---|---|---|---|
| | | Effusion | Biopsy or surgical specimen | Autopsy |
| Behebani et al. (2) | 1 | 1 | | |
| Hsu et al. (3) | 2 | 2 | | |
| Klominek et al. (4) | 2 | 2 | | |
| Lauber et al. (5) | 1 | 1 | | |
| Manning et al. (6) | 5 | 5 | | |
| Masuda et al. (7) | 1 | 1 | | |
| Pelin-Enlund et al. (8) | 9 | 3 | 6 | |
| Popescu et al. (9) | 1 | 1 | | |
| Schmitter et al. (10) | 7 | 3 | 4 | |
| Shanfang et al. (11) | 1 | | 1 | |
| Versnel et al. (1) | 17 | 10 | 2 | 5 |

[a]Abstracts from meetings were not included.

available in the literature on patient material used for the establishment of 47 malignant mesothelioma cell lines are summarized (1–11). More than 60% (29/47) of the malignant mesothelioma cell lines were established from pleural effusion cells. Data on the success rate of the isolation of malignant mesothelioma cell lines from the various sources of patient material are listed in Table 2 (1,3,6). The overall success rate of the establishment of malignant mesothelioma cell lines from pleural effusions is 28%. Establish-

**Table 2** Establishing Rate of Human Malignant Mesothelioma Cell Lines from Patient Material

| Author (Ref.) | Successful isolation of a cell line/ no. of specimens | | |
|---|---|---|---|
| | Effusion | Biopsy | Autopsy |
| Hsu et al. (3) | 2/4 | | |
| Manning et al. (6) | 11/33 | | |
| Versnel et al. (1) | 10/46 | 2/9 | 2/6[a] |

[a]From one autopsy four cell lines were isolated from the primary tumor and metastases.

ment of cell lines from thoracoscopic biopsy material is frequently unsuccessful owing to the absence of tumor tissue in the specimen used. Autopsy material has a low viability, and is frequently not sterile, but nevertheless, gave rise to five cell lines in our hands. An advantage of autopsy material is that the primary tumor and metastases outside the thoracic cavity can be used for the establishment of cell lines. By this approach we have isolated cell lines from the primary tumor and from three different metastases (1).

### A.  Processing of Patient Material

Pleural fluid has to be collected in a vial with heparin to prevent clotting. After immediate transportation to the laboratory, the cells are harvested by centrifugation, washed with sterile saline, and plated at high density. We remove the medium after overnight incubation to eliminate the nonadherent cells, such as lymphocytes and erythrocytes (1). However, density gradient centrifugation through Ficoll-Paque (6) or lysis by an ammonium chloride buffer (5,10) was also used.

Solid tumor tissue was obtained under sterile conditions and, subsequently, fat, necrotic, and lung tissues were removed. After mincing with scissors, we incubate the pieces overnight with collagenase and plated the dissociated cells only (1). Other investigators successfully used an explant technique (8) or finely minced tumor tissue in medium and collected the dissociated cells (10).

### B.  Culture Conditions

In our laboratory, F10 medium, supplemented with 15% fetal calf serum (FCS) and antibiotics, was used for the establishment of malignant mesothelioma cell lines. Other investigators successfully employed RPMI 1640, supplemented with 5, 10, or 15% FCS. The addition of epidermal growth factor (EGF) and hydrocortisone (HC), or EGF alone, increases the chance of a successful isolation of a malignant mesothelioma cell line from pleural effusion cells (1). However, the effect on the isolation of cell lines from individual samples is unpredictable. Interestingly, the proliferation of two established malignant mesothelioma cell lines was inhibited by EGF plus HC in the presence of FCS, whereas EGF alone increased the proliferation (12). For the detachment of malignant mesothelioma cells, trypsin, trypsin-EDTA, or edetate sodium (Versene) was used. In summary, it seems that the choice of the culture medium used for the establishment of malignant mesothelioma is not particularly critical, as routinely used media, such as RPMI and F10, are found to be appropriate, although sometimes chemically defined media in the absence of FCS are employed. The doubling time of many malignant mesothelioma cell lines has been determined and, in most cell lines, was approximately 30 h (range 25–145 h). There seems to be no correlation between the doubling time, the histological subtype, or any other feature of the cell line.

## IV. Isolation of Normal Human Mesothelial Cell Lines

For investigation of the biological properties involved in the malignant transformation of mesothelial cells, a comparison of the features of normal and malignant mesothelial cells is important. Studies with cultured human mesothelial cells are difficult for several reasons. First, patient material suitable for the isolation of normal mesothelial cell cultures is difficult to obtain. Mostly, pleural effusions of noncancerous patients, such as those with congestive heart failure, were used. As these reactive pleural effusions can have a variety of causes, these patients frequently are not in the pulmonary department of the hospital, and good organization is needed to obtain such pleural effusions. Furthermore, the cultivation of normal mesothelial cells is hampered by the limited growth potential. In our hands mesothelial cells can be cultured for about 15 passages, but the variation between different patients is considerable (1).

### A. Processing of Patient Material

Most normal mesothelial cell cultures were isolated from pleural effusions (1,13,14). The method used for isolation of these cell lines is the same as described for malignant mesothelioma cell lines from pleural effusions. Alternatively, pieces of mesothelium from the pleura derived from thoracic surgery can be used. After removal of fat and lung tissue, the mesothelium is cut into small pieces and covered with a small film of medium. When the pieces have adhered to the culture dish, more medium is added. As this material is always sterile and definitely does not contain malignant cells, in our hands, this approach was always successful in obtaining primary mesothelial cell lines (Versnel, unpublished results). Others employed a comparable method using omental specimens as a source of mesothelial cells (15). Pleural or omental tissue specimens can also be digested with trypsin-EDTA or collagenase before plating (15,16).

### B. Culture Conditions

We always culture normal mesothelial cells on F10 medium (1), but other culture media, such as a mixture of M199 and MCDB202 (1:1), M199, and LHC are also used (13,14,17). Depending on the medium used, a supplementation with FCS or fetal bovine serum (FBS) can be used. Epithelial growth factor (EGF) and hydrocortisone (HC) were found to stimulate the proliferation of normal mesothelial cells (17). Extensive studies of the proliferative response of normal mesothelial cells to a variety of growth factors have been performed (14,18,19). Sustained growth of normal meso-thelial cells was found in LHC medium with 3% chemically denatured serum (CDS), HC, insulin, transferrin, and any one of the following growth factors: EGF, transforming growth factor (TGF)-α, TGF-β1, TGF-β2, platelet-derived growth factor (PDGF)-AB, PDGF-BB, acidic fibroblast growth factor (FGF), basic FGF, interleukin (IL)-1α, IL-1β, IL-2, inter-feron (IFN)-γ, IFN-β, or cholera toxin (14). However, in cultured normal mesothelial cells of 57 donors, an enormous interindividual variation in response to different growth factors was observed (19). Furthermore, the proliferation of these cultures in a routinely used medium varied consider-ably (19). Normal mesothelial cells can be cultured in serum-supplemented medium in culture flasks without a coating with extracellular matrix but, under serum-free conditions, a coating is advisable. A comparison of [$^3$H]TdR incorporation into normal mesothelial cells grown in serum-free medium on dishes coated with various coating mixtures of basement mem-brane constituents revealed that the growth rate was optimal using a fibro-nectin coating (14).

## V.  Characterization of Normal and Malignant Mesothelial Cell Lines

Careful characterization of normal mesothelial and malignant mesotheli-oma cell lines is essential, as they will be used as a tool for the study of the properties of malignant transformation of mesothelial cells. The criteria generally used are cytomorphology, electron microscopy, immunocyto-chemistry, tumorigenicity in nude mice, and cytogenetics. The results ob-tained by us and others will be summarized and discussed.

### A.  Morphology

Malignant mesothelioma cell lines display a heterogeneity in morphological features. The cells can be spindle-shaped, or more epithelial-like as cobble-stones (Fig. 1). Contact inhibition has been observed in several cell lines (8,10). All malignant mesothelioma cell lines have an adherent phenotype, but a single malignant mesothelioma cell line AL5 has been described with both adherent and floating cells (5). The floating cells were able to again form a population of adherent and floating cells after reseeding. In our own panel of malignant mesothelioma cell lines, some also always contain floating cells, independent of the density of the culture, but reseeding exper-iments were not performed (Versnel, personal observation). Interestingly,

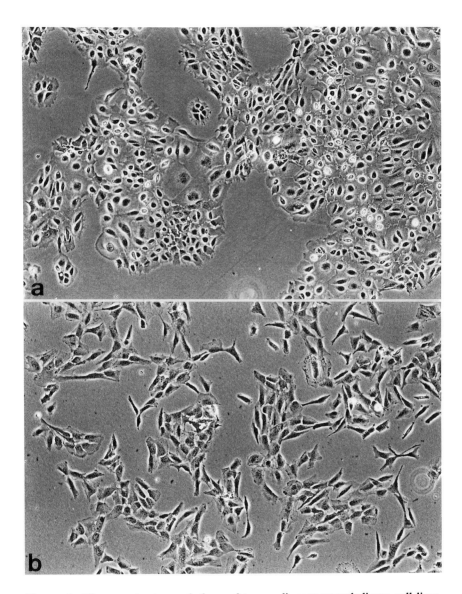

**Figure 1** Phase-contrast morphology of two malignant mesothelioma cell lines. (a) Mero-25 with an epithelial morphology and (b) Mero-82 with a more fibroblastoid morphology.

two malignant mesothelioma cell lines in vitro changed their morphology from fibroblastlike to epithelioid, when the medium supplemented with FCS was replaced by medium supplemented with human serum (HS) (4). Addition of EGF, PDGF, or insulin-like growth factor-1 (IGF-1) to medium supplemented with FCS did not influence the morphological appearance of the cells (4). However, the observed phenomenon could still be due to a difference in growth factor composition of FCS versus HS, because combinations of growth factors were not examined.

Normal human mesothelial cells can change their morphological appearance when grown on medium supplemented with different growth factors. In medium with FCS and HS, normal mesothelial cells form a simple epithelium at saturation density (17). When EGF was added to the culture medium, the cells grew more rapidly, had a fibroblastoid morphology, and formed multilayers of cells. This morphological change was accompanied by a change in the intermediate filament composition, from high keratin and low vimentin to low keratin and high vimentin contents (17). Retinoic acid (RA) had a reversible effect on human mesothelial cells, switching the cells from low keratin and abundant vimentin to high keratin and low vimentin content (20). The feature of cultured normal mesothelial cells to switch their morphological structure after addition of EGF has been used by several authors for the characterization of normal mesothelial cell cultures (12,21).

### B.  Electron Microscopy

The ultrastructural features of malignant mesothelioma cell lines have been investigated by several authors. Consistent with malignant mesothelioma are microvilli, glycogen granules, perinuclear intermediate filaments, and tight junctions. These properties can be used only to establish consistency with a mesothelial origin. There are no specific electron microscopic characteristics available for the discrimination between cultured malignant and normal mesothelial cells. To distinguish cultured mesothelial cells from fibroblasts, which can be relevant when the cells were cultured from solid tissues, the presence of tight junctions is indicative of cells of epithelial origin and excludes fibroblasts.

### C.  Immunocytochemistry

As yet, there is no single marker that is characteristic for malignant mesothelioma cell lines only. Malignant mesothelioma cell lines can be characterized and distinguished from adenocarcinomas, normal mesothelial cells, and fibroblasts by staining with several antibodies. Normal and malignant mesothelial cell lines can be characterized using antibodies against the intermediate filaments, keratin and vimentin. For the characterization of malignant mesothelioma cell lines, several antibodies against glycoproteins, such as epithelial membrane antigens (EMA) and carcinoembryonic antigen (CEA) are employed. Application of these antibodies for characterization of cell lines is discussed in this section and summarized in Table 3.

In solid tumor specimens, coexpression of keratin and vimentin is considered distinctive for malignant mesotheliomas rather than adenocarcinomas. Also normal and malignant mesothelial cells in vitro coexpress keratin and vimentin (22). However, epithelial cells in pleural effusions, as well as in culture, expressed vimentin, whereas in the solid tumor, no vimentin was detected (23). This indicates that vimentin expression can be induced in tissue culture, and that coexpression of vimentin and keratin in cultured cells is not useful for discrimination between cultured adenocarcinoma cells and malignant mesothelioma cells. The expression of keratin is a feature of epithelial cells in general and, in this context, is useful only for the differentiation between epithelial (or mesothelial) cells and fibroblasts. More detailed analysis of the individual cytokeratin polypeptides can be performed by immunofluorescence or immunoblotting with chain-specific monoclonal antibodies, or with two-dimensional gel electrophoresis. Comparison of the intermediate filament cytoskeleton of malignant mesothelioma and lung adenocarcinoma revealed that malignant mesothelioma cells expressed cytokeratin 5, which was absent in lung adenocarcinomas (24). With two-dimensional gel electrophoresis and immunoblotting with an antibody against cytokeratins 5 and 8, no cytokeratin 5-like protein was detected in the three malignant mesothelioma cell lines investigated (12). Moll et al. described an antibody that selectively recognized cytokeratin 5 and

**Table 3** Staining Pattern of Various Cultured Cell Types with Antibodies Relevant for Characterization of Malignant Mesothelioma Cell Lines

| Antibody | Malignant mesothelioma | Normal mesothelium | Adenocarcinoma | Fibroblasts |
|---|---|---|---|---|
| Keratin[a] | + | + | + | − |
| Vimentin | + | + | + | + |
| EMA | +[b] | −/(+)[c] | + | − |
| CEA | −/(+)[d] | − | + | − |
| ME1 | + | + | − | − |

[a]Pankeratin marker.
[b]Not all malignant mesotheliomas were EMA-positive.
[c]Occasionally EMA-positive reactive mesothelial cells were described.
[d]Occasionally CEA expression has been found in malignant mesothelioma cells.

stained most malignant mesotheliomas (25). This antibody could be useful for the discrimination between malignant mesothelioma cell lines and adenocarcinoma cell lines, but it has not yet been used for this purpose.

The antigens EMA and CEA are markers that, in many specimens, are helpful for a cytological diagnosis of malignant mesothelioma (26). Malignant mesothelioma cells are frequently EMA-positive; however, EMA cannot discriminate between malignant epithelial cells and malignant mesothelial cells. Incidentally, reactive normal mesothelial cells express EMA, and malignant mesothelioma cell lines also express EMA (1,6). Expression of EMA on cultured cells can be applied to distinguish malignant epithelial or mesothelial cells and fibroblasts. Expression of CEA is seldom found on malignant mesothelioma cells, whereas adenocarcinomas are frequently positive. Most malignant mesothelioma cell lines investigated for CEA were negative (6,10), but one CEA-positive malignant mesothelioma cell line has been described (6).

To establish the mesothelial nature of normal and malignant cell lines, the antibody ME1 has been used by several groups. ME1 recognizes a mesothelial membrane antigen on malignant and normal mesothelial cells and discriminates between malignant mesothelioma tissues and adenocarcinomas (27). All 12 investigated malignant mesothelial cell lines express ME1 (6,10).

### D. Cytogenetics

Detailed cytogenetic analysis of malignant mesothelioma cell lines has been performed on numerous cell lines (1,4,6,8,9). The reported malignant mesothelioma cell lines had a highly aneuploid karyotype, with clearly clonally rearranged chromosomes. Comparison of karyotypes of cell lines with those in the original patient material revealed that the chromosomal abnormalities were the same as those in the original patient material. In cell lines, the modal chromosomal number varies between 28 and 140, with a peak in the hypotriploid number. In patient material we described types of clustered aberrations, the most frequent showing hypodiploid karyotype with nonrandom loss of chromosomes 4, 22, 9p, and 3p (28). Evidence was found for clonal progression by tetraploidization, followed by random loss of chromosomes to a hypotriploid modal chromosomal number (1,28). Neither comparison of karyotypes of different malignant mesothelioma cell lines, nor studies of the cytogenetics of patient material of malignant mesotheliomas, have yet resulted in the detection of specific abnormalities characteristic for malignant mesothelioma that are useful for diagnostic application (28).

Cytogenetic analysis is an important step to establish the identity of a cell line, and during the isolation procedure of a malignant mesothelioma cell line, it is useful to establish whether the proliferating cells have normal or abnormal karyotype and, consequently, are normal or malignant cells. When a mixture of normal and malignant cells is detected by cytogenetics immediate subcloning has been useful to prevent overgrowth of malignant mesothelial cells by normal mesothelial cells. Sequential cytogenetic studies have occasionally shown a good stabilization of the aneuploid karyotype, with only a few or no variations between different passages. In other instances, the cytogenetic picture was still evolving owing to gain and loss of chromosomes, but the characteristic markers attesting to the origin of the line were always retained. Furthermore, correlation of karyotypic abnormalities with biological features, such as oncogene expression, might indicate which of the many cytogenetic abnormalities found in malignant mesotheliomas are primarily involved in oncogenesis and which are secondary changes. It has been investigated whether the elevated expression of the PDGF A- and B-chain genes in malignant mesothelioma cell lines, compared with normal mesothelial cell lines, and the observed pattern of PDGF $\alpha$- and $\beta$-receptor expression in normal and malignant mesothelial cells correlated with cytogenetic abnormalities in the chromosomes on which these genes have been mapped (29,30). However, no correlation with a numerical or structural abnormality was found. In conclusion cytogenetic analysis of growing cultures is suitable for discrimination between normal and malignant cells.

In vitro-growing normal mesothelial cell lines have a normal karyotype. Sequential studies after several passaging may show minor abnormalities (trisomy, translocation, deletion), apparently "spontaneously" acquired in vitro. As far as our experience is concerned, these changes did not affect the finite life span or other characteristics of the cell lines. The only exception is the TM-2 cell line (34).

### E. Tumorigenicity

The incidence of tumors after subcutaneous inoculation of malignant mesothelioma cell lines in nude mice varies greatly between the different investigated panels of cell lines. From the 32 malignant mesothelioma cell lines investigated for tumorigenicity in nude mice, 14 (44%) produced tumors with histological features consistent with a mesothelioma. It seems that tumorigenicity in nude mice is not a general feature of malignant mesothelioma cell lines.

### VI. Transformed Human Mesothelial Cell Lines

To obtain mesothelial cell lines that are less susceptible to senescence and useful as models for the study of malignant transformation, mesothelial cells have been transfected with the cancer-derived c-H-*ras* mutation EJ-*ras*, SV40 early region DNA, or both. Normal human mesothelial cells transfected with EJ-*ras* gene became EGF-independent, senescent at the same age as their untransfected parental strain, and were not tumorigenic in nude mice (31). Furthermore, the EJ-*ras*-transformed cells produced EGF-like activity (31). Transfection of SV40 large T antigen resulted in colonies of transformed mesothelial cells, with a greatly extended life span of 60–70 population doubling (PD) versus 15 PD in untransfected cells (21). A single transfected culture escaped senescence and became immortal (21). This MeT5A cell line was nontumorigenic. The mesothelial nature of MeT5A was convincingly established by demonstration of expression of the mesothelial markers ME1 and ME2, variation in cytokeratin expression under different growth conditions, and mitogenic response to the same growth factors as untransfected mesothelial cells (21). When the MeT5A cell line was subsequently transfected with the EJ-*ras* oncogene, the cell line became tumorigenic (32). However, working with SV40 T–antigen-transformed cells can be risky, as it was recently described that in SV40 T–antigen-transformed embryonic lung fibroblasts, PDGF receptor expression is suppressed (33). As there are indications that PDGF chain and receptor expression is involved in the malignant transformation of mesothelial cells, the use of SV40-transformed lines for the study of PDGF chain and receptor expression in the malignant transformation of mesothelial cells should be avoided. We recently described the cell line TM-2, which was derived by spontaneous in vitro transformation from the normal mesothelial cell culture NM-7. TM-2 has an indefinite life span, an abnormal karyotype, and proliferates independently of the addition of growth factors (34). The expression pattern of PDGF chains and receptors strongly resembled the pattern described for malignant mesothelioma cell lines (29,30,35). The establishment of more mesothelial cell lines transformed by transfection seems a good approach for the study of the malignant transformation of mesothelial cells; however, comparative studies with untransformed mesothelial cells still are essential, as transformed mesothelial cell lines are an artificial system.

## VII. Discussion

In this chapter we have summarized the data available on the establishment and characterization of human malignant mesothelioma cell lines. Although the success rate for establishing these lines is not very high, several newly established ones have been described. There is as yet no single specific feature for discrimination between malignant mesothelioma cells, reactive mesothelial cells, and adenocarcinoma cells in vivo as well as in vitro. Consequently, the characterization of newly established cell lines as malignant mesothelioma is difficult, and the data presented are not always convincing. An illustration of the difficulty in characterization of newly established cell lines was recently reported. Two earlier-described lung cancer cell lines from the American Type Culture Collection (ATCC) were investigated for their immunostaining pattern with a number of markers to establish the tissue of origin. The results indicated that one cell line exhibited a marker pattern indicating that this cell line is a malignant mesothelioma cell line, rather than a cell line from a pleural metastasis of a squamous carcinoma (36).

Recent investigations of malignant mesothelioma cell lines have revealed several characteristics that seem consistent features for malignant mesothelioma cell lines and might be useful for characterization of newly established cell lines. Eighteen human malignant mesothelioma cell lines express elevated levels of PDGF A- and B-chain mRNA, compared with 17 normal mesothelial cell lines (29,35). The PDGF $\beta$-receptor mRNA was found in all 12 investigated cell lines, suggesting an autocrine growth stimulation of PDGF-BB, acting through the PDGF $\beta$-receptor in malignant mesothelioma cells (30). Normal mesothelial cells express preponderantly PDGF $\alpha$-receptor mRNA (30). This consistent expression pattern of PDGF chain and receptor genes in normal and malignant mesothelial cell lines might be useful for characterization of newly established normal and malignant mesothelial cell lines. As the establishment of the diagnosis of malignant mesothelioma is still difficult, newly found characteristics of normal and malignant mesothelial cells must be evaluated for application in diagnostic procedures. Improvement of diagnosis of malignant mesothelioma on pleural effusion cells is especially important, as more invasive diagnostic procedures can then be avoided. The expression of PDGF and PDGF receptors in vivo and their diagnostic relevance is currently under investigation in our laboratory.

Normal mesothelial cell lines can be established easily, but are difficult to handle and characterize. However, in our opinion, the comparison of malignant mesothelioma cell lines with untransformed normal mesothelial cells is important for the application of an in vitro model to study the malignant transformation of mesothelial cells. Although transformed mesothelial cell lines are easier to culture than normal mesothelial cell lines, and these cells might represent an intermediate stage between normal and malignant cells, there are several indications that in vitro-transformed cells can exhibit features different from cultured normal mesothelial cells. This was illustrated by an observation on production of IL-6 by all seven investigated malignant mesothelioma cell lines. In contrast with the malignant mesothelioma cell lines, the SV40-transformed mesothelial cell line MeT5A did not secrete IL-6 (10). This observation led to speculations on aberrant IL-6 expression in malignant mesothelioma. However, recently IL-6 expression has also been found in all five investigated human peritoneal mesothelial cell lines (37).

Currently, in vitro model systems for malignant mesothelioma are mostly used for the study of the expression of growth factors and their receptors. These studies resulted in a variety of new characteristics of normal and malignant mesothelioma cells. The possibility of manipulating normal and malignant mesothelial cell lines by transfection with expression vectors of characteristic growth factors and growth factor receptors, is a great advantage of an in vitro model. In the near future, this approach will lead to more insight into the involvement of these growth factors in the malignant transformation of mesothelial cells.

Interesting are the studies using malignant mesothelioma cell lines as targets for immunotherapy. Malignant mesothelioma cell lines were resistant to natural killer cell lysis and susceptible to lysis by lymphokine-activated killer cells (38,39). Until now, an in vitro model of malignant mesothelioma has not been employed for the screening of newly developed drugs. After a primary screening in vitro, only the drugs that have been effective have to be tested in nude mice. Malignant mesothelioma cell lines that are tumorigenic in nude mice are especially valuable for this approach.

In conclusion, during the last decade, in vitro models for malignant mesothelioma have been developed and characterized extensively, but so far these studies have been rather descriptive. In the future, manipulation of in vitro growing cells will reveal the role of growth factors and their receptors in the malignant transformation of mesothelial cells. The possibilities for intervention in these processes will ultimately lead to new therapeutic approaches.

## Acknowledgments

We are grateful to professor Dr. R. Benner for his continuous support and Ms. P.A.J.M. de Laat, Dr. A.W. Langerak, Mrs. M.J. Bouts, Ms. E. Franken-Postma, and Mr. M. Delahaye for their advice and technical assistance. Mr. T.M. van Os is acknowledged for excellent photographic assistance and Ms. A.C. de Vries is acknowledged for typing the manuscript.

## References

1.  Versnel MA, Bouts MJ, Hoogsteden HC, van der Kwast TH, Delahaye M, Hagemeijer A. Establishment of human malignant mesothelioma cell lines. Int J Cancer 1989; 44:256–260.

2.  Behebani AM, Hunter WJ, Chapman AL, Lin F. Studies of human mesothelioma. Hum Pathol 1982; 13:862–866.
3.  Hsu S-M, Hsu P-L, Zhao X, Kao-Shan CS, Whang-Peng J. Establishment of human mesothelioma cell lines (MS-1, -2) and production of a monoclonal antibody (anti-MS) with diagnostic and therapeutic potential. Cancer Res 1988; 48:5228–5236.
4.  Klominek J, Robert K-H, Hjerpe A, Wickstrom B, Gahrton G. Serum-dependent growth patterns of two, newly established human mesothelioma cell lines. Cancer Res 1989; 49:6118–6122.
5.  Lauber B, Leuthold M, Schmitter D, Cano-Santos J, Waibel R, Stahel RA. An autocrine mitogenic activity produced by a pleural human mesothelioma cell line. Int J Cancer 1992; 50:943–950.
6.  Manning LS, Whitaker D, Murch AR, Garlepp MJ, Davis MR, Musk AW, Robinson BWS. Establishment and characterization of five human malignant mesothelioma cell lines derived from pleural effusions. Int J Cancer 1991; 47: 285–290.
7.  Masuda N, Fukuoka M, Takada M, Kudoh S, Kusunoki Y. Establishment and characterization of 20 human non-small cell lung cancer cell lines in a serum-free defined medium (ACL-4). Chest 1991; 100:429–438.
8.  Pelin-Enlund K, Husgafvel-Pursiainen K, Tammilehto L, Klockars M, Jantunen K, Gerwin BI, Harris CC, Tuomi T, Vanhala E, Mattson K, Linnainmaa K. Asbestos-related malignant mesothelioma: growth, cytology, tumorigenicity and consistent chromosome findings in cell lines from five patients. Carcinogenesis 1990; 11:673–681.
9.  Popescu NC, Chahinian AP, DiPaolo JA. Nonrandom chromosome alterations in human malignant mesothelioma. Cancer Res 1988; 48:142–147.
10. Schmitter D, Lauber B, Fagg B, Stahel RA. Hematopoietic growth factors secreted by seven human pleural mesothelioma cell lines: interleukin-6 production as a common feature. Int J Cancer 1992; 51:296–301.
11. Shanfang W, Enzhong W, Jianzhong S, Huixuan X, Zhenqiong L, Gifu S, Changwen X, Ruiming C, Xuizhen Y, Dehou Z, Zhenghong Y. Establishment and characterization of human malignant pleural mesothelioma cell line SMC-1. Sci Sin 1985; 28:281–286.
12. Versnel MA, Hoogsteden HC, Hagemeijer A, Bouts MJ, van der Kwast TH, Delahaye M, Schaart G, Ramaekers FCS. Characterization of three human malignant mesothelioma cell lines. Cancer Genet Cytogenet 1989; 42:115–128.
13. Lechner JF, Tokiwa T, La Veck M, Benedict WF, Banks-Schlegel S, Yeager H, Banerjee A, Harris CC. Asbestos-associated chromosomal changes in human mesothelial cells. Proc Natl Acad Sci USA 1985; 82:3884–3888.
14. La Veck MA, Somers ANA, Moore LL, Gerwin BI, Lechner JF. Dissimilar peptide growth factors can induce normal human mesothelial cell multiplication. In Vitro Cell Dev Biol 1988; 24:1077–1084.
15. Stylianou E, Jenner LA, Davies MD, Coles GA, Williams JD. Isolation, culture and characterization of human peritoneal mesothelial cells. Kidney Int 1990; 31:1563–1570.
16. Hinsbergh VWM, Kooistra T, Scheffer MA, van Bockel JH, van Muijen

GNP. Characterization and fibrinolytic properties of human omental tissue mesothelial cells. Comparison with endothelial cells. Blood 1990; 75:1490–1497.

17. Connell ND, Rheinwald JG. Regulation of the cytoskeleton in mesothelial cells: reversible loss of keratin and increase in vimentin during rapid growth in culture. Cell 1983; 34:245–253.

18. Gabrielson EW, Gerwin BI, Harris CC, Roberts AB, Sporn MB, Lechner JF. Stimulation of DNA synthesis in cultured primary human mesothelial cells by specific growth factors. FASEB J 1988; 2:2717–2721.

19. Lechner JF, La Veck MA, Gerwin BI, Matis EA. Differential responses to growth factors by normal human mesothelial cultures from individual donors. J Cell Physiol 1989; 139:295–300.

20. Kim KH, Stellmach V, Javors J, Fuchs E. Regulation of human mesothelial cell differentiation: opposing roles of retinoids and epidermal growth factor in the expression of intermediate filament proteins. J Cell Biol 1987; 105: 3039–3051.

21. Ke Y, Reddel RR, Gerwin BI, Reddel HK, Somers ANA, McMenamin MG, La Veck MA, Stahel RA, Lechner JF, Harris CC. Establishment of a human in vitro mesothelial cell model system for investigating mechanisms of asbestos-induced mesothelioma. AM J Pathol 1989; 134:979–991.

22. LaRocca PJ, Rheinwald JG. Coexpression of simple epithelial keratins and vimentin by human mesothelium and mesothelioma in vivo and in culture. Cancer Res 1984; 44:2991–2999.

23. Ramaekers FCS, Haag D, Kant A, Moesker O, Jap PHK, Vooijs GP. Coexpression of keratin- and vimentin-type intermediate filaments in human metastatic carcinoma cells. Proc Natl Acad Sci USA 1983; 80:2618–2622.

24. Blobel GA, Moll R, Franke WF, Kayser KW, Gould VE. The intermediate filament cytoskeleton of malignant mesotheliomas and its diagnostic significance. Am J Pathol 1985; 121:235–247.

25. Moll R, Dhouailly D, Sun T-T. Expression of keratin 5 as a distinctive feature of epithelial and biphasic mesotheliomas. Virchows Archiv [B] 1989; 58:129–145.

26. van der Kwast TH, Versnel MA, Delahaye M, de Jong A, Zondervan PE, Hoogsteden H. Expression of epithelial membrane antigen on malignant mesothelioma cells. Acta Cytol 1988; 32:169–174.

27. Stahel RA, O'Hara CJ, Waibel R, Martin A. Monoclonal antibodies against mesothelial membrane antigen discriminate between malignant mesothelioma and lung adenocarcinoma. Int J Cancer 1988; 41:218–223.

28. Hagemeijer A, Versnel MA, van Drunen E, Bouts MJ, van der Kwast TH, Hoogsteden HC. Cytogenetic analysis of malignant mesothelioma. Cancer Genet Cytogenet 1990; 47:1–28.

29. Versnel MA, Hagemeijer A, Bouts MJ, van der Kwast TH, Hoogsteden HC. Expression of c-sis (PDGF B-chain) and PDGF A-chain genes in ten human malignant mesothelioma cell lines derived from primary and metastatic tumors. Oncogene 1988; 2:601–605.

30. Versnel MA, Claesson-Welsh L, Hammacher A, Bouts MJ, van der Kwast

TH, Eriksson A, Willemsen R, Weima SM, Hoogsteden HC, Hagemeijer A, Heldin C-H. Human malignant mesothelioma cell lines express PDGF β-receptors whereas cultured normal mesothelial cells express predominantly PDGF α-receptors. Oncogene 1991; 6:2005–2011.

31. Tubo RA, Rheinwald JG. Normal human mesothelial cells and fibroblasts transfected with the EJ-*ras* oncogene become EGF-independent, but are not malignantly transformed. Oncogene Res 1987; 1:407–421.

32. Reddel RR, Malan-Shibley L, Gerwin BI, Metcalf RA, Harris CC. Tumorigenicity of human mesothelial cell line transfected with EJ-*ras* oncogene. JNCI 1989; 81:945–948.

33. Wang J-L, Nister M, Ponten J, Westermark B. Suppression of PDGF alpha and beta receptor mRNA expression by SV40 T/t antigen. J Cell Biochem 1992; 166.

34. Langerak AW, Vietsch H, Bouts MJ, Hagemeijer A, Versnel MA. A spontaneously in vitro transformed mesothelial cell line has a similar pattern of PDGF chain and PDGF receptor expression to malignant mesothelioma cell lines. Eur Respir Rev 1994; 3:170–174.

35. Gerwin BI, Lechner JF, Reddel RR, Roberts AB, Robbins KC, Gabrielson EW, Harris CC. Comparison of production of transforming growth factor-β and platelet-derived growth factor by normal human mesothelial cells and mesothelioma cell lines. Cancer Res 1987; 47:6180–6184.

36. Daniel MR, Burnett HE. Immunocytochemical investigation of the tissue of origin of two lung cancer cell lines. Int J Exp Pathol 1991; 72:397–405.

37. Lanfrancone L, Boraschi D, Ghiara P, Falini B, Grignani F, Peri G, Mantovani A, Pelicci PG. Human peritoneal mesothelial cells produce many cytokines (G-CSF; GM-CSF; IL-1; IL-6) and are activated and stimulated to grow by IL-1. Blood 1992; 11:2835–2842.

38. Manning LS, Bowman RV, Darby SB, Robinson BWS. Lysis of human malignant mesothelioma cells by natural killer (NK) and lymphokine-activated killer (LAK) cells. Am Rev Respir Dis 1989; 139: 1369–1374.

39. Manning LS, Bowman RV, Davis MR, Musk AW, Robinson BWS. Indomethacin augments lymphokine-activated killer cell generation by patients with malignant mesothelioma. Clin Immunol Immunopathol 1989; 53:68–77.

# 10

## Experimental and Spontaneous Mesotheliomas

**JOHN M. G. DAVIS**

Institute of Occupational Medicine
Edinburgh, Scotland

## I. Introduction

Mesotheliomas, tumors developing from the cells lining the pleural or peritoneal cavities, have been known for over 200 years, being reported by Lieutaad in 1767, according to Wolff (1), and a detailed description of such tumors was published by Laenec (2). Mesotheliomas were always considered extremely rare tumors, however, and some pathologists believe that those described were, in fact, secondary deposits of unrecognized primary tumors from other sites, and this view was still expressed as late as the 1960s (3,4). They were considered as of little real importance until Wagner, in 1960 (5), reported that industrial exposure to blue asbestos or crocidolite was associated with a relatively high incidence of mesotheliomas in the South African mining areas, and studies in all parts of the world rapidly confirmed that the industrial use of at least the amphibole asbestos types was causally associated with the accounts of mesotheliomas in asbestos workers.

Mesotheliomas are still rare tumors in humans, with numbers reported being a matter of a few hundreds each year worldwide. However, their association with an industrial exposure has given them great prominence. This has been enhanced by one characteristic of the mesothelioma: namely, the induction period between first exposure to asbestos and tumor development is usually extremely long, often up to 40 years. Thus, although extremely strict controls of fiber levels in asbestos mines and factories have now been enforced for some time in most countries and, indeed, the industrial use of asbestos has greatly diminished, mesotheliomas from past exposures are still occurring and will continue to do so for at least another decade. Since 1960, the association of mesotheliomas with what used to be an extremely important industry has resulted in much study of the condition clinically, epidemiologically, and experimentally, but even today, there are many aspects of mesothelioma development that are not understood.

## II. Experimental Studies of Mesotheliomas

For the study of any disease, it is important to duplicate the condition in experimental animals so that experimental manipulation is possible. Following his discovery of the association between asbestos exposure and mesotheliomas in 1960 (5), Wagner quickly achieved this, reporting in 1962 (6) that rats would develop pleural mesotheliomas if asbestos dust was injected directly into the pleural cavities. This technique is artificial, in that it bypasses many of the body's defense mechanisms, since asbestos fibers are normally inhaled and must survive in the lung tissue long enough to be moved to the pleura if they are to affect the mesothelial tissues. In 1974, Wagner (7) reported that rats could indeed develop mesotheliomas following asbestos inhalation and, since then, baboons and hamsters have also produced mesotheliomas in experimental inhalation studies (8–10). Apart from rats, rabbits, hamsters, and mice have produced mesotheliomas following the injection of asbestos or other mineral fibers (11–13).

Both pleural and peritoneal mesotheliomas in humans have structural characteristics that set them apart from other tumors, in that they frequently contain highly variable histological features, with cells and cellular growth patterns characteristic of both epithelial and connective tissues. Some mesotheliomas show the histological patterns of sarcomas, whereas, in others, cells of the epithelial type may form papillary or tubulopapillary patterns (14,15). Examination of human mesotheliomas by transmission electron microscopy (TEM) has demonstrated that the epithelial-type cells from mesotheliomas have two particular characteristics. Frequently, the outer membranes of these cells are covered with unusually long cylindrical microvilli and, also, the cells often contain intracytoplasmic vacuoles lined with similar microvilli. Connective tissue elements of human mesotheliomas have cells with extremely well-developed and active granular endoplasmic reticulium, and on their surface membranes, there are extremely long and irregularly shaped processes stretching away among the connective tissue fibers for as much as 10–15 $\mu$m in any direction (16–20). These characteristics are closely matched by mesotheliomas produced in experimental animals both by the inhalation and injection of asbestos and as seen both by normal light microscope examination of histological sections (7,12,21–25).

Davis examined the early stages of development of both pleural and peritoneal mesotheliomas in the rat following the injection of crocidolite (23,24). For peritoneal mesotheliomas, the earliest discernible neoplastic stage consisted of many small pedunculated nodules scattered over the surfaces of the viscera, diaphragm, and body wall. These nodules contained a central core of reticulin or collagen, surrounded by layers of pleomorphic connective tissue cells. The surfaces of the nodules were covered by a single layer of epithelial cells, similar to normal mesothelium. In later stages, some nodules remained distinct and increased in size (Fig. 1), but often the tumor spread over the peritoneal surfaces as a uniform sheet. The cells found in sheets were mostly the same type as those in large nodules: pleo-

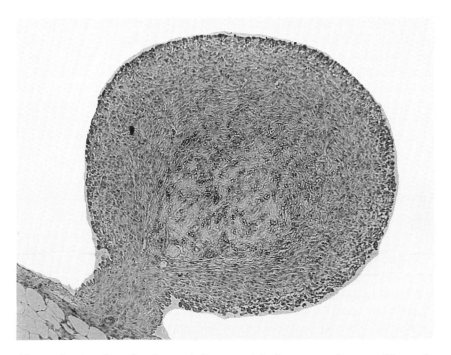

**Figure 1** A pedunculated mesothelioma nodule from rat peritoneum 18 months after the injection of crocidolite. Magnification × 50. (From Ref. 23.)

morphic connective tissue cells in the central regions and epithelial cells on the surface. In some advanced tumors, however, the cells had a spindle-cell pattern, similar to a fibroma or fibrosarcoma. In this form the neoplasms were locally invasive.

Electron microscopic examination of the smallest nodules showed that the single layer of cells on the surface appeared to be normal mesothelial cells, although they were more rounded than usual. These cells had the characteristic elongated microvilli of normal mesothelium on their free surfaces, but on their lower surfaces were only occasional irregular cytoplasmic projections. The cell cytoplasm contained many short lengths of granular endoplasmic reticulum, which were often dilated and filled with amorphous material. The mesothelial cells were firmly attached to one another with membrane tight junctions, and occasional desmosomes, but they were not associated with a basement membrane. Below the mesothelial layer, the cells were unevenly arranged in a thin network of reticulin or collagen. They were more irregularly shaped and showed many cytoplasmic projections on their surface membranes. These projections were similar to the phagocytic processes of macrophages and, in their simplest form, had a diameter of 1000 A. The cytoplasm of the submesothelial cells always contained much granular endoplasmic reticulum, with the sacs sometimes dilated and filled with amorphous material (Fig. 2). Toward the center of the older tumor nodules, the collagen and reticulin network became more dense and the cells more flattened. They still retained their well-differentiated endoplasmic reticulum, but the number of complex surface processes was reduced. As the nodules enlarged, the distinct surface layer of normal mesothelial cells was lost, and the surfaces of the nodules consisted of layers of loose, rounded cells, with a structure intermediate between normal mesothelial cells and the deeper-lying tumor cells. At this stage, the surface cells often contained intracellular cysts lined by elongated microvilli, similar to those on the outer cell membranes.

Mesotheliomas developing in rats as the result of intrapleural injections of fibers also demonstrated a biphasic pattern and were similar to peritoneal mesotheliomas in that some areas were sarcomatous (Fig. 3). They differed, however, in more frequently having the epithelial element of the tumors preponderant. Some tumors were papillomatous, consisting mainly of columns of cells of epithelial type, whereas others showed a cystic pattern, with large spaces supported by a loose connective tissue. These spaces were lined by extremely extended epithelial-type cells. The cells forming the main papillomatous areas were large and rounded with numerous elongated microvilli on their surfaces and were closely attached to one another by desmosomes (Fig. 4). These cells frequently contained internal spaces lined by microvilli similar to those on the cell surfaces (Fig. 5).

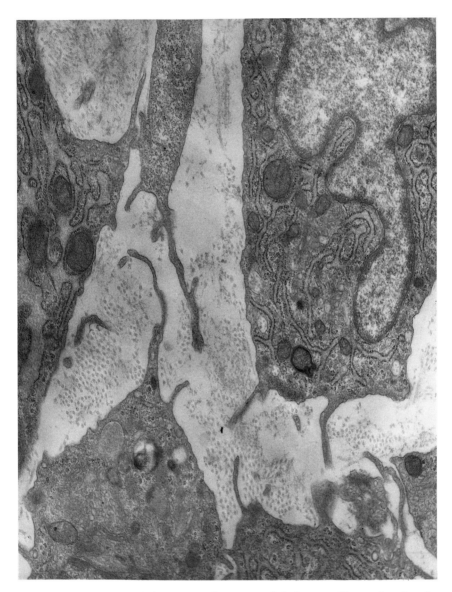

**Figure 2**   Areas of cells from a small tumor nodule in a rat 10 months after the injection of crocidolite asbestos. Cells are of connective tissue type and surface membranes are modified to form long cytoplasmic processes. A network of collagen or reticulin fibers is present between the cells. Magnification × 15,000.

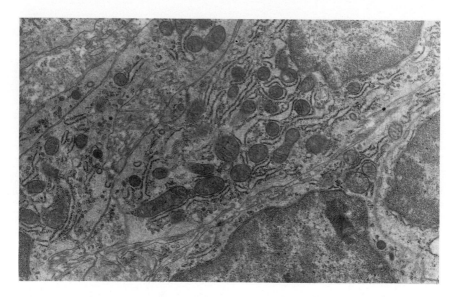

**Figure 3** A group of closely packed spindle-shaped cells from a rat pleural meso-thelioma. No surface processes are present on the cell membranes, although the cells are separated in some places by small amounts of collagen or reticulin fibers. Magnification × 12,000. (From Ref. 24.)

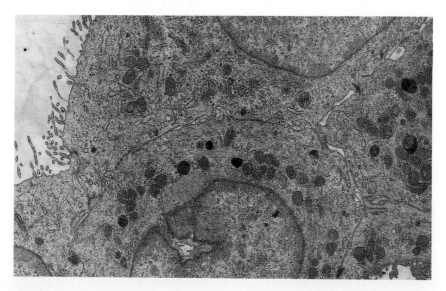

**Figure 4** Rounded cells from a papillomatous mesothelioma in a rat. A few micro-villi are present between the closely packed cells, but these processes are numerous on free cell surfaces and lining intracellular spaces. Magnification × 7500. (From Ref. 24.)

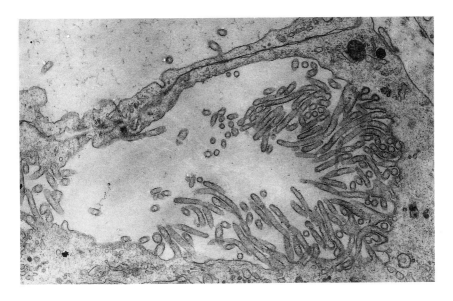

**Figure 5** Intracellular spaces within the cytoplasm of two mesothelioma cells. In some areas the cytoplasm lining the spaces is thick and contains normal cell organelles. In other areas it forms a layer with a depth of only about 0.2 μm. Magnification × 12,000. (From Ref. 24.)

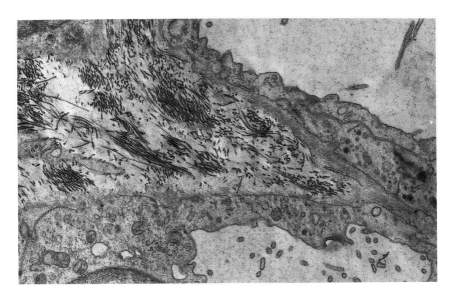

**Figure 6** Tissue spaces in a rat mesothelioma. In this instance the cells lining spaces are supported by collagen and reticulin fibers which are surfaced by basement membrane material. Magnification × 10,000. (From Ref. 24.)

Cystic areas usually had the tissue spaces supported by loose connective tissue, and the flattened mesothelial cells lining the spaces were separated from the connective tissue fibers by a clear basement membrane (Fig. 6). In some sites, however, the cystic structure had no obvious support, and spaces were separated from one another merely by two layers of extended mesothelial cell cytoplasm, with no obvious basement membrane between them (Fig. 7).

Experimental mesotheliomas produced by injection of fibers are artificial, but those mesotheliomas that develop in rats following dust inhalation do show the same variations in histological structure. At autopsy, the visceral and parietal pleural surfaces may be fused to one another by tumor masses or, alternatively, small tumor deposits may be scattered over both surfaces (Fig. 8). The histological pattern of these mesotheliomas may be papillomatous, with columns of cells of epithelial type supported by loose connective tissue (Fig. 9); they may show sarcomatous areas, or tumor masses may contain cystic spaces lined by flattened cells (Fig. 10). In some cases, all of these patterns may be found in one small area of tumor (Fig. 11).

There are many points concerning the development of mesotheliomas that still remain uncertain, even after many years of study and experimentation. It is believed that asbestos fibers inhaled and deposited in the pulmo-

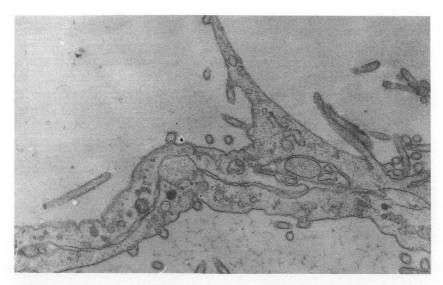

**Figure 7**  Intracellular spaces within the cytoplasm of rat mesothelioma cells. The two upper spaces are within the same cell and separated by a cytoplasmic layer only 0.1 μm thick. Magnification × 21,000. (From Ref. 24.)

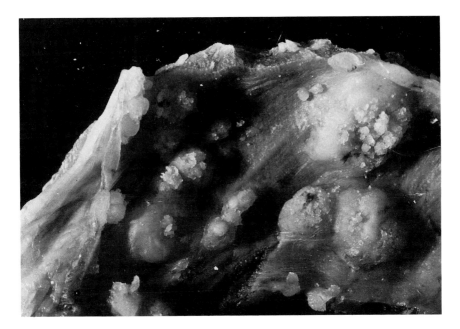

**Figure 8** Macroscopic photograph of the external wall of a rat thoracic cavity. This animal had inhaled amosite asbestos and developed a pleural mesothelioma. Tumor nodules are scattered over the parietal pleural surface. Magnification × 15.

nary parenchyma must be moved at least to the area of the visceral pleura to affect the mesothelial cells, but whether or not they have to penetrate the pleural surface remains uncertain. There have been suggestions that the buildup of fibers immediately beneath the pleural surfaces might cause a chronic inflammatory response, characterized by the release of growth factors from cells, such as macrophages, that could diffuse across the pleura and to which mesothelial cells might be particularly susceptible (26). Much asbestos dust is certainly removed from the lung parenchyma by the lymphatic channels, and the pulmonary-associated lymph nodes can become heavily laden. Some fibers obviously penetrate much farther than the first major lymph node they reach. Many human mesotheliomas appear to develop on the parietal pleural surface, and Jones (27) suggested that this results from fibers being "milked around the subpleural lymphatics until they reach a point of stasis." It must be assumed that peritoneal mesotheliomas result from transport of fibers from the lungs to some site within the peritoneal cavity, and lymphatic transport appears the most likely mechanism for this occurrence. In general, however, fiber transport from the

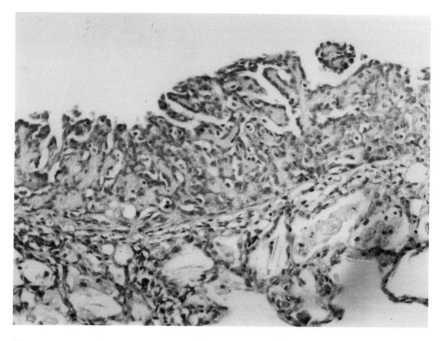

**Figure 9**   Mesothelioma growing on the visceral pleural surface of a rat treated with chrysotile and quartz by inhalation. The tumor exhibits a tubulopapillary pattern. Magnification × 200. (From Ref. 21.)

lung has been inadequately researched in experimental studies; it is even uncertain whether or not the process is sufficiently similar in all species to extrapolate results obtained to the human situation. Rats have produced mesotheliomas in most experimental inhalation studies so far published, but the proportion of animals affected has always been small in spite of dose levels often as high as several thousand fibers per milliliter or air (Table 1). It may be considered that this pattern repeats the human situation in which mesothelioma proportions in populations of asbestos workers have seldom been higher. Recent studies using hamsters, however, have reported 35% of pleural mesotheliomas following the inhalation of thin ceramic fibers at dose levels of 200 fibers per milliliter (10). This observation needs to be supported by studies using other fiber types, but might indicate that the hamster would be a more useful experimental model for mesothelioma studies than the rat. Rats have, however, produced mesotheliomas in almost 100% of animals inhaling erionite fibers, which are also unusually carcinogenic to humans (28,29), but this may indicate that erio-

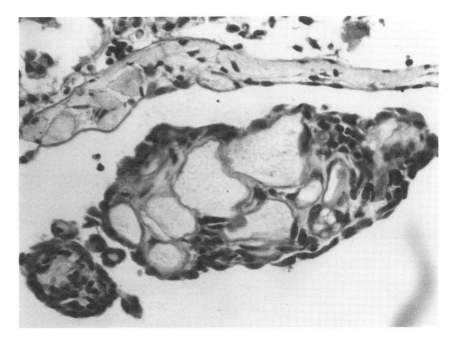

**Figure 10**   An area of mesothelioma within the pleural cavity of a rat with chrysotile and quartz. Spaces within the tumor are lined with flattened "mesothelial" cells but the cells at the surface of the tumor are rounded. Magnification × 400. (From Ref. 21.)

nite produces mesotheliomas by a somewhat different process than chrysotile and amphibole fibers and, moreover, its carcinogenicity to hamsters has not been tested. High incidence of mesotheliomas in hamsters could be because these animals transfer fibers more effectively to their pleural surfaces than do rats, or merely that hamster mesothelial cells are more susceptible to transformation. Davis (26) reported that rats inhaling large doses of pure asbestos fibers often have dense subpleural deposits of fiber just within the external elastic lamina of the lung, but that fibers cannot be found actually penetrating the pleural surface. However, the presence of some types of particulate dusts in the rat lung at the same time as asbestos fibers can aid pleural penetration. It had been noted that, in rat inhalation studies using coal mine dusts containing high levels of quartz, granulomas containing both quartz and coal dust particles developed on the visceral pleural surface (26). In addition, more quartz particles of coal mine dusts were preferentially transported to the lymphatics of rats than were other dust components (30). It had seemed likely that quartz penetrating the

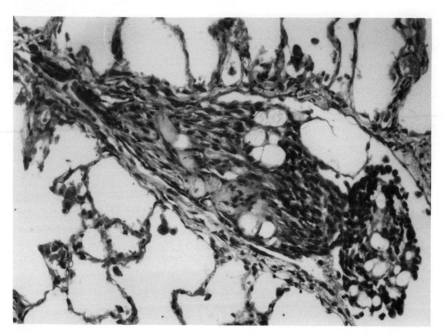

**Figure 11**  Pleural mesothelioma growing in a fissure between two pulmonary lobes. Much of this tumor consists of spaces line by flattened type, but on the surface, cells are rounded and of epithelial pattern. Magnification × 200. (From Ref. 21.)

visceral pleural surface also facilitated the transport of coal and other particulate minerals so that mixed granulomas resulted, and studies using mixtures of asbestos and quartz were undertaken to see if the phenomenon applied to all dust types. These rat inhalation studies did result in granulomas containing quartz and asbestos fibers on their visceral pleural surface, and the study reported the highest proportion of mesotheliomas in this species of any study using the main varieties of asbestos (21). In view of the recent findings with ceramic fibers, the pleural penetration of fibers in hamsters needs to be examined; and the possible existence of a "quartz effect" determined. One human epidemiological study does suggest that the presence of quartz in the lung could affect mesothelioma development in humans. Finkelstein (31) reported 10 cases of mesothelioma within a group of only 328 workers in the asbestos cement industry, and this is an unusually high figure for any type of asbestos exposure. The asbestos used was mainly chrysotile, with a small amount of crocidolite, but in addition to asbestos and cement, the mix for pipemaking was recorded as involving the

**Table 1** Proportions of Rats Developing Mesotheliomas in Rat Inhalation Studies Using Asbestos Dose 10 mg/m³ of Respirable Dust Administered for 12 Months

| Ref. | Dust | Mesotheliomas |
|------|------|---------------|
| 7 | Amosite (UICC) | 0/24 |
|   | Anthophyllite (UICC) | 1/28 |
|   | Crocidolite (UICC) | 2/26 |
|   | Chrysotile (Canadian UICC) | 3/23 |
|   | Chrysotile (Rhodesian UICC) | 0/27 |
| 65 | Chrysotile (SFA) | 0/22 |
|   | Chrysotile (grade 7) | 0/24 |
|   | Chrysotile (UICC) | 0/23 |
| 66 | Chrysotile (Rhodesian UICC) | 0/40 |
|   | Amosite (UICC) | 0/43 |
|   | Crocidolite (UICC) | 0/40 |
| 67 | Tremolite | 2/39 |
| 38 | Amosite | 3/40 |
| 39 | Chrysotile (Canadian) | 3/40 |

addition of "silica." The necessity of transporting fiber from the pulmonary parenchyma to the pleural surfaces and beyond for mesothelioma development may have resulted in one important curiosity with these tumors. Doll and Peto (32) have pointed out that, in asbestos-exposed workers, there does not appear to be an age effect for mesothelioma development, in contrast with other types of human tumors. However, Berry and Wagner (33) demonstrated that rats injected with asbestos in middle age developed mesotheliomas more rapidly than did those injected while young. Berry and Wagner's results, obtained by implanting dust directly into the pleural cavity, suggested that the lack of a clear age effect in humans may well be due to the very variable transport of dust from lung parenchyma to pleura. Once fibers have accumulated in the pleural tissues, it does appear that mesothelioma development shows a clear age effect, at least in the rat.

The small number of mesotheliomas occurring in most experimental inhalation studies with rats have precluded the use of this experimental system for examining which characteristics of a fiber sample are most potent in mesothelioma development, and the artificial injection of dust directly into the pleural or peritoneal cavities has been used instead. With this system, by using high dust doses rats can develop pleural mesotheliomas in up to 60% of animals and peritoneal mesotheliomas in almost 100%.

The most important information to result from injection studies has been the relation between fiber geometry and tumorigenicity. Work in two laboratories demonstrated that long, thin fibers were the most carcinogenic with the best correlation with mesothelioma development being found with a number of fibers longer than 8 $\mu$m and smaller than 0.25 $\mu$m in diameter (34–37). Unfortunately, an exact determination of the effect of fiber length on mesothelioma production has yet to be made because of the limitations of the dust samples available for experimentation. Most fibrous dust samples are a mixture of all fiber lengths, with even highly carcinogenic asbestos samples having over 95% of fibers shorter than 5 $\mu$m. Certainly, very short asbestos fibers have little or no carcinogenic potential (38,39), but crucial issues remaining to be solved are whether carcinogenic potential increases at all above 8 $\mu$m in length and whether or not there is gradual and regular reduction below this figure. It may be that all fibers have some limited potency or, alternatively, there could be a threshold length below which there is no potential at all to initiate mesothelioma development. The clarification of these important questions will require the production of a series of fiber specimens of different lengths, with little variation between the individual fibers. This has not yet proved possible.

Injection studies have also been used to demonstrate that mesothelioma production is closely related to dose for any fiber sample considered. Both intrapleural and intraperitoneal injection studies have demonstrated a clear dose–response for several asbestos types (36,40–42). The intraperitoneal model particularly is very sensitive, with high dose producing tumors in almost 100% of animals. Lower doses produced progressively fewer tumors, but the tumor induction period becomes progressively longer. Most studies have used doses estimated by mass, but we have demonstrated (42) that where comparisons between the dose–response for different dust types are concerned, doses injected should be matched for numbers of long, thin fibers. When considered by mass, crocidolite, amosite, chrysotile, and erionite showed similarly shaped, but widely separated, dose–responses. When considered by fiber number, however, crocidolite, amosite, and chrysotile showed a very similar response, with only erionite appearing significantly more carcinogenic at any fiber number, a fact that matches the known extreme carcinogenic potency of this material (28,29). Experimental studies have as yet been unable to answer the question of whether there is a threshold dose of any fiber type below which mesotheliomas will not occur. We found no mesotheliomas with any dust for doses of fewer than 150,000 fibers longer than 8 $\mu$m (42). With groups of only 50 rats, however, the possibility of an occasional mesothelioma at doses lower than this could not be excluded. Demonstration of whether or not there is a threshold for mesothelioma development will probably have to wait for experimental studies that can elucidate the actual mechanisms of carcinogenesis involved.

The experimental studies, and particularly injection studies, that have produced controversial data on mesothelioma development concern the carcinogenic potency of different mineral types. This is most probably because experimental studies are unable to reproduce the effects of "fiber durability" in human lungs. To produce disease, it is believed that fibers must accumulate in the pulmonary tissues until a dangerous level is reached. However, after deposition, many inhaled fibers are cleared by the phagocytic ability of pulmonary macrophages and, in addition, some fibers will undergo chemical dissolution, which may result in their complete disappearance, or result in their fracture to shorter and less harmful material (43). For mesothelioma production, fibers must survive long enough in the lung to be transported to pleural or peritoneal sites where they can accumulate and cause cell transformation. Lack of correlation between experimental studies and human information results because fiber dissolution is mainly a chemical process and will occur at similar speeds in all species, whereas tumor production is a factor of the species lifespan. Two years is sufficient to produce a mesothelioma in a rat, but 20 years or more is usually required in a human. Thus, a fiber with a tissue survival time of 2 years would be highly carcinogenic in rats and have no significant carcinogenic potential in the human species. With mesothelioma production, the best example of this so far demonstrated is chrysotile asbestos. Chrysotile has a relatively low durability in lung tissue (26,44) and, in humans, only a very few mesotheliomas have been reported from supposedly pure chrysotile exposure. These studies, from the Canadian chrysotile mining industry are now considered by many to be due to the contamination of the chrysotile ore bodies with tremolite, which is an amphibole fiber with durability similar to crocidolite. No mesotheliomas have yet been reported from the chrysotile mines in southern Africa, which are reported to be free of tremolite. In experimental inhalation and injection studies, however, chrysotile has repeatedly produced as many mesotheliomas as other asbestos types. This finding probably indicates that the carcinogenic potential of chrysotile to cells is as high as the other asbestos types, and it is just sufficiently durable to exert its maximum effect in rats, although it is unable to survive long enough to do so in humans.

Although experimental inhalation studies in short-lived rodent species allowed little time for fiber dissolution, injection studies have the added disadvantage that they largely eliminate macrophage clearance. Moreover, even tissue dissolution may be much less than in the lung, since fibers deposited as a massive bolus largely remain closely packed and not dispersed as they are in lung tissue following deposition after inhalation. It is not surprising, therefore, that in injection studies, almost all long, thin fibers tested have produced large numbers of mesotheliomas. Care must be taken not to assume that this automatically indicates a human hazard from any material, and even the relatively short-term animal inhalation studies can often be used to eliminate this possibility. This situation has arisen with many man-made mineral fibers, particularly those of fine glass. These will regularly produce mesotheliomas following injection in rats (34,37), yet appear to have no carcinogenic potential following inhalation by the same species (45–48). Where both injection and inhalation studies in animals produce mesotheliomas, as with some ceramic fibers (10,49), there is greater need for concern, and data will be needed on the durability of these materials over 20 years in human lungs before the human hazard can be accurately predicted.

## III.  Spontaneous Mesotheliomas

Although asbestos is obviously a major cause of mesothelioma development in humans, most series of cases reported in the literature contain a significant proportion, perhaps 30%, for whom no exposure to asbestos can be traced. Some of these are likely to be due to other extraneous agents, but some will result from spontaneous neoplastic transformation of mesothelial cells, as occurs with all tumor types, both in humans and in animal species (50).

Among nonfibrous agents believed to have caused mesotheliomas in humans are petrochemicals (51), copper and nickel (52), beryllium (53), radiation (54), and even infectious agents that result in chronic inflammation (55,56). Similarly, many nonfibrous agents have produced mesotheliomas when administered to experimental animals, such as ethylene oxide (57), aluminum (58), cadmium, ferric oxide and nickel (59), polymers (60), hormones (61), many hydrocarbons, and even viruses (62).

In experimental studies, extraneous agents, other than that under test, can be excluded, but spontaneous mesotheliomas can be of great importance, especially when response rates are low. Spontaneous mesotheliomas have been reported in several animal species, but particularly in seven different strains of laboratory rat (50), and they have been present in the control groups of all major studies utilizing asbestos or other mineral fibers, and different authors have suggested different response levels for accepting the study as positive. Over many experiments undertaken in Stanton's laboratory (36,58,63), it was reported that spontaneous pleural mesotheliomas were found in 4–5% of untreated controls and animals subjected to pleurectomy alone, and it was considered that a 30% response to any implanted material was necessary for a study to be considered positive. However, Wagner et al. (64) reported that, in their laboratory, spontaneous mesotheliomas in rats rarely exceeded 2% and considered that a response of over 10% with any material was "cause for concern." Pott has found the highest proportion of spontaneous mesotheliomas in rats often as high as 10% of animals (59).

This regular occurrence of spontaneous mesotheliomas has to be taken into account when examining the results of all animal experiments. The use of high test doses and careful analysis of differences in tumor numbers between control and test populations can eliminate error when a study is undertaken simply to demonstrate a possible hazard from any material. However, the occurrence of significant numbers of spontaneous mesotheliomas in such species as the rat makes it extremely difficult to satisfactorily examine the effects of very low doses of all but the most potent of materials or the existence of a safety threshold below which mesotheliomas will not be caused. It is doubtful if any species has a rate of spontaneous mesotheliomas low enough for this problem to be properly examined, and this includes humans.

### Acknowledgments

The author would like to thank the editors of the *Journal of the National Cancer Institute*, the *British Journal of Experimental Pathology*, and the *International Journal of Experimental Pathology* for permission to reproduce illustrations originally published in their journals.

### References

1. Wolff A. Lehre Krebskrank 1911; 2:834.
2. Laennec RTH. Traitè de l'auscultation Mediate 1819; 2:368.
3. Robertson HE. J Cancer Res 1924; 8:317–375.
4. Willis RA. The pathology of tumours, 4th ed. London: Butterworths, 1967.
5. Wagner JC, Sleggs CA, Marchand P. Br J Ind Med 1960; 17:260.
6. Wagner JC. Nature 1962; 196:180.
7. Wagner JC, Berry G, Skidmore JW, Timbrell V. Br J Cancer 1974; 29:252.
8. Goldstein B, Webster I, Rendall REG. Biological effects of man-made mineral fibres. Proceedings of a WHO/IARC conference. Copenhagen: World Health Organization, 1984: 273.
9. Smith DM, Oritz LW, Archuleta RF, Johnson NF. Ann Occup Hyg 1987; 31: 731.
10. Hesterberg TW, Mast R, McConnell EE, Chevalier J, Bernstein DM, Burn WB, Anderson R. Chronic inhalation toxicity of refractory ceramic fibers in Syrian hamsters. In: Brown RC, Hoskins JA, Johnson NF, eds. Mechanisms of fiber carcinogenesis. NATO ASI Ser. [A] 1992; 223:519–539.
11. Reeves AL, Puro HE, Smith RG, Vorwald AJ. Environ Res 1971; 4:496.
12. Smith WE, Miller L, Elsasser RE, Hubert DD. Tests for carcinogenicity of asbestos. Ann NY Acad Sci 1965; 132:456.

13. Pott F, Friedrichs KH, Huth F. Ergebnisse aus Tierversuchen zur Kanzerogenen Wirkung faserformiger Staube und ihre Deutung im Hinblick auf die Tumorentstehung beim Menschen. Zentralbl Bakteriol Parasitenkde Infecionskr Hyg 1976; 162:467–505.
14. McCaughey WTE. Ann NY Acad Sci 1965; 132:603.
15. Churg J, Rosen SH, Moolten S. Ann NY Acad Sci. 1965; 132:614.
16. Stoebner P, Miech G, Sengel A. Notions d'ultrastructure pleurale les mesotheliomas. Presse Med 1970; 24:1403–1408.
17. Kay S, Silverberg SG. Ultrastructural studies of a malignant fibrous mesothelioma of the pleura. Arch Pathol 1971; 92:449–455.
18. Wang NS. Electron microscopy in the diagnosis of pleural mesotheliomas. Cancer 1973; 31:1046–1054.
19. Suzuki Y, Kannerstein M, Churg J. Electron microscopy of normal, hyperplastic and neoplastic mesothelium. In: Bogovski P, ed. Biological effects of asbestos. IARC Sci Publ 8: 1973; 74–80.
20. Davis JMG. JNCI 1974; 52:1715.
21. Davis JMG, Jones AD, Miller BG. Experimental studies in rats on the effects of asbestos inhalation coupled with the inhalation of titanium dioxide or quartz. Int J Exp Pathol 1991; 72:501–525.
22. Shin MD, Firminger MD. Acute and chronic effects of intraperitoneal injection of two types of asbestos in rats with a study of histopathogenesis and ultrastructure of resulting mesotheliomas. Am J Pathol 1973; 70:291–307.
23. Davis JMG. JNCI 1974; 52:1823.
24. Davis JMG. The histopathology and ultrastructure of pleural mesotheliomas produced in the rat by injections of crocidolite asbestos. Br J Exp Pathol 1979; 60:642.
25. Suzuki Y, Kohyama N. Malignant mesothelioma induced by asbestos and zeolite in the mouse peritoneal cavity. Environ Res 1984; 35:277.
26. Davis JMG. Mineral fibre carcinogenesis: experimental data relating to the importance of fibre type, size, deposition, dissolution and migration. In: Bignon J, Peto J, Saracci R, eds. Nonoccupational exposure to mineral fibres. IARC Publ 1989; 90:33–46.
27. Jones JSP. Pathology of the mesothelium. New York: Springer-Verlag, 1987: 123.
28. Wagner JC, Skidmore JW, Hill RJ, Griffiths DM. Erionite exposure and mesothelioma in rats. Br J Cancer 1985; 51:727.
29. Baris YI, Artvinli M, Sahin AA. Ann NY Acad Sci 1979; 330:423.
30. Vincent JH, Jones AD, Johnston AM, McMillan C, Bolton RE, Cowie H. Accumulation of inhaled mineral dust in the lung and associated lymph nodes: implications for exposure and dose in occupational lung disease. Ann Occup Hyg 1987; 31:375–393.
31. Finkelstein MM. Mortality among long-term employees of an Ontario asbestos-cement factory. Br J Ind Med 1983; 40:138–144.
32. Doll R, Peto J. Asbestos: effects on health of exposure to asbestos, pp. 1–58. Health and Safety Commission, London: Her Majesty's Stationery Office, 1985.
33. Berry G, Wagner JC. Effects of age at inoculation of asbestos on occurrence of mesothelioma in rats. Int J Cancer 1976; 17:477–483.

34. Pott F, Friedrichs KH. Tumours in rats after intraperitoneal injection of asbestos dusts. Naturwissenschaften 1972; 59:318–332.
35. Pott F. Some aspects of the dosimetry of the carcinogenic potency of asbestos and other fibrous dusts. Staub-Reinholt Luft 1978; 38:486–490.
36. Stanton MF, Wrench C. JNCI 1972; 48:797.
37. Stanton MF, Layard M, Tegeris A, Miller M, Kent E. JNCI 1977; 58:587.
38. Davis JMG, Addison J, Bolton RE, Donaldson K, Jones AD, Smith T. The pathogenicity of long versus short fibre samples of amosite asbestos administered to rats by inhalation and intraperitoneal injection. Br J. Exp Pathol 1986; 67:415.
39. Davis JMG, Jones AD. Comparisons of the pathogenicity of long and short fibres of chrysotile asbestos in rats. Br J Exp Pathol 1988; 69:717.
40. Smith WE, Hubert DD, Miller L, Badollet MS, Churg J. Tests for levels of carcinogenicity of asbestos. In: Biologische wirkungen des asbestos. International conference, Dresden. Berlin: Deutches Zentralinstitut ftlr Arbeitsmedizin, 1968:240–242.
41. Wagner JC, Berry G, Timbrell V. Br J Cancer 1973; 28:173.
42. Davis JMG, Bolton RE, Miller BG, Niven K. Mesothelioma dose response following intraperitoneal injection of mineral fibres. Int J Exp Pathol 1991; 72:263–274.
43. Bignon J, Sarracci R. Biopersistence of respirable synthetic fibres and minerals. Report of a workshop sponsored by the International Agency for Research on Cancer, Lyon 1992 (in press).
44. Gylseth B, Mowe G, Wannag A. Fibre type and concentration in the lungs of workers in an asbestos cement factory. Br J Ind M 1983; 40:375–379.
45. Wagner JC, Berry GB, Hill RJ, Munday DE, Skidmore JW. Animal experiments with MMM(V)F. Effects of inhalation and intraperitoneal inoculation in rats. In: Biological effects of man-made mineral fibres. Report of a WHO/IARC meeting. Copenhagen: WHO, 1984:207–233.
46. McConnell EE, Wagner JC, Skidmore JW, Moore JA. A comparative study of the fibrogenic and carcinogenic effects of UICC Canadian chrysotile B asbestos and glass microfibre (JM100). In: Biological effects of man-made mineral fibres. Report of a WHO/IARC meeting. Copenhagen: WHO, 1984: 234–252.
47. Le Bouffant L, Daniel H, Henin JP, Martin JC, Normand C, Tichoux G, Trolard F. Experimental study on long-term effects of inhaled MMMF on the lungs of rats. Ann Occup Hyg 1987; 31:765–791.
48. Muhle H, Pott F, Bellman B, Takenaka S, Ziem V. Inhalation and injection experiments in rats to test the carcinogenicity of MMMF. Ann Occup Hyg 1987; 31:755–765.
49. Davis JMG, Addison J, Bolton RE, Donaldson K, Jones AD, Wright A. The pathogenic effects of fibrous ceramic aluminum silicate glass administered to rats by inhalation or peritoneal injection. In: Biological effects of man-made mineral fibres. Proceedings of a symposium 1982. Copenhagen: WHO, 1984: 303–322.
50. Ilgren EB, Wagner JC. Background incidence of mesothelioma; animal and human evidence. Regul Toxicol Pharmacol 1991; 13:133–149.

51. Roggle V, McGauran M, Subach J, Syberts H, Greenberg S. Pulmonary asbestos body counts and electron probe analysis of asbestos body coves in patients with mesotheliomata. A study of 25 cases. Cancer 1982; 50:2423-2432.
52. McDonald A, Harper A, El Attar O, McDonald J. Epidemiology of primary malignant mesothelial tumours in Canada. Cancer 1970; 26:914-919.
53. Oels H, Harrison E, Carr D, Bernatz P. Diffuse malignant mesothelioma of the pleura: a review of 37 cases. Chest 1971; 60:564-570.
54. Pelnar P. Further evidence of non-asbestos-related mesothelioma. Scand J Work Environ Health 1988; 14:141-144.
55. Brown J, Kristensen K, Monroe L. Peritoneal mesothelioma following pneumoperitoneum maintained for twelve years: report of a case. Am J Dig Dis 1968; 13:830-835.
56. Chakinian A, Pajak T, Holland J, Norton L, Ambinder R, Mandel E. Diffuse malignant mesothelioma. Ann Intern Med 1982; 96:746-755.
57. Lynch D, Lewis T, Moorman W, Burg J, Groth D, Khan A, Ackerman L, Cockrell B. Carcinogenic and toxicologic effects of inhaled ethylene oxide and propylene in F344 rats. Toxicol Appl Pharmacol 1984; 76:69-84.
58. Stanton M, Layard M. The carcinogenicity of fibrous minerals. Nat Bureau Stand Spec Publ 1977; 506:143-151.
59. Pott F, Ziem U, Reiffer F, Huth F, Ernst H, Mohr U. Carcinogenicity studies on fibres, metal compounds and some other dusts in rats. Exp Pathol 1987; 32:129-152.
60. Autian J, Singh A, Turner J, Hung G, Nunez L, Lawrence W. Carcinogenesis from polyurethane. Cancer Res 1975; 35:1591-1596.
61. McClure H, Graham C. Malignant uterine mesotheliomas in squirrel monkeys following diethylstilbesterol administration. Vet Rec 1973; 35:468-471.
62. Chabot J, Beard D, Langlois A, Beard JW. Mesotheliomas of peritoneum, epidardium and pericardium induced by strain MC29 avian leukosis virus. Cancer Res 1970; 30:1287-1308.
63. Stanton M, Lauyard M, Tegeris A, Miller E, May M, Morgan M, Smith A. JNCI 1981; 48:797.
64. Wagner JC, Griffith D, Munday D. Experimental studies with palygorskite dusts. Br J Ind Med 1987; 44:749-753.
65. Wagner JC, Berry G, Skidmore JW. The comparative effects of three chrysotiles by injection and inhalation in rats. In: Wagner JC, ed. Biological effects of mineral fibres. IARC Publ 1980; 30:363-373.
66. Davis JMG, Beckett ST, Bolton RE, Collings P, Middleton AP. Mass and number of fibres in the pathogenesis of asbestos-related lung disease in rats. Br J Cancer 1978; 37:673-688.
67. Davis JMG, Bolton RE, Donaldson K, Jones AD, Miller B. Inhalation studies on the effects of tremolite and brucite dust in rats. Carcinogenesis 1985; 6:667-674.

# 11

## Neoplastic Transformation of Mesothelial Cells

**MARIE-CLAUDE JAURAND**

Institut National de la Santé et de la
  Recherche Médicale
Créteil, France

**J. CARL BARRETT**

National Institute of Environmental Health
  Sciences
National Institutes of Health
Research Triangle Park, North Carolina

## I.  Introduction

Cancer is fundamentally a cellular disease. The classic experiments of Furth showed that transplantation of a single cell into a new host could completely recapitulate the disease (1). Therefore, an understanding of the cellular and molecular alterations in the cancer cell, compared with the normal cell from which it was derived, can yield insights into the cancer process and etiology. In mesothelioma, the target cell for neoplastic transformation, the mesothelial cell, is an unusual cell in terms of its differentiative capacity, as discussed elsewhere in this volume. Understanding the neoplastic changes in mesotheliomas may provide further insights into the normal functions of these cells.

In this review, we discuss different aspects of neoplastic transformation of mesothelial cells. The cytogenetic and molecular genetic changes in mesotheliomas are discussed, as well as alterations in growth factor expression and response. Finally, the ability to transform normal mesothelial cells in culture by known etiological agents (e.g., asbestos) and to follow the multistep process of neoplastic transformation is presented.

## II. Cytogenetic Changes Associated with Mesothelial Cell Transformation

Identification of specific cytogenetic alterations associated with many human and rodent tumors has yielded useful knowledge about the developmental mechanisms of these tumors (2–4). Two types of genes are involved in neoplastic transformation: oncogenes and tumor suppressor genes (5). Activation of cellular oncogenes can occur as a result of point mutations, chromosomal rearrangements, or amplification of portions of chromosomes on which these genes are located (6). Chromosomal deletion can result in the loss of a normal allele of a tumor suppressor gene (7,8). The presence of chromosomal abnormalities can be an indicator of the involvement of either oncogenes, tumor suppressor genes, or both, in the transformation process.

Specific nonrandom chromosomal alterations have been observed in transformed mesothelial cells, both in humans (9–17) and rodents. These findings are also discussed in detail in Chapter 13. Of particular interest are alterations involving human chromosomes 1, 3, 5, and 7. Deletions or rearrangements involving chromosome 1 have been reported in several studies involving human mesothelial cells (10–17); in one report, these aberrations have been reported to occur with a frequency of more than 60% (10). A gene important for cellular senescence is thought to be located on human chromosome 1 (18). Alterations of this gene may play a role in cellular immortalization and, thus, may be critical for development or progression of the neoplastic phenotype. Aberrations involving chromosome 1 are frequently observed in many other types of human cancer (19,20).

A second commonly observed cytogenetic alteration in human mesothelioma cells is deletion or monosomy of chromosome 3 (9,11–13,21,22). Although alterations of 3p are frequently observed in mesotheliomas, mesothelial cells directly exposed to asbestos did not exhibit this alteration in one report (14), suggesting that it may be a secondary event occurring late in mesothelioma development. A tumor suppressor gene involved in several human cancers, including lung cancer (23), renal cell carcinoma (23–25), and cervical carcinoma (26), is located on chromosome 3p. Alterations in this region of chromosome 3 in mesotheliomas suggest that this same tumor suppressor gene could be involved in mesothelioma development. However, a direct role for this tumor suppressor gene in the genesis of mesothelioma has not yet been demonstrated.

Polysomy (gains) of chromosome 7 (14,15,22) has been observed frequently in human mesotheliomas, suggesting that increased dosage of a gene on chromosome 7 may play a role in transformation of mesothelial cells. Chromosome 7 is the site of the protooncogene *HER-1*, which encodes the epidermal growth factor receptor (EGF-R) (27). Trisomy or polysomy of chromosome 7 has been observed in other types of human cancer (24,27–29) and may be responsible for altered expression of the EGF-R in melanoma cells (30). To date, the role of EGF-R expression in the development of mesothelioma has not been thoroughly investigated. In addition, platelet-derived growth factor alpha (PDGF-$\alpha$) is located on human chromosome 7 (31), and a role for this growth factor in the development of mesothelioma has been suggested (see later discussion).

Pelin-Enlund and co-workers recently reported an excess of the short arm of chromosome 5 in six of seven human mesothelioma cell lines (17). In addition, monosomy of chromosome 13, which contains the retinoblastoma (*Rb*) tumor suppressor gene (4), was cited in this report (17). Loss of normal *Rb* gene function has been observed in human lung tumors (32–35), but no direct evidence exists for a role for this gene in mesothelioma development.

Less information is available on cytogenetic alterations associated with mineral fiber-induced mesothelioma in rodents. Several alterations involving rat chromosomes that correspond to human chromosomes altered in transformed mesothelial cells have been reported. Polysomy and structural alterations of rat chromosome 1 have been observed (36–38). Chromosome 1 of the rat is homologous with chromosome 11 of humans and chromosome 3 of the hamster (39). Chromosome 11 is frequently altered in transformed human mesothelial cells (14,40–42), and asbestos-transformed Syrian hamster embryo (SHE) cells exhibit polysomy of chromosome 3, chromosome 8, and chromosome 11 (43). In addition, rat chromosomes 5, 8, 10, and 16, which are altered in rat mesotheliomas, contain linkage groups located on human chromosomes 1 and 9, 3, 7q, and 17, respectively (39), which are frequently altered in human mesothelioma. In addition, chromosome 8, which is altered in asbestos-transformed hamster cells, contains a linkage group syntenic with human chromosome 12 (39), which is altered in human mesothelioma.

Aberrations in chromosomal regions syntenic between rodents and humans suggest that molecular alterations in the same genes may be responsible for mesothelioma in diverse species. However, this hypothesis has not been tested because the majority of the genes have not been cloned. The involvement of specific, cloned genes in mesotheliomas is discussed in the next section.

## III. Role of Oncogenes and Tumor Suppressor Genes in Mesothelial Cell Transformation

### A. Involvement of Oncogenes

Few studies have investigated modifications of oncogenes and tumor suppressor genes in mesothelial cell transformation. Mutations of Ki-*ras* were studied in 20 human mesothelioma cell lines, mainly obtained from subjects exposed to asbestos (44). Following polymerase chain reaction (PCR) amplification of genomic DNA, all cell lines exhibited a wild-type sequence of the gene, suggesting that an alteration of Ki-*ras* is not a critical step in the development of mesothelioma, at least in tumors resulting from asbestos exposure. From three human mesothelioma cell lines, Lamb et al. (45) reported that transforming genes were detected, using the nude mouse tumor assay, following transfection of tumor cell DNA into NIH 3T3 cells. Although not yet identified, these genes are not members of the *ras* family.

Gene transfer methods can be useful tools to determine the effects of specific genes in neoplastic transformation. Transfection of normal pleural mesothelial cells, obtained from 14 donors, with a construct containing SV40 early region resulted in the appearance of morphologically transformed clones in all cases (41). After further growth, cells exhibited an increased number of population doublings, but still senesced. Only one culture yielded an immortalized cell line, MeT-5A, suggesting that the SV40 early region is insufficient to produce immortal cells with indefinite life span and that additional events are necessary.

Plasmids containing activated forms of c-Ha-*ras* transform human bronchial epithelial cells as well as some rodent cells (46,47). The EJ-*ras*, a mutated form of the c-Ha-*ras* protooncogene, was transfected into MeT-5A at passage 70 (48); this transfection resulted in the formation of neoplastic cells, as demonstrated by the ability to form tumors in nude mice. These results show that EJ-*ras* is able to achieve human mesothelial cell transformation of previously immortalized cells. This is in agreement with previous findings on the role of EJ-*ras* in other cell types (46). However, it does not necessarily imply that mesothelial cell transformation in vivo results from the activation of such genes.

The effect of EJ-*ras* has also been studied in another mesothelial cell strain, LP-9, which is a peritoneal cell strain cultured from ascite fluids of a patient with ovarian carcinoma (49). Interestingly, EJ-*ras* did not induce immortalization nor neoplastic transformation of these cells. The only consistent change observed was in growth factor-dependence of cell proliferation; whereas epidermal growth factor (EGF) was necessary for the proliferation of the original cell strain, the transfected cells grew without EGF. In addition, these transfected cells produced mitogenic factors that could replace the EGF requirement for normal cells (50).

The results obtained following *ras* transfection of human mesothelial cells are in agreement with the findings that several events are necessary to produce complete neoplastic transformation of these cells. The MeT-5A cells described earlier exhibit a large range of chromosomal abnormalities (hypodiploidy, structural chromosomal aberrations, and marker chromosomes), which may contribute to the expression of the neoplastic phenotype following gene transfer (41). However, these authors noted that these changes were not specific to mesothelial cell transfection, but are features observed in other SV40-transformed cells.

Attempts to transfect normal rat pleural mesothelial cells with a EJ-*ras* plasmid, containing a selection marker, were reported (51). Early passages of rat pleural mesothelial cells were very resistant to transfection with all methods used (calcium and strontium precipitation, polybrene, lipofection, electroporation, microinjection). This may be due to the low replication rate of early passages of normal cells, because cells at later passages formed stably transfected colonies; however, even with older cells, the transfection rate still remained low (51). Because the transfection rate is generally low (in the order of $10^{-4}$ and $10^{-6}$) with both rodent and human cells (41,48,50,51), clones from these experiments might not be representative of the initial population or may have additional changes necessary for increased transfection efficiency. Therefore, the conclusions on the role of a given oncogene, based on transfection experiments, should be drawn with caution, taking into consideration both cell characteristics and technical features.

### B. Involvement of Tumor Suppressor Genes

The involvement of specific tumor suppressor genes in malignant mesothelioma has been studied, including the retinoblastoma gene and *p53* gene. No abnormalities in retinoblastoma protein or mRNA expression were found in human mesothelioma cell lines (52). Investigations of *p53* alterations from two laboratories have given different results. In a study by Cote et al. (53), two of four cell lines had *p53* mutations, whereas in a study by Metcalf et al. (44), only 10% of mesotheliomas had *p53* alterations. In this latter study, 20 cell lines were examined by direct sequencing of genomic DNA after PCR amplification, and point mutations were observed in only two cell lines. Differences between the two studies are difficult to explain. They do not seem related to asbestos exposure of patients because most cases were considered as exposed in both studies. However, the characteristics of the exposure may differ. More likely, the different number of cases studied may account for the different results.

Only one study in rodents has investigated the alterations of the *p53* gene in mesothelioma cell lines derived from tumors after inoculation of crocidolite fibers (54). The results showed rearrangements of the *p53* gene in 76% of neoplastic mouse cell lines. However, mouse fibroblastlike cell lines in culture spontaneously acquire *p53* mutations, and it will be necessary to verify if these mutations are in the tumors before cell culture establishment.

In conclusion, none of the known tumor suppressor genes yet examined are clearly involved in mesotheliomas. However, as discussed under the previous section, cytogenetic evidence for tumor suppressor genes involvement is provided by nonrandom deletions of specific chromosomes. As more genes are cloned, tumor suppressor gene involvement in mesotheliomas is likely to become more evident.

## IV. Role of Growth Factors in Mesothelial Cell Transformation

### A. Platelet-Derived Growth Factor

As suggested by several authors, platelet-derived growth factor (PDGF) plays a role in human mesothelial cell transformation; its expression is critical for mesothelial cell growth, and deregulation of PDGF expression is associated with mesothelial cell transformation (55–58). Detailed results are given in Chapter 12. To summarize, normal human mesothelial cells do not produce PDGF B-chain, whereas PDGF A-chain expression has been found. No data are available on receptor $\alpha$ expression, but the protein has been detected (58). In contrast, $\beta$-receptor expression for PDGF-B chain has been described (56,58).

Normal mesothelial cells transfected with large T antigen of SV40 express enhanced levels of PDGF B-chain in comparison with normal cells, suggesting that this factor may be associated with loss of control of limited life span (41). Transfection of the PDGF A-chain into immortalized mesothelial cells (Met-5A) is associated with the expression of PDGF A-chain results in tumorigenic conversion of the cells (59).

Only one study has reported the expression of receptors and peptide for both PDGF-A and PDGF-B directly in tumor samples (56). Concerning mesothelioma cell lines, no clear-cut situation is observed; mesothelioma cells express different levels of mRNA specific for both A- and B-chains of PDGF (55,57,58). However, PDGF seems to play a role in the stimulation of cell growth, because antisense oligonucleotides suppress cell proliferation (56). Expressions and both $\alpha$- and $\beta$-receptor proteins have been reported in tumorigenic cells (56,58).

These results suggest a role of PDGF, especially PDGF-A, in human mesothelial cell transformation. Results obtained following transfection of PDGF-A suggest that PDGF-A is more likely a cause than a consequence of cell transformation. However, extrapolations should be made with caution because of the multiple events necessary to accomplish transformation.

Although the transformation of mice cells may be dependent on PDGF expression (63), a different situation arises with rat mesothelial cells, in which no $\alpha$-receptor expression in normal cells nor in transformed cells has been found (61,62). This may indicate that rat cells have different mechanisms or pathways of transformation than human cells (63).

### B. Other Growth Factors

Platelet-derived growth factor is not the only growth factor involved in mesothelial cell transformation. Epidermal growth factor (EGF) is mitogenic for normal human mesothelial cells (50), but is inhibitory for the growth of normal rat pleural mesothelial cells (64). Neoplastic rat pleural mesothelial cells do not respond to EGF, suggesting a switch in the sensitivity to EGF following neoplastic transformation (65).

Several lines of evidence suggest that EGF plays a critical role in mesothelial cell transformation. First, EGF in association with other factors, is necessary to support human mesothelial cell growth (49,50,66). Human parietal mesothelial cells have been obtained from consecutive thoracic surgeries carried out for lung pathologies (Jaurand MC, et al., unpublished). Mesothelial cell layers were scraped from the normal part of the thorax and immediately grown in a culture medium supplemented only with 10% fetal bovine serum (FBS), which is poor in EGF-like factors. Only primary cultures were obtained from these cells, and the cells failed to exhibit serial growth; after subculture, senescent binucleated and multinucleated cells were formed. A second line of evidence is that EGF supports the growth of normal human mesothelial cells in semisolid medium (66), which is generally permissive only for the growth of transformed cells. In contrast, EGF might act as a differentiation factor, because growth of rat mesothelial cells is blocked by EGF (64), and normal pericardial mesothelial cells from rabbits produce hyaluronic acid, a normal component of the pleura, in the presence of EGF (67).

The EGF receptor (EGF-R) is present in normal rat mesothelial cells (64) and in rabbit mesothelial cells (67), and it has been detected in human normal pleura and in malignant mesothelioma (68,69). Although EGF-R expression cannot distinguish between malignant and benign tissue (69), the role of EGF-R has been poorly investigated with human mesothelioma cells.

Mesothelioma cell lines produce factors that stimulate the growth of other mesothelioma cell lines (70). A possible key event in the transformation of mesothelial cells is the ability of the cells to produce these cytokines (71), a feature that is also observed following stimulation of normal mesothelial cells both in vivo and in vitro (72,73). However, the role of specific cytokines in stimulation of mesothelioma cell growth remains undetermined (71).

### C. Questions Related to the Responses of Mesothelial Cells to Growth Factors

In spite of the foregoing results, no generalization can be made on the exact role of PDGF or other growth factors in mesothelial cell transformation.

The characteristics of normal versus transformed mesothelial cells are difficult to establish because of the variability of the features of both cell types.
One typical peculiarity is the great heterogeneity among mesothelial cells in
the expression of growth factors and also in the response to growth factors.
This may partly be due to the heterogeneity of normal mesothelial cells or
of mesotheliomas as well as to technical problems.

Great differences exist between the origin of the cells under investigation, which are obtained from pleural or pericardial effusions or from
peritoneal ascites. The physiological activity of mesothelial cells in different
parts of the body may differ. For example, differences exist between pleural
and omental mesothelial cells in their fibrinolytic potential (74,75). Differentiation capacity changes during development, and mesothelial cell characteristics may change, depending on the microenvironment and the functions
exerted by other cells. In addition, normal human mesothelial cells for
study are generally obtained from tissue effusions. Cell populations obtained from these procedures may be enriched for malignant or premalignant cells. Furthermore, fluid in the cavities of the body is not a normal
situation, and the mesothelial cells recovered may have biological changes
related to cellular responses to the pathological nature of the agent creating
the pleural effusion. Lechner et al. reported that the divergence of sensitivity of normal pleural mesothelial cells to growth factors is not dependent
on the clinical context (73). However, such divergence between cells from a
given tissue are not known for other tissues. Thus, the recovery of many
responsive mesothelial cells may reflect a difference in their stage of evolution from well-differentiated resident mesothelial cells into dedifferentiated
or reactive circulating cells.

Finally, use of defined culture media supplements may modulate the
response to growth factors. For example, PDGF expression was modulated
by hydrocortisone in a mesothelioma cell line (76); this agent is used in
some culture mediums. Normal human mesothelial cells cultured for several
passages are generally grown in the presence of EGF and other factors
that might select EGF-dependent cells and, consequently, modulate growth
factor sensitivity. Moreover, interactions between several growth factors
may also be important. However, Lechner et al. have noted the different
responses of normal pleural mesothelial cells to growth factors are not
dependent on the culture procedure (73).

## V.  Transformation of Mesothelial Cells

Malignant mesotheliomas are produced in humans following exposure to
asbestos fibers and also other forms of natural mineral fibers. However,

not all mesothelioma cases are related to asbestos exposure and other environmental agents may induce malignant mesothelioma. No epidemiological study has yet shown an association between malignant mesothelioma and the exposure to agents other than asbestos, but some evidence exists that radiation or chemicals (e.g., pesticides) may be involved (77).

### A.  Induction of Cell Transformation by Asbestos Fibers

The mechanisms whereby mesothelial cells are transformed by asbestos are not completely understood, but chromosomal mutations seem to play a critical role (78). As discussed before, nonrandom chromosomal changes are observed in human and rodent mesotheliomas. Multiple origins of these chromosomal changes may exist, but asbestos exposure can induce such changes in mesothelial and other cell types in culture.

Aneuploidy induction has been observed following treatment of mesothelial cells with asbestos. Lechner et al. reported hypodiploidy after amosite treatment of human cells (40), and anaphase aberrations were observed in Met-5A cells treated with several types of asbestos (79). Similar results were obtained with rat mesothelial cells following treatment with chrysotile asbestos; aneuploidy characterized by an excess of chromosomes was observed (80). Aneuploidy has also been induced after crocidolite exposure, but the cells were more often hypodiploid (81). This latter observation was also made with human cells (40). Complete neoplastic transformation following treatment of rat mesothelial cells with chrysotile has been reported (82,83).

The results show that asbestos, a known pleural carcinogen, produces chromosomal changes in cultured mesothelial cells. Taking into consideration the observations that nonrandom karyotypic alterations are observed in malignant mesothelial cells and asbestos fibers can induce these changes in normal mesothelial cells, it is reasonable that chromosomal mutations play an important role in mesothelial cell transformation by asbestos. This is in agreement with observations made in other cell systems (43,84), suggesting that the mechanisms of transformation are related to the neoplastic agent. Whether such a mechanism operates in vivo is unknown, but the nonrandom cytogenetic changes observed both in human and in rat mesotheliomas suggest that these events are relevant.

Cell transformation may be described in terms of initiation and promotion (85). Chromosomal mutations provide a mechanism for initiation of these cancers. A promotional effect of asbestos on mesothelial cells has not yet been demonstrated. Events associated with tumor promotion include increased cell proliferation and production of oxygen radicals (85). Proliferation of cells of the parietal pleura has been reported in human organ cultures treated with crocidolite (86); however, it is not clear if only mesothelial cells are involved. Thymidine incorporation into cells of the rat visceral pleura has also been observed following intratracheal instillation of chrysotile (87). However, no stimulation of cell proliferation has been found in vitro (88,89). These data suggest that either cell proliferation occurs to repair damaged tissue, or it is the consequence of the production of growth factors by nontarget cells, which stimulates the proliferation of pleural cells. Conflicting results on other effects associated with the action of tumor promoters, such as production of oxygen radicals, have been observed with mesothelial cells. Rat pleural mesothelial cells form oxygen derivatives after asbestos treatment that produce DNA damage (unpublished data), but human mesothelial cells do not (90). Taken together, these results are too limited to draw conclusions on the possible promotional effects of asbestos and other fibers on mesothelial cell transformation.

### B.  Agents Other Than Asbestos

Numerous chemical carcinogens must be metabolically activated to mutagenic intermediates. Cytochrome P-450 enzymes and reductases transform xenobiotics into metabolites that interact with DNA (91). Little is known about the metabolic capabilities of xenobiotics from human mesothelial cells. However, cultures of rat pleural mesothelial cells possess the metabolic systems to activate polycyclic aromatic hydrocarbons (92). This accounts for the ability of benzo[a]pyrene to produce, at least in vitro, neoplastic transformation of these cells. Rat pleural mesothelial cells transformed by benzo[a]pyrene have the ability to form abnormal colonies in liquid medium (93), to grow in semisolid medium, and to produce tumors in nude mice (83), which are phenotypes exhibited by other transformed cells. The karyotypes of the cells remain nearly diploid after transformation (80,94). Several forms of cytochrome P-450, including 1A1 and 2E1, have been described in cultures of rat pleural mesothelial cells. Interestingly, the metabolic capabilities of the cells are maintained following multiple passages (92). This suggests that mesothelial cells can be transformed by chemical carcinogens, and several chemicals in rodent bioassays induce mesotheliomas (95–97).

### VI.  Conclusions

The finding of nonrandom cytogenetic changes in mesotheliomas suggests that these cancers, like other human cancers, arise as a consequence of multiple genetic changes. However, the nature of the changes in mesotheliomas is still undefined. The most commonly altered genes in other human malignancies, including *p53*, *RB*, and *ras*, are not mutated frequently in these tumors. Nonrandom losses of other chromosomes implicate still un-identified tumor suppressor genes in mesotheliomas. The cloning of these tumor suppressor genes should yield important new insights into mesothelial cell transformation.

Gains of specific chromosomes are also common in mesotheliomas and suggest gene dosage effects, such as increases of growth factors or growth factor receptors. Some data support the concept that PDGF, EGF, or other growth factors, are important in these cancers, although a clear and consistent model has not emerged. This may be due to the heterogeneity or the plasticity of the cells in culture. Future studies on the growth control of cells in vivo may help elucidate the role of growth factors and cytokines in mesotheliomas.

The genetic changes observed in mesotheliomas are consistent with the known mechanisms of action of asbestos, the major etiological agent for this cancer. Because asbestos fibers induce chromosomal alterations in human and rodent cells (78), deletions and gains of specific chromosomal regions could result. In addition, asbestos fibers might elicit inflammatory and other tissue responses that could alter cytokine and growth factor production, which could then influence tumor promotion. The exact mechanisms for the latter events are poorly understood and will require further studies, particularly of mesothelial cells in vivo following asbestos exposure.

### References

1.  Furth J, Kahn MC. Am J Cancer 1937; 31:276.
2.  Yunis JJ. Science 1983; 221:227.
3.  Sandberg AA, Turc-Carel C, Gemmill RM. Cancer Res 1988; 48:1049.
4.  Knudson AG Jr. Annu Rev Genet 1986; 20:231.
5.  Boyd J, Barrett JC. Mol Carcinogen 1990; 3:325.
6.  Bishop JM. Science 1987; 235:305.
7.  Weinberg RA. Science 1991; 254:1138.
8.  Lasko D, Cavenee W, Nordenskjold M. Annu Rev Genet 1991; 25:281.
9.  Mark J. Acta Cytol (Praha) 1978; 22:398.
10. Gibas A, Li FP, Antman KH, Bernal S, Stahel R, Sandberg AA. Cancer Genet Cytogenet 1986; 20:191.
11. Bello MJ, Rey JA, Aviles MJ, Arevalo M, Benitez J. Cancer Genet Cytogenet 1987; 29:75.
12. Popescu NC, Chahinian AP, DiPaolo JA. Cancer Res 1988; 48:142.
13. Flejter WL, Li FP, Antman KH, Testa JR. Genes Chromosom Cancer 1989; 1:148.
14. Olofsson K, Mark J. Cancer Genet Cytogenet 1989; 41:33.
15. Tiainen M, Tammilehto L, Rautonen J, Tuomi T, Mattson K, Knuutila S. Br J Cancer 1989; 60:618.

16. Versnel MA, Bouts MJ, Hoogsteden HC, van der Kwast TH, Delahaye M, Hagemeijer A. Int J Cancer 1989; 44:256.
17. Pelin-Enlund K, Husgafvel-Pursiainen K, Tammilehto L, Klockars M, Jantunen K, Gerwin BI, Harris CC, Tuomi T, Vanhala E, Mattson K, Linnainmaa K. Carcinogenesis 1990; 11:673.
18. Sugawara O, Oshimura M, Koi M, Annab LA, Barrett JC. Science 1990; 247: 707.
19. Atkin NB. Cancer Genet Cytogenet 1986; 21:275.
20. Olah E, Baloghh E, Kovacs I, Kiss A. Cancer Genet Cytogenet 1989; 43:179.
21. Stenman G, Olofsson K, Mansson T, Hagmar B, Mark J. Hereditas 1986; 105:233.
22. Hagemeijer A, Versnel MA, Van Drunen E, Moret M, Bouts MJ, van der Kwast TH, Hoogsteden HC. Cancer Genet Cytogenet 1990; 47:1.
23. Zbar B. Important Adv Oncol 1989; 22:41.
24. Walter TA, Berger CS, Sandberg AA. Cancer Genet Cytogenet 1989; 43:15.
25. Kovacs G. J Cancer Res Clin Oncol 1990; 116:318.
26. Yokota J, Tsukada Y, Nakajima T, Gotoh M, Shimosato Y, Mori N, Tsunokawa Y, Sugimura T, Terada M. Cancer Res 1989; 49:3598.
27. Carpenter G. Cell 1984; 37:357.
28. Becher R, Gibas Z, Sandberg AA. Cancer Genet Cytogenet 1983; 3:329.
29. Rey JA, Bello MJ, de Campos JM, Kusak ME, Moreno S. Cancer Genet Cytogenet 1987; 29:323.
30. Trent JM, Leong SP, Meyskens FL. Carcinog Compr Surv 1989; 11:165.
31. Betsholtz, C, Johnson A, Heldin C-H, Westmark B, Lind P, Urdea MS, Eddy R, Shows TB, Philpott K, Mellor AL, Knott TJ, Scott J. Nature 1986; 320: 695.
32. Harbour JW, Lai SL, Whang-Peng J, Gazdar AF, Minna JD, Kaye FJ. Science 1988; 241:353.
33. Yokota J, Akiyama T, Fung Y-KT, Benedict WF, Namba Y, Hanaoka M, Wada M, Terasaki T, Shimosato Y, Sugimura T, Terada M. Oncogene 1988; 3:471.
34. Mori N, Yokota J, Akiyama T, Sameshima Y, Okamoto A, Mizoguchi H, Toyoshima K, Sugimura T, Terada M. Oncogene 1990; 5:1713.
35. Rygaard K, Sorenson GD, Pettengill OS, Cate CC, Spang-Thomsen M. Cancer Res 1990; 50:5312.
36. Libbus BL, Craighead JE. Cancer Res 1988; 48:6455.
37. Palekar LD, Eyre JF, Coffin DL. Chromosomal changes associated with tumorigenic mineral fibers. In: Wehner AP, Felton DL, eds. Biological interaction of inhaled mineral fibers and cigarette smoke. Proceedings of an international symposium workshop, Seattle, Washington, 1988:355–372.
38. Funaki K, Everitt J, Bermudez E, Walker C. Cancer Res 1991; 51:4059.
39. Lalley PA, Davisson MT, Graves JAM, O'Brien SJ, Womack JE, Roderick TH, Creau-Goldberg N, Hillyard AL, Doolittle DP, Rogers JA. Cytogenet Cell Genet 1989; 51:503.
40. Lechner JF, Tokiwa T, LaVeck M, Benedict WF, Banks-Schlegel S, Yeager H, Barnerjee A, Harris CC. Proc Natl Acad Sci USA 1985; 82:3884.

41. Ke Y, Reddel RR, Gerwin BI, Reddel HK, Somers ANA, McMenamin MG, LaVeck MA, Stahel RA, Lechner JF, Harris CC. Am J Pathol 1989; 134:979.
42. Tiainen M, Tammilehto L, Mattson K, Knuutila S. Cancer Genet Cytogenet 1988; 33:251.
43. Oshimura M, Hesterberg TW, Barrett JC. Cancer Genet Cytogenet 1986; 22: 225.
44. Metcalf RA, Welsh JA, Bennett WP, Seddon MB, Lehman TA, Pelin K, Linnainmaa K, Tammilehto L, Mattson, K, Gerwin BI, Harris CC. Cancer Res 1992; 52:2610.
45. Lamb P, Wiseman R, Ozawa N, Suzuki Y, Chahinian P, Barrett JC. Proc Am Assoc Cancer Res 1988; 29:142A.
46. Land H, Chen AC, Morgenstern JP, Parada LF, Weinberg RA. Mol Cell Biol 1986; 6:1917.
47. Yoakum GH, Lechner JF, Gabrielson EW, Korba BE, Malan-Shibley L, Willey JC, Valerio MG, Shamsuddin AM, Trump BF, Harris CC. Science 1985; 227:1174.
48. Reddel RR, Malan-Shibley L, Gerwin BI, Metcalf RA, Harris CC. JNCI 1989; 81:945.
49. Wu YJ, Parker LM, Binder NE, Beckett MA, Sinard JH, Griffiths CT, Rheinwald JG. Cell 1982; 31:693.
50. Tubo RA, Rheinwald JG. Oncogene Res 1987; 1:407.
51. Moritz S, Salmons B, Renier A, Günzburg W, Barrett JC, Jaurand MC. Eur Respir Rev 1993; 3:167.
52. Van der Meeren A, Seddon MB, Kispert J, Harris CC, Gerwin BI. Eur Respir Rev 1993; 3:177.
53. Cote RJ, Jhanwar SC, Novick S, Pellicer A. Cancer Res 1991; 51:5410.
54. Cora EM, Kane AB. Eur Respir Rev 1993; 3:148.
55. Gerwin BI, Lechner JF, Reddel RR, Roberts AB, Robbins KC, Gabrielson EW, Harris CC. Cancer Res 1987; 47:6180.
56. Garlepp MJ, Christmas TI, Manning LS, Mutsaers SE, Dench J, Leong C, Robinson BWS. Eur Respir Rev 1993; 3:189.
57. Langerak AW, Vietsch H, Bouts MJ, Hagemeijer A, Versnell MA. Eur Respir Rev 1993; 3:170.
58. Versnel MA, Langerak AW, van der Kwast TH, Hoogsteden HC, Hagemeijer A. Eur Respir Rev 1993; 3:186.
59. Van der Meeren A, Seddon MB, Betsholtz CA, Lechner JF, Gerwin BI. Eur Respir Rev 1993; 3:180.
60. Garlepp MJ, Christmas TI, Mutsaers SE, Manning LS, Davis MR, Robinson BWS. Eur Respir Rev 1993; 3:192.
61. Bermudez E, Everitt J, Walker C. Exp Cell Res 1990; 190:91.
62. Walker C, Bermudez E, Stewart W, Bonner J, Molloy CJ, Everitt J. Cancer Res 1992; 52:301.
63. Walker C, Bermudez E, Bonner J, Everitt J. Eur Respir Rev 1993; 3:153.
64. Van der Meeren A, Levy F, Renier A, Katz A, Jaurand MC. J Cell Physiol 1990; 144:137.
65. Van der Meeren A, Levy F, Bignon J, Jaurand MC. Biol Cell 1988; 62:293.

66. La Rocca PJ, Rheinwald JG. In Vitro Cell Dev Biol 1985; 21:67.
67. Honda A, Noguchi N, Takehara H, Ohashi Y, Asuwa N, Mori Y. J Cell Sci 1991; 98:91.
68. Haeder M, Rotsch M, Bepler G, Hennig C, Havemann E, Heimann B, Moelling K. Cancer Res 1988; 48:1132.
69. Dazzi H, Hasleton PS, Thatcher N, Wilkes S, Swindell R, Chatterjee AK. Br J Cancer 1990; 61:924.
70. Lauber B, Leuthold M, Schmitter D, Canosantos J, Waibel R, Stahel RA. Int J Cancer 1992; 50:943.
71. Schmitter D, Lauber B, Fagg B, Stahel RA. Int J Cancer 1992; 51:296.
72. Boylan AM, Ruegg C, Kim KJ, Hebert CA, Hoeffel JM, Pytela R, Sheppard D, Goldstein IM, Broaddus VC. J Clin Invest 1992; 89:1257.
73. Lechner JF, Laveck MA, Gerwin BI, Matis EA. J Cell Physiol 1989; 139:295.
74. Hinsbergh VWM, Kooistra T, Scheffer MA, Van Bockel JH, Van Muijen GNP. Blood 1990; 75:1490.
75. Idell S, Zwieb C, Kumar A, Koenig KB, Johnson AR. Am J Respir Cell Mol Biol 1992; 7:414.
76. Versnel MA, Bouts MJ, Langerak AW, van der Kwast TH, Hoogsteden HC, Hagemeijer A, Heldin CH. Exp Cell Res 1992; 200:83.
77. Peterson JT, Greenberg SD, Buffler PA. Cancer 1984; 54:951.
78. Barrett JC, Lamb PW, Wiseman RW. Environ Health Perspect 1989; 81:81.
79. Pelin K, Husgafvelpursiainen K, Vallas M, Vanhala E, Linnainmaa K. Toxicol In Vitro 1992; 6:445.
80. Jaurand MC, Buard A, Zeng L, Laurent P, Fleury J, Kheuang L. Eur Respir Rev. 1993; 3:126.
81. Yegles M, Saint-Etienne L, Renier A, Janson X, Jaurand MC. Am J Respir Cell Mol Biol 1993; 9:186.
82. Jaurand MC, Saint-Etienne L, Van der Meeren A, Endo-Capron S, Renier A, Bignon J. Neoplastic transformation of rodent cells. In: Lechner JF, Brinkley BR, Harris CC, eds. Cellular and molecular aspects of fiber carcinogenesis. Current communications in cell and molecular biology, vol 2. Cold Spring Harbor, NY: Cold Spring Harbor Laboratory Press, 1991;131.
83. Saint-Etienne L, Endo-Capron S, Jaurand MC. Eur Respir Rev 1993; 3:141.
84. Hei TK, Piao CQ, He ZY, Vannais D, Waldren CA, Cancer Res 1992; 52: 6305.
85. Walker C, Everitt J, Barrett JC. Am J Ind Med 1992; 21:253.
86. Rajan KT, Wagner JC, Evans PH. Nature 1972; 238:346.
87. Bryks S, Bertalanffy FD. Arch Environ Health 1971; 23:469.
88. Jaurand MC, Bastie-Sigeae I. Bignon J, Stoebner P. Environ Res 1983; 30: 255.
89. Gabrielson EW, Van der Meeren A, Reddel RR, Reddel H, Gerwin BI. Carcinogenesis 1992; 13:1359.
90. Gabrielson EW, Rosen GM, Grafstrom C, Strauss KE, Harris CC. Carcinogenesis 1986; 7:1161.
91. Gonzalez FJ. Pharmacol Rev 1989; 40:243.

92. Buard A, Beaune PH, Renier A, Jaurand MC, Bignon J, Laurent P. Eur Respir Rev 1993; 3:138.
93. Patérour MJ, Bignon J, Jaurand MC. Carcinogenesis 1985; 6:523.
94. Medrano L, Kheuang L, Patérour MJ, Bignon J, Jaurand MC. Chromosomal changes in cultured rat mesothelial cells treated with benzo 3-4 pyrene and/or chrysotile asbestos. In: Beck EG, Bignon J, eds. In vitro effects of mineral dusts 1985;511.
95. Huff J, Cirvello J, Haseman J, Bucher J. Environ Health Perspect 1991; 93: 247.
96. Berhan JJ, Rice JM. Vet Pathol 1979; 16:574.
97. Ogiu T, Fukami H, Mackawa A. J Cancer Res Clin Oncol 1988; 114:259.

# 12

## Mesothelial Carcinogenesis
## Possible Avenues of Growth Factor Promotion

**BRENDA I. GERWIN**

National Cancer Institute
National Institutes of Health
Bethesda, Maryland

## I. Introduction

Studies of cellular growth regulation provide the framework within which carcinogenesis studies seek to position the genetic and epigenetic alterations that correlate with the deregulated growth state termed cancer. It has become clear that malignant cells have acquired multiple alterations from "normal" in which a cell loses suppressor gene activity and gains growth-potentiating activity, eventually accumulating sufficient alteration to escape normal regulatory processes (1). Cancer research attempts to delineate these changes by comparing normal and tumorigenic examples of a given cellular lineage. Molecular analyses of tumor material strongly suggest that multiple pathways, even within a given cell type (2), may lead to cancer, as defined by the ability of altered cell populations to kill their host by overwhelming normal cell function and uncontrolled growth. The revolution of molecular biology allows precise definitions of gene products, the alterations of which are associated with cancer, as well as the critical testing of hypotheses concerning the role of such alterations in carcinogenesis. Genes can be manipulated and transferred to create cells and animals with specific changes from normal, and the consequences of these changes in relation to tumorigenicity can be defined relative to the disease or replicative status of the altered animal or cell.

In any tumor type, the specific progenitor cell will likely define the most probable route to tumorigenic conversion, since its normal state expresses a unique constellation of "active" genes that are essential for its function. Thus, each organ and cell type provides a unique target for genetic and epigenetic alteration, whereas its position within the organism subjects it to a characteristic spectrum of endogenous and exogenous "carcinogenic" compounds. The adult animal is largely a differentiated creature in which few cells are actively dividing. Thus, some of the critical stages of the carcinogenesis pathway for any cell are likely to consist of the inappropriate expression or disregulation of gene products, such as growth factors and their receptors, that can convert that cell from a nondividing to a proliferative state. Wounding and healing generally induce the appropriate expression of multiple growth promoters. When these stimuli are not appropriately regulated, the altered cell(s) achieve a growth advantage over the surrounding normal cells (3).

Since mesothelioma is a cancer that develops from mesothelial cells in animals exposed to carcinogenic fibers (4,5), much research has focused on defining the consequences of exposing cells to such fibers. Such studies have indicated that fiber exposure can induce DNA damage (6,7), perhaps mediated by active oxygen species (AOS) (8), or association with chromosomes (9) after entering the nucleus and associating with spindle fibers (10–12). In a newt epithelial cell model, Cole and co-workers showed that only crocidolite fibers shorter than 5 $\mu$m undergo translocation to the perinuclear region by cytoplasmic microtubule-dependent saltatory transport. These short fibers are membrane-encapsulated. In contrast, fibers longer than 5 $\mu$m did not undergo saltatory transport. The authors speculated that long fibers may be unencapsulated and also less efficiently translocated by astral microtubules. Therefore, long fibers might be preferentially positioned to interfere with spindle formation and chromosomal movement (13). Such physical interaction would be likely to induce large, multilocus chromosomal alterations (14) that could both activate growth enhancers and cause loss of tumor suppressor genes. In a complementary approach, investigators (15,16) have defined in vitro growth conditions for mesothelial cells that allow examination of growth factor responsiveness and production. Perhaps in this cancer, induced by a known class of carcinogens from normal mesothelial cells, comparison of growth controls and responses of the normal and tumor cells, coupled with analysis of the response to the carcinogen, will lead to the mapping of the most likely routes of carcinogenesis and suggest means to block or reverse this path.

## II. Growth Factor Responsiveness of Normal Human Mesothelial Cells

Growth media formulated for optimal growth of normal human mesothelial (NHM) cells contained hydrocortisone (HC) as well as both high levels of fetal bovine serum (FBS) (10–20%) and exogenous epidermal growth factor (EGF) (15,17). When serum was removed from the culture medium leaving only the components of LHC basal medium (18), a basal level of sustained growth required supplementation by high-density lipoproteins as well as transferrin, insulin, and one of several peptide growth factors (16,19). Also, addition of either EGF or fibroblast growth factor (FGF; acidic or basic) plus another of a wide range of factors, resulted in more rapid replication (16). Interestingly, the effects of EGF and FGF were not additive, suggesting that growth stimulatory signals from these factors share a common downstream pathway in NHM cells. In addition, comparison of NHM cells from different donors revealed interindividual differences in replication rate and patterns of growth factor responsiveness. Thus, cells from a given individual exhibited an innate pattern of stimulation or inhibition by specific factor combinations that were not altered by the selection pressure applied by growth in nonoptimal media formulations (20). Table 1 lists those factors that were generally stimulatory to NHM cells, with the caveat that interferon gamma (IFN-$\gamma$) and interleukin-2 (IL-2) were cytotoxic to some NHM cells (20). In addition to interindividual differences among humans, data that indicate that normal rat pleural mesothelial cells are inhibited by EGF (26) suggest that major interspecies differences also exist. Human peritoneal mesothelial cells show a proliferative

**Table 1** Factors Stimulating Normal Mesothelial Cell Growth

| Growth factors | Cytokines | Other |
| --- | --- | --- |
| TGF-$\beta_1$[a,b] | IL-1$\alpha$[b,e] | Insulin[b,c] |
| TGF-$\beta_2$[b] | IL-1$\beta$[b,e] | Transferrin[b] |
| FGF(a)[h] | IFN-$\alpha$[b] | Hydrocortisone[c] |
| FGF(b)[b] | IFN-$\beta$[b] | High-density lipids[b,d] |
| TGF-$\alpha$[b] | IFN-$\gamma$[b] | Cholera toxin[b] |
| EGF[b,c] | IL-2[b] | 200-kD[a] gp[f,g] |
| PDGF-AB[a,b,d] | | |
| PDGF-BB[b,d] | | |
| IGF-1[h] | | |

*Sources*: Refs. [a]19; [b]16; [c]15; [d]21; [e]22; [f]23; [g]24; [h]25.

response to both IL-1α and IL-1β and express the IL-1 receptor type 1 (IL-1R1) (22). Recent detection of responsiveness to and receptors for insulin-like growth factor 1 (IGF-1) (27) indicates that this growth factor also is a stimulator of this cell type.

### III. Growth Factor and Cytokine Production by Normal Human Mesothelial Cells

Several laboratories have described the production of endogenous growth factors by NHM cells in culture. With use of growth of ovarian tumor cells in soft agar as an assay, Wilson isolated NHM cells from the malignant ascites and tested them as a feeder layer (28). The NHM cells were growth stimulatory when present at equal or greater numbers than the tumor cells. Stimulation decreased with increasing distance between cell layers, suggesting a diffusible factor(s). Breborowicz et al. who used NHM cells from omentum, found that medium conditioned by these cells increased the growth rate of similar NHM cells in M199 medium supplemented with hydrocortisone (HC) and 10% fetal calf serum (FCS). This stimulatory activity was partially heat-labile at 60°C (29). Donna and co-workers have purified a 200-kDa glycoprotein, from serous effusions of mesothelioma patients, that increases the growth rate of NHM cells as well as mesothelioma cells, but was not stimulatory for a lung adenocarcinoma cell line (23). By using a polyclonal antibody to this protein, they have been able to neutralize growth stimulation, demonstrate specificity for cells of mesothelial origin, and localize the protein to endoplasmic reticulum and plasma membrane (24). Further characterization and cloning of this molecule will be of great interest. Additional evidence that NHM cells can produce autocrine factors is provided by the observation that NHM cells transfected with the EJ-*ras* gene remain nontumorigenic, but become independent of EGF while producing neither EGF nor transforming growth factor (TGF)-α (30; Reinwald JG, personal communication). In addition, the density-dependence of keratin synthesis (31) may indicate an autocrine effect regulating the expression of intermediate filament proteins.

The production of known growth factors by NHM cells has also been documented (Table 2). Northern analysis for TGF-β1 and platelet-derived growth factor (PDGF) A- and B-chains indicated the consistent production of TGF-β mRNA (33), but not PDGF by normal cells (33,39) in culture. The NHM cells also respond to mitogenic signals from IGF-1 and produce both IGF-1 and IGF-binding protein type 3 (IGFBP-3), suggesting an identity for some of the autocrine activity of NHM cells (27). Treatment of human cells with PDGF (40) or combined exposure to IGF-1 and EGF in

**Table 2** Factors Produced by Normal Mesothelial Cells

| Factor | mRNA basal | mRNA stimulated | Bioassay/protein |
|---|---|---|---|
| PDGF | | a,b | a |
| TGF-$\beta$1 | c | | c |
| 200-kD$^a$ gp | | | d,e |
| IL-1$\alpha$ | f | | f |
| IL-1$\beta$ | f | g | f |
| IL-6 | f | g | f,k |
| IL-8 | k | i,j,k | i,j,k |
| MCP-1 | k | k | k |
| M-CSF | f,g | g | f |
| G-CSF | f | g | g,f |
| GM-CSF | f | g | g,f |

*Sources*: Data from Refs. [a]3; [b]25; [c]33; [d]23; [e]24; [f]22; [g]34; [h]35; [i]36; [j]37; [k]38.

rabbit mesothelial cells (41) stimulates hyaluronic acid synthetase. Apparently, endogenous IGF-1 synthesis is ineffective in the absence of EGF. This stimulation is dependent on tyrosine phosphorylation, suggesting that it is mediated by receptor-dependent signaling processes.

In addition to these cytokines, a long-term culture of NHM cells has been shown to produce colony-stimulating factors (CSF) in vitro (34). In a basal medium containing 7% FCS, NHM cells expressed macrophage (M)-CSF mRNA, whereas addition of EGF, *Escherichia coli* lipopolysaccharide (LPS), or tumor necrosis factor (TNF) induced the production of granulocyte (G)-CSF mRNA and biological activity as well as IL-1$\beta$ mRNA. Interestingly, the combination of TNF and EGF was needed to induce a low level of granulocyte–macrophage (GM)-CSF mRNA and biological activity. These CSF activities are unlikely to be the autocrines described by others, since they were unable to substitute for EGF in supporting growth of NHM cells (34) and were not mitogenic (42) for the T–antigen-immortalized NHM model cell, MeT-5A (21). Production of CSFs has also been observed in primary peritoneal mesothelial cell cultures (22). Normal human peritoneal mesothelial cells without added activators produced M-CSF, G-CSF, GM-CSF, IL-6, IL-1$\alpha$, and IL-1$\beta$ spontaneously, with GM-CSF being detectable only after 70–90 days in culture. Transcripts for IL-2, IL-3, IL-4, IL-5, and IL-7 were not detected. Interestingly, these workers showed that both IL-1$\alpha$ and IL-1$\beta$ were produced by the cells and that these factors were able to stimulate the expression of GM-CSF and G-CSF as well as their own transcripts (22).

Asbestos inhalation can lead to a benign pleurisy in some subjects. In a rabbit model using crocidolite inoculated into the pleural space, Shore and co-workers (43) found that an influx of polymorphonuclear lymphocytes was secondary to production of chemotactic activity from sources other than complement. In experiments designed to detect products of mesothelial cells after asbestos exposure, Antony et al. showed that crocidolite and chrysotile fibers induced production of a complement-independent chemoattractant for neutrophils in rabbit mesothelial cells (35). This activity has subsequently been identified as interleukin-8 (IL-8) (37), and it has been shown that NHM cells from pleural effusions produce a low level of chemotactic activity in vitro but are induced to produce IL-8 mRNA and increased chemotactic activity by TNF-$\alpha$, IFN-$\gamma$, and IL-1$\alpha$. Use of LPS did not increase the basal level of chemotactic activity produced (36). Human peritoneal mesothelial cells also express IL-8 as well as monocyte chemotactic protein 1 (MCP-1) (38).

The possibility exists that asbestos or cytokine exposure might induce production of other growth factors in NHM cells. Antony et al. have recently reported that rat pleural mesothelial cells produce a PDGF-like activity that can be neutralized by anti-PDGF IgG (32). This induction by asbestos exposure has been observed in NHM cells (25) and suggests a partial mechanism for mesothelial regeneration after injury. Normal human mesothelial cells contain both $\alpha$- and $\beta$-PDGF receptors (PDGFR) (44).

## IV. Growth Factor Production and Responsiveness of Mesothelioma Cell Lines

The breadth of mitogenic responsiveness shown by NHM cells when coupled with their expected exposure to cytokines expressed by activated macrophages suggested that paracrine factors might provide a mitogenic stimulus for these cells, promoting the eventual selection of clones that had accumulated sufficient alterations to achieve growth factor-independence or tumorigenic conversion. Investigators have established that medium conditioned by mesotheliomas contains growth stimulating activities. Donna and co-workers have shown that the 200-kDa protein isolated from mesothelioma effusions is mitogenic for mesotheliomas, as well as NHM cells (33). Autocrine activity, which was not PDGF, TGF-$\beta$, or EGF, was observed in conditioned medium from the mesothelioma line ZL5 (45), and mitogenic activity for mesothelioma cells was observed in media conditioned by six other mesothelioma cell lines (42).

Many known growth factors and cytokines have been detected in mesothelioma cell lines and conditioned medium. The TGF-$\beta$1 protein and mRNA are produced by mesothelioma cell lines that express TGF-$\beta$ receptors, but there is no evidence for greater than normal expression of the growth factor(s) or activation of the latent form in tumorigenic cells (33). The production of both PDGF-A and PDGF-B mRNA in human mesotheliomas has been demonstrated (33,39), and PDGF A-chain protein has been detected in medium conditioned by mesothelioma cell lines (46). In addition, the nontumorigenic, but immortalized, human mesothelial cell line, MeT-5A (21) was converted to tumorigenicity after transfection with a PDGF A-chain vector (46). The mechanism of this conversion cannot be a simple autocrine stimulation by the secreted AA homodimer, since the expression of $\alpha$-PDGFR, which is the major PDGFR species in NHM cells, was not detected in mesotheliomas (44), except by RNase protection assays (47). However, antisense oligonucleotides for PDGF A-chain, but not for B-chain, inhibited the growth of mesothelioma cell lines, but not of MeT-5A cells (47). Interestingly, MeT-5A cells also become tumorigenic after transfection with EJ-*ras* (48), but Northern analysis shows that they do not express PDGF-A mRNA (46). This finding is especially interesting, since transfection of the same *ras* vector into the longlived human mesothelial cell line, LP-9, produced EGF-independent cells that were not tumorigenic (30). Furthermore, in agreement with the suggestions of Donna et al. concerning the pluripotent nature of mesothelial cells (49), the *ras*-transfected MeT-5A cells induced epithelial tumors in athymic nude mice, whereas the PDGF-A-transfected cells induced spindeloid tumors (Fig. 1). This finding indicates that a single mesothelial cell clone can produce tumors of the common pathological types and suggests that mixed morphology tumors may be nonclonal. These findings are in agreement with the report of Cardiff et al. (50) showing that characteristic histopathology of tumors could be predicted from the oncogene, the effects of which generated the tumor. In addition to the "competence" effects of PDGF (51), the production of the "progression" growth factor IGF-1 and IGFBP-3 have been demonstrated in mesotheliomas as well as NHM cells (27). These findings predict an increased hyaluronic acid synthase activity, based on the activation seen in normal mesothelial cells (40,41; Lee TC, personal communication).

Hematopoietic growth factor production by mesothelioma cells has been documented. Demetri and co-workers (34) showed that all mesotheliomas as well as NHM cells produced M-CSF, whereas two of the four lines analyzed spontaneously expressed G-CSF and GM-CSF mRNA and biological activity. The JMN1B subclone of JMN cells spontaneously produced IL-1$\beta$ and IL-6 transcripts, whereas the parental JMN culture expressed

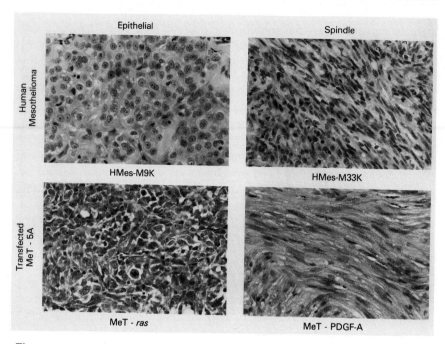

**Figure 1** Tumors induced by mesothelial cell lines.

these genes under the same conditions as NHM cells. However, Schmitter et al. found no mitogenic activity of IL-6, GM-CSF, or G-CSF for MeT-5A or mesothelioma cells (42). These authors examined medium conditioned by seven mesothelioma cell lines and MeT-5A grown in RPMI/10% FCS for colony-stimulating activity and immunoreactivity in enzyme-linked immunosorbentassay (ELISA) tests for IL-6, GM-CSF, and G-CSF. One of the seven lines secreted colony-stimulating activity that correlated with production of both GM-CSF and G-CSF, whereas all seven produced IL-6. The MeT-5A cells produced neither CSF nor IL-6, suggesting that this production is not associated with nonactivated mesothelial cells. Thus, the growth factors produced by mesotheliomas is, at present, a complex list of factors (Table 3), which may reflect interindividual variation among progenitors or may present a pattern not readily discernible with the information now available.

**Table 3** Factors Produced by Mesotheliomas

| Factor | mRNA | Protein | Bioassay | Ref. |
|---|---|---|---|---|
| TGF-$\beta$ | + | | + | 33 |
| PDGF-A | + | + | +[a] | 33,39,46 |
| PDGF-B | + | | +[a] | 33,39 |
| IGF-1 | + | + | + | 25,27 |
| 200-kD[a] gp | | + | + | 23,24 |
| IL-1$\beta$ | + | | | 34 |
| IL-6 | + | | + | 34,42 |
| G-CSF | + | | + | 34,42 |
| GM-CSF | + | | + | 34,42 |
| M-CSF | + | | + | 34,42 |

[a]Mitogenic activity for fibroblasts inhibited by polyclonal anti-PDGF-AB heterodimer antiserum (34).

## V. Possible Cellular Interactions

Development of mesothelioma in response to asbestos exposure occurs after a long latency. Before tumor development, an exposed individual would be subject to more acute responses to fiber exposure and wounding that would involve and recruit other cell types (52,53). Thus, any discussion of growth factor involvement in mesothelial carcinogenesis must consider the products of the activated macrophages and other lung cells (54) that would be induced on asbestos exposure. Indeed, as cited earlier, activated mesothelial cells, themselves, generate the chemoattractant IL-8 (36,37), which would intensify a mesothelial cell–fibroblast–macrophage interaction (Fig. 2), and peritoneal mesothelial cells produce this protein as well as monocyte chemotactic protein-1 (MCP-1) (37). Furthermore, the production of colony-stimulating factors (22,34,36) suggests that mesothelial cells may modulate the nature of hematopoietic cells in their environment. Such interactions have been studied in a culture system that used intact membranous mesentery, which contained mast cells, some macrophages, fibroblasts, and mesothelial cells. Activation of mast cells for histamine release, resulted in an increased proliferation of fibroblasts and mesothelial cells (55). A greater effect of long asbestos fibers, compared with short fibers or silica, on stimulating fibroblast growth and collagen synthesis in the interstitium was seen in vivo, but was not found when these agents were used to treat alveolar or interstitial macrophages in vitro (56).

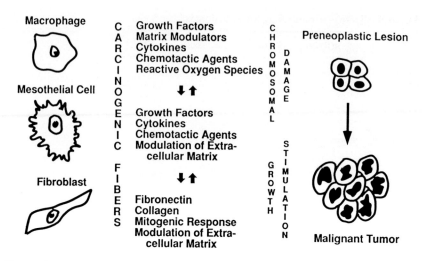

**Figure 2**   Hypothesis of multistage mesothelial cell carcinogenesis.


## VI.   Inoculation or Inhalation Studies in Animal Models

Studies, in which asbestos fibers were inoculated intraperitoneally into mice, demonstrated acute inflammatory reactions and mesothelial cell death (57) in response to crocidolite. After the acute reaction, these workers observed regeneration of the mesothelium, but retention of clusters of fibers that, although partially covered with mesothelium, were foci for macrophages and regenerating mesothelial cells. In addition, Kane and co-workers (58) have shown that weekly intraperitoneal inoculation of crocidolite, which resulted in mesothelioma after 30–50 weeks, induced capillary networks in 30% of the fiber-containing foci after 6 weeks. This result contrasted with values of 8 and 9%, respectively, for injection of nontumorigenic fibers or silica particles (58).

Studies of animals and humans after asbestos inhalation have shown the development of inflammatory lesions consisting of mixed cell types (59–63). In a study employing morphometric techniques (63) to analyze first alveolar duct bifurcations after 1 h of chrysotile inhalation, the authors found significant increases in the numbers of macrophages and epithelial cells within 2 days and, after a month, increased interstitial matrix volume with persistently high numbers of macrophages and fibroblasts. In vivo and in vitro studies show that many particulates, including asbestos, activate complement to produce chemotactic activity, stimulating an influx of macrophages (64). In addition, silica particles or asbestos fibers can induce leukotriene-B$_4$ (LTB$_4$) from macrophages (65), and alveolar macrophages collected by lavage from asbestos-exposed patients produce increased levels of this arachidonic acid lipoxygenase metabolite (66). Thus, after inhalation or inoculation, exposure to carcinogenic asbestos fibers is associated with fiber deposits that stimulate inflammatory reactions, such as those seen in patients with asbestos exposure.

### VII. Macrophage Mitogenic Activities

Macrophages found at wound sites or in inflammatory reactions are known to produce both characterized growth factors and cytokines and "activities" that may reflect combinations of factors or uncharacterized molecules involved in the inflammatory reaction and tissue repair. These have been described in numerous reports and are the subject of extensive reviews (54, 67–71). Of special interest relative to pleural mesothelioma, alveolar macrophages from patients with lung disease, associated with inhalation of inorganic dust, release elevated levels of active oxygen species (AOS) as well as fibronectin and other growth-promoting activities (72). Furthermore, macrophages from asbestos-exposed subjects showed an elevated population capable of DNA synthesis (73). Presumably, some of the growth factor activity released on asbestos exposure contributes to these findings. In addition, asbestos exposure induces rapid and persistent production of growth-stimulatory activity to which fibroblasts can respond (74).

In inhalation experiments in rats, asbestos exposure produces a mitogenic response in epithelial cells and interstitial fibroblasts (75), in the bronchiolar–alveolar regions as well as in endothelial and smooth-muscle cells of small vessels in the same loci (76). It would be expected that mesothelial cells exposed to asbestos would also be subject to the influence of these macrophage products, as well as to reactive oxygen species and products of lipid peroxidation that are generated by interaction of asbestos with macrophages and epithelial cells (8,77–81). Thus, mesothelial cells, altered by asbestos, or by the products of its cellular interactions, would be exposed to growth factors, cytokines, and AOS in a microenvironment that would be changing owing to the effects of such factors on fibroblastic, endothelial, and smooth-muscle cells in the region. Since it is clear that the microenvironment has a major role in modulating the effects of such factors on a given cell and tissue (82), an evolving environment might interact with altered cells to favor selection of those that were especially sensitive to growth-stimulatory signals. The multiplicity of factors that modulate human mesothelial cell growth (16) suggests that they would provide a responsive target for such effectors.

## VIII.   Induction of Specific Growth Factors by Fibers

Studies on the interaction of asbestos fibers with macrophages have demonstrated the induction of factors that stimulate the growth of human mesothelial cells. Asbestos exposure is only one of many stimuli that induce macrophages to produce such activities. When mRNA from adherent cells, isolated from subepidermal wound cylinders, was studied by reverse transcription and PCR amplification, transcripts for TGF-$\alpha$, TGF-$\beta$, PDGF-A, EGF, and IGF-1 were detected consistently, and IL-1$\alpha$ was frequently found (83). Macrophages stimulated with LPS in vitro produced and secreted TGF-$\alpha$, PDGF, TGF-$\beta$, and basic FGF (83). The constitutive production of TGF-$\beta$ observed would provide a chemotactic stimulus for monocytes, dependent on its degree of activation. Also, TGF-$\beta$ has been implicated in induction of TNF-$\alpha$ from monocytes (84) and of PDGF from epithelial cells (85). All of these growth factors are mitogenic for human mesothelial cells in vitro (15,16,19; Lee TC, personal communication). It has been directly shown that alveolar macrophages, activated by chrysotile, secrete IGF-1 (86), and that chrysotile can stimulate IGF-1 expression in bone marrow-derived macrophages (87). Furthermore, this factor should provide autocrine stimulation of activated alveolar macrophages that, in contrast with unstimulated cells or those isolated from disease-free individuals, showed expression of the IGF-1 receptor or specific binding of the growth factor (88).

The production of PDGF activity and expression of PDGF mRNAs have been documented in human alveolar macrophages from both normal persons and from those with interstitial lung diseases (89). Activation of macrophages by various stimuli (88) both increases the amount of activity produced and the steady-state level of mRNAs for the A- and B-chain genes. Interestingly, LPS activation stimulates the transcription of both genes threefold, without altering the 10 : 1 ratio of B/A chains observed in unstimulated cells. This in vitro activation reproduces the levels of these genes expressed by macrophages from persons with interstitial lung disease (90). Particulate exposure of macrophages induces PDGF expression. Carbonyl iron spheres or chrysotile asbestos fibers induce production of a PDGF-type molecule by rat alveolar macrophages when treated in vitro (91) or when studied after inhalation exposure (92). The increment in PDGF secretion at optimal induction was dependent on both the time and dose of exposure to iron or asbestos, and induction was at least tenfold. In the rat system, it was observed that most secreted PDGF activity was bound to $\alpha_2$-macroglobulin (93). Thus, direct evidence indicates that exposure to asbestos and other particulates will induce production of PDGF.

## IX. Summary

Asbestos fibers are able to act as a complete carcinogen in the development of mesothelioma. In the two-stage model of carcinogenesis, this implies that they supply both initiation and promotion function, causing initial mutations and, then, stimulating the growth of altered cells. The mutagenic potential of fibers has been demonstrated directly in an assay designed to detect large deletions and rearrangements (14), and indirect damage could well be mediated through the AOS generated by the fibers (94).

It is now understood that the two-stage model represents a process in which genetic and epigenetic changes accumulate until a cell is sufficiently altered to be considered "malignant" (2). In most tumor types, alterations have been defined, which include the gain of oncogenic function and the loss of regulatory, tumor suppressor function. Although *p53* mutations have been described in mesothelioma cell lines (95,96), they could not be considered characteristic of the disease as is loss of the *Rb* gene for retinoblastoma. Furthermore, recent studies find normal Rb protein and mRNA expression in 20 mesothelioma cell lines surveyed (97). Thus, it can be expected that loss of function associated with other tumor suppressor genes may also be associated with development of mesothelioma. Changes involving gain of oncogenic function in lung cancer have often included mutations in K-*ras* (98–101), but no mutations at codons 12, 13, or 61 were found in 20 mesothelioma cell lines studied (96).

In this context, the presence of paracrine stimulation is a growth-promoting alteration. The presence of asbestos fibers might be considered to provide a chronic inflammatory stimulus, resulting in an environment providing constant paracrine growth signals through growth factor production by macrophages. Such an environment might eventually result in "inappropriate expression" (3) of growth factors and receptors in mesothelial cells. This category of molecules constitutes a class of oncogenes associated with tumorigenesis when disregulated (102–105). In mesothelioma, overexpression of PDGF species has been associated with tumor cell lines (33,39) as well as changes in the ratio of $\beta$- to $\alpha$-PDGF receptors from normal mesothelial cells that primarily express the $\alpha$-PDGFR, to mesotheliomas in which the $\beta$-, but not the $\alpha$-PDGFR, is detectable by Northern or immunoprecipitation analysis (44). It is known that the different isoforms of PDGF have different consequences and expression patterns in biological systems (106–111), and this altered expression pattern in mesotheliomas may be a clue to the carcinogenic pathway of this disease. It is probable that the effects of growth factors may be cell-type or environment-specific (67) and that multiple factors will interact. Indeed, whereas in some systems TGF-$\beta$

induces PDGF expression (85), in others, PDGF induces the expression of TGF-$\beta$ (112). Clearly, the situation is complex and can be expected to evade generalization. It has already been demonstrated that normal mesothelial cells can produce growth stimulators, chemotactic agents, and molecules involved in hematopoietic growth regulation. It is hoped that the rapidly increasing amount of information concerning growth factor and receptor production and function in normal and diseased states will help clarify the pathogenesis and perhaps lead to treatment of the asbestos-produced diseases.

### Acknowledgments

It is the author's pleasure to acknowledge the critical reading and helpful suggestions of Dr. John F. Lechner and Dr. Curtis C. Harris. The encouragement and support of the Laboratory of Human Carcinogenesis has been crucial for these studies. In addition, the expert editorial and graphic talents of Ms. Dorothea Dudek are greatly appreciated.

### References

1. Harris CC. Chemical and physical carcinogenesis: advances and perspectives. Cancer Res 1991; 51:5023s–5044s.
2. Fearon ER, Vogelstein B. A genetic model for colorectal tumorigenesis. Cell 1990; 61:759–767.
3. Antoniades HN. Linking cellular injury to gene expression and human proliferative disorders: examples with the PDGF genes. Mol Carcinog 1992; 6: 175–181.
4. Wagner JC, Sleggs CA, Marchand P. Diffuse pleural mesothelioma and asbestos exposure in the North Western Cape Province. Br J Ind Med 1960; 17:260–271.
5. Craighead JE, Mossman BT. The pathogenesis of asbestos-associated diseases. N Engl J Med 1982; 306:1446–1455.
6. Jackson JH, Schraufstatter IU, Hyslop PA, Vosbeck K, Sauerheber R, Weitzman SA, Cochrane CG. Role of oxidants in DNA damage. Hydroxyl radical mediates the synergistic DNA damaging effects of asbestos and cigarette smoke. J Clin Invest 1987; 80:1090–1095.
7. Libbus BL, Illenye SA, Craighead JE. Induction of DNA strand breaks in cultured rat embryo cells by crocidolite asbestos as assessed by nick translation. Cancer Res 1989; 49:5713–5718.
8. Mossman BT, Marsh JP. Evidence supporting a role for active oxygen species in asbestos-induced toxicity and lung disease. Environ Health Perspect 1989; 81:91–94.
9. Wang NS, Jaurand MC, Magne L, Kheuang L, Pinchon MC, Bignon J.

The interactions between asbestos fibers and metaphase chromosomes of rat pleural mesothelial cells in culture. A scanning and transmission electron microscopic study. Am J Pathol 1987; 126:343–349.

10. Haugen A, Schafer PW, Lechner JF, Stoner GD, Trump BF, Harris CC. Cellular ingestion, toxic effects, and lesions observed in human bronchial epithelial tissue and cells cultured with asbestos and glass fibers. Int J Cancer 1982; 30:265–272.

11. Ruttner JR, Lang AB, Gut DR, Wydler MU. Morphological aspects of interactions between asbestos fibers and human mesothelial cell cytoskeleton. Exp Cell Biol 1987; 55:285–294.

12. Somers ANA, Mason EA, Gerwin BI, Harris CC, Lechner JF. Effects of amosite asbestos fibers on the filaments present in the cytoskeleton of primary human mesothelial cells. In: Brown RC, et al., eds. Mechanisms in fibre carcinogenesis. New York: Plenum Press, 1991:481–490.

13. Cole RW, Ault JG, Hayden JH, Reider CL. Crocidolite asbestos fibers undergo size-dependent microtubule-mediated transport after endocytosis in vertebrate lung epithelial cells. Cancer Res 1991; 51:4942–4947.

14. Hei TK, Piao CQ, He ZY, Vannais D, Waldren CA. Chrysotile fiber is a strong mutagen in mammalian cells. Cancer Res 1992; 52:6305–6309.

15. Connell ND, Rheinwald JG. Regulation of the cytoskeleton of mesothelial cells: reversible loss of keratin and increase of vimentin during rapid growth in culture. Cell 1983; 34:245–253.

16. LaVeck MA, Somers ANA, Moore LL, Gerwin BI, Lechner JF. Dissimilar peptide growth factors can induce normal human mesothelial cell multiplication. In Vitro 1988; 24:1077–1084.

17. LaRocca PJ, Rheinwald JG. Anchorage-independent growth of normal human mesothelial cells: a sensitive bioassay for EGF which discloses the absence of this factor in fetal calf serum. In Vitro 1985; 21:67–72.

18. Lechner JF, Haugen A, McClendon IA, Pettis EW. Clonal growth of normal adult human bronchial epithelial cells in a serum-free medium. In Vitro 1982; 18:633–642.

19. Gabrielson EW, Gerwin BI, Harris CC, Roberts AB, Sporn MB, Lechner JF. Stimulation of DNA synthesis in cultured primary human mesothelial cells by specific growth factors. FASEB J 1988; 2:2717–2722.

20. Lechner JF, LaVeck MA, Gerwin BI, Matis EA. Differential responses to growth factors by normal human mesothelial cultures from individual donors. J Cell Physiol 1989; 139:295–300.

21. Ke Y, Reddel RR, Gerwin BI, Reddel HK, Somers ANA, McMenamin MG, LaVeck MA, Stahel R, Lechner JF, Harris CC. Establishment of a human in vitro mesothelial cell model system for investigating mechanisms of asbestos-induced mesothelioma. Am J Pathol 1989; 134:979–991.

22. Lanfrancone L, Boraschi D, Ghiara P, Falini B, Grignani F, Peri G, Mantovani A, Pelicci PG. Human peritoneal mesothelial cells produce many cytokines (granulocyte colony-stimulating factor [CSF], granulocyte monocyte-CSF, macrophage-CSF, interleukin-1 [IL-1], and IL-6) and are activated and stimulated to grow by IL-1. Blood 1992; 80:2835–2842.

23.  Donna A, Betta PG, Cosimi MF, Robutti F, Bellingeri D, Marchesini A. Putative mesothelial cell growth-promoting activity of a cytoplasmic protein expressed by the mesothelial cell. A preliminary report. Exp Cell Biol 1989; 57:193–197.

24.  Donna A, Betta PG, Ribotta M, Maran E, Mazzucco G, Mollo F, Bellingeri D, Libener R. Mitogenic effects of a mesothelial cell growth factor: evidence for a potential autocrine regulation of normal and malignant mesothelial cell proliferation. Int J Exp Pathol 1992; 73:193–202.

25.  Lee TC, Jagirdar J, Guillemin B, Zhang Y, Rom WN. Insulin-like growth factor gene expression by normal and malignant human mesothelial cells [abstr]. Am Rev Respir Dis 1992; 145:A124.

26.  Van der Meeren A, Levy F, Renier A, Katz A, Jaurand MC. Effect of epidermal growth factor on rat pleural mesothelial cell growth. J Cell Physiol 1990; 144:137–143.

27.  Lee TC et al. Cancer Res 1993; 53:2858–2864.

28.  Wilson AP. Mesothelial cells stimulate the anchorage-independent growth of human ovarian tumour cells. Br J Cancer 1989; 59:876–882.

29.  Breborowicz A, Rodela H, Pagiamtzis J, Oreopoulos DG. Stimulation of mesothelial cells proliferation by endogenous growth factor(s). Peritoneal Dial Int 1991; 11:228–232.

30.  Tubo RA, Rheinwald JG. Normal human mesothelial cells and fibroblasts transfected with the EJras oncogene become EGF-independent, but are not malignantly transformed. Oncogene Res 1987; 1:407–421.

31.  Kim KH, Stellmach V, Javors J, Fuchs E. Regulation of human mesothelial cell differentiation: opposing roles of retinoids and epidermal growth factor in the expression of intermediate filament proteins. J Cell Biol 1987; 105:3039–3051.

32.  Antony VB, Godbey SW, Sparks JA, Hott JW. Pleural mesothelial cells release a growth factor for fibroblasts. Eur Respir Rev 1993; 3:156–158.

33.  Gerwin BI, Lechner JF, Reddel RR, Roberts AB, Robbins KC, Gabrielson EW, Harris CC. Comparison of production of transforming growth factor-beta and platelet-derived growth factor by normal human mesothelial cells and mesothelioma cell lines. Cancer Res 1987; 47:6180–6184.

34.  Demetri GD, Zenzie BW, Rheinwald JG, Griffin JD. Expression of colony-stimulating factor genes by normal human mesothelial cells and human malignant mesothelioma cells lines in vitro. Blood 1989; 74:940–946.

35.  Antony VB, Owen CL, Hadley KJ. Pleural mesothelial cells stimulated by asbestos release chemotactic activity for neutrophils in vitro. Am Rev Respir Dis 1989; 139:199–206.

36.  Goodman RB, Wood RG, Martin TR, Hanson-Painton O, Kinasewitz GT. Cytokine-stimulated human mesothelial cells produce chemotactic activity for neutrophils including NAP-1/IL-8. J Immunol 1992; 148:457–465.

37.  Boylan AM, Ruegg C, Kim KJ, Hebert CA, Hoeffel JM, Pytela R, Sheppard D, Goldstein IM, Broaddus VC. Evidence of a role for mesothelial cell-derived interleukin 8 in the pathogenesis of asbestos-induced pleurisy in rabbits. J Clin Invest 1992; 89:1257–1267.

38. Jonjic N, Peri G, Bernasconi S, Sciacca FL, Colotta F, Pelicci P, Lanfrancone L, Mantovani A. Expression of adhesion molecules and chemotactic cytokines in cultured human mesothelial cells. J Exp Med 1992; 176:1165–1174.

39. Versnel MA, Hagemeijer A, Bouts MJ, van der Kwast TH, Hoogsteden HC. Expression of c-*sis* (PDGF B-chain) and PDGF A-chain genes in ten human malignant mesothelioma cell lines derived from primary and metastatic tumors. Oncogene 1988; 2:601–605.

40. Heldin P, Asplund T, Ytterberg D, Thelin S, Laurent TC. Characterization of the molecular mechanism involved in the activation of hyaluronan synthetase by platelet-derived growth factor in human mesothelial cells. Biochem J 1992; 283:165–170.

41. Honda A, Noguchi N, Takehara H, Ohashi Y, Asuwa N, Mori Y. Cooperative enhancement of hyaluronic acid synthesis by combined use of IGF-I and EGF, and inhibition by tyrosine kinase inhibitor genistein, in cultured mesothelial cells from rabbit pericardial cavity. J Cell Sci 1991; 98:91–98.

42. Schmitter D, Lauber B, Fagg B, Stahel RA. Hematopoietic growth factors secreted by seven human pleural mesothelioma cell lines: interleukin-6 production as a common feature. Int J Cancer 1992; 51:296–301.

43. Shore BL, Daughaday CC, Spilberg I. Benign asbestos pleurisy in the rabbit. A model for the study of pathogenesis. Am Rev Respir Dis 1983; 128:481–485.

44. Versnel MA, Claesson-Welsh L, Hammacher A, Bouts MJ, van der Kwast TH, Eriksson A, Willemsen R, Weima SM, Hoogsteden HC, Hagemeijer A, et al. Human malignant mesothelioma cell lines express PDGF beta-receptors whereas cultured normal mesothelial cells express predominantly PDGF alpha receptors. Oncogene 1991; 6:2005–2011.

45. Lauber B, Leuthold M, Schmitter D, Cano-Santos J, Waibel R, Stahel RA. An autocrine mitogenic activity produced by a pleural human mesothelioma cell line. Int J Cancer 1992; 50:943–950.

46. Van der Meeren A, Seddon MB, Betsholtz CA, Lechner JF, Gerwin BI. Tumorigenic conversion of human mesothelial cells as a consequence of platelet-derived growth factor-A chain overexpression. Am J Respir Cell Mol Biol 1993; 8:214–221.

47. Garlepp MJ, Christmas TI, Manning LS, Mutsaers SE, Dench J, Leong C, Robinson BWS. The role of platelet-derived growth factor in the growth of human malignant mesothelioma. Eur Respir Rev 1993; 3:189–191.

48. Reddel RR, Malan-Shibley L, Gerwin BI, Metcalf R, Harris CC. Tumorigenicity of a human mesothelial cell line transfected with the EJ-*ras* oncogene. JNCI 1989; 81:945–948.

49. Donna A, Betta PG, Bianchi V, Ribotta M, Bellingeri D, Robutti F, Marchesini A. A new insight into the histogenesis of 'mesodermomas' — malignant mesotheliomas. Histopathology 1991; 19:239–244.

50. Cardiff RD, Sinn E, Muller W, Leder P. Transgenic oncogene mice. Tumor phenotype predicts genotype. Am J Pathol 1991; 139:495–501.

51. Pledger WJ, Stiles CD, Antoniades HN, Scher CD. Induction of DNA synthesis in BALB/c 3T3 cells by serum components: reevaluation of the commitment process. Proc Natl Acad Sci USA 1977; 74:4481–4485.

52. Rom WN, Travis WD, Brody AR. Cellular and molecular basis of the asbestos-related diseases [see comments]. Am Rev Respir Dis 1991; 143:408–422.

53. Mantovani A, Bottazzi B, Colotta F, Sozzani S, Ruco L. The origin and function of tumor-associated macrophages. Immunol Today 1992; 13:265–270.

54. Kelley J. Cytokines of the lung [see comments]. Am Rev Respir Dis 1990; 141:765–788.

55. Druvefors P, Norrby K. Molecular aspects of mast-cell-mediated mitogenesis in fibroblasts and mesothelial cells in situ. Virchows Arch [B] 1988; 55:187–192.

56. Adamson IY, Letourneau HL, Bowden DH. Comparison of alveolar and interstitial macrophages in fibroblast stimulation after silica and long or short asbestos. Lab Invest 1991; 64:339–344.

57. Moalli PA, MacDonald JL, Goodglick LA, Kane AB. Acute injury and regeneration of the mesothelium in response to asbestos fibers. Am J Pathol 1987; 128:426–445.

58. Branchaud RM, MacDonald JL, Kane AB. Induction of angiogenesis by intraperitoneal injection of asbestos fibers. FASEB J 1989; 3:1747–1752.

59. Wagner JC. The sequelae of exposure to asbestos dust. Ann NY Acad Sci 1965; 132:691–697.

60. Wagner JC, Berry G, Skidmore JW, Timbrell V. The effects of the inhalation of asbestos in rats. Br J Cancer 1974; 29:252–269.

61. Craighead JE, Abraham JL, Churg A, Green FH, Kleinerman J, Pratt PC, Seemayer TA, Vallyathan V, Weill H. The pathology of asbestos associated diseases of the lungs and pleural cavities: diagnostic criteria and proposed grading schema. Report of the Pneumoconiosis Committee of the College of American Pathologists and the National Institute for Occupational Safety and Health. Arch Pathol Lab Med 1982; 106:544–596.

62. Begin R, Rola-Pleszczynski M, Masse S, Lemaire I, Sirois P, Boctor M, Nadeau D, Drapeau G, Bureau MA. Asbestos-induced lung injury in the sheep model: the initial alveolitis. Environ Res 1983; 30:195–210.

63. Chang LY, Overby LH, Brody AR, Crapo JD. Progressive lung cell reactions and extracellular matrix production after a brief exposure to asbestos. Am J Pathol 1988; 131:156–170.

64. Warheit DB, Overby LH, George G, Brody AR. Pulmonary macrophages are attracted to inhaled particles through complement activation. Exp Lung Res 1988; 14:51–66.

65. Dubois CM, Bissonnette E, Rola-Pleszczynski M. Asbestos fibers and silica particles stimulate rat alveolar macrophages to release tumor necrosis factor. Autoregulatory role of leukotriene B$_4$. Am Rev Respir Dis 1989; 139:1257–1264.

66. Garcia JG, Griffith DE, Cohen AB, Callahan KS. Alveolar macrophages from patients with asbestos exposure release increased levels of leukotriene B$_4$. Am Rev Respir Dis 1989; 139:1494–1501.

67. Nathan CF. Secretory products of macrophages. J Clin Invest 1987; 79:319–326.

68. Knighton DR, Fiegel VD. Macrophage-derived growth factors in wound heal-

ing: regulation of growth factor production by the oxygen microenvironment. Am Rev Respir Dis 1989; 140:1108–1111.

69. Brandes ME, Finkelstein JN. The production of alveolar macrophage-derived growth-regulating proteins in response to lung injury [discussion]. Toxicol Lett 1990; 54:3–22.

70. Cromack DT, Porras-Reyes B, Mustoe TA. Current concepts in wound healing: growth factor and macrophage interaction. J Trauma 1990; 30:S129–S133.

71. Sunderkotter C, Goebeler M, Schulze-Osthoff K, Bhardwaj R, Sorg C. Macrophage-derived angiogenesis factors. Pharmacol Ther 1991; 51:195–216.

72. Rom WN, Bitterman PB, Rennard SI, Cantin A, Crystal RG. Characterization of the lower respiratory tract inflammation of nonsmoking individuals with interstitial lung disease associated with chronic inhalation of inorganic dusts. Am Rev Respir Dis 1987; 136:1429–1434.

73. Spurzem JR, Saltini C, Rom W, Winchester RJ, Crystal RG. Mechanisms of macrophage accumulation in the lungs of asbestos-exposed subjects. Am Rev Respir Dis 1987; 136:276–280.

74. Lemaire I, Beaudoin H, Masse S, Grondin C. Alveolar macrophage stimulation of lung fibroblast growth in asbestos-induced pulmonary fibrosis. Am J Pathol 1986; 122:205–211.

75. Brody AR, Overby LH. Incorporation of tritiated thymidine by epithelial and interstitial cells in bronchiolar–alveolar regions of asbestos exposed rats. Am J Pathol 1989; 134:133–140.

76. McGavran PD, Moore LB, Brody AR. Inhalation of chrysotile asbestos induces rapid cellular proliferation in small pulmonary vessels of mice and rats. Am J Pathol 1990; 136:695–705.

77. Mossman BT, Landesman JM. Importance of oxygen free radicals in asbestos-induced injury to airway epithelial cells. Chest 1983; 83:50S–51S.

78. Kouzan S, Brody AR, Nettesheim P, Eling T. Production of arachidonic acid metabolites by macrophages exposed in vitro to asbestos, carbonyl iron particles, or calcium ionophore. Am Rev Respir Dis 1985; 131:624–632.

79. Goodglick LA, Kane AB. Role of reactive oxygen metabolites in crocidolite asbestos toxicity to mouse macrophages. Cancer Res 1986; 46:5558–5566.

80. Goodglick LA, Pietras LA, Kane AB. Evaluation of the causal relationship between crocidolite asbestos-induced lipid peroxidation and toxicity to macrophages. Am Rev Respir Dis 1989; 139:1265–1273.

81. Kamp DW, Graceffa P, Pryor WA, Weitzman SA. The role of free radicals in asbestos-induced diseases. Free Radical Biol Med 1992; 12:293–315.

82. Nathan C, Spron M. Cytokines in context. J Cell Biol 1991; 113:981–986.

83. Rappolee DA, Mark D, Banda MJ, Werb Z. Wound macrophages express TGF-alpha and other growth factors in vivo: analysis by mRNA phenotyping. Science 1988; 241:708–712.

84. Wiseman DM, Polverini PJ, Kamp DW, Leibovich SJ. Transforming growth factor-beta (TGF beta) is chemotactic for human monocytes and induces their expression of angiogenic activity. Biochem Biophys Res Commun 1988; 157:793–800.

85. Leof EB, Proper JA, Goustin AS, Shipley GD, DiCorleto PE, Moses HL. Induction of c-*sis* nRNA and activity similar to platelet-derived growth factor by transforming growth factor beta: a proposed model for indirect mitogenesis involving autocrine activity. Proc Natl Acad Sci USA 1986; 83:2453–2457.

86. Rom WN, Basset P, Fells GA, Nukiwa T, Trapnell BC, Crysal RG. Alveolar macrophages release an insulin-like growth factor I-type molecule. J Clin Invest 1988; 82:1685–1693.

87. Noble PW, Henson PM, Riches DW. Insulin-like growth factor-1 (IGF1) mRNA expression in bone marrow derived macrophages is stimulated by chrysotile asbestos and bleomycin. A potential marker for a reparative macrophage phenotype. Chest 1991; 99:79S–80S.

88. Rom WN, Paakko P. Activated alveolar macrophages express the insulinlike growth factor-I receptor. Am J Respir Cell Mol Biol 1991; 4:432–439.

89. Mornex JF, Martinet Y, Yamauchi K, Bitterman PB, Grotendorst GR, Chytil-Weir A, Martin GR, Crystal RG. Spontaneous expression of the c-*sis* gene and release of a platelet-derived growth factorlike molecule by human alveolar macrophages. J Clin Invest 1986; 78:61–66.

90. Nagaoka I, Trapnell BC, Crystal RG. Upregulation of platelet derived growth factor-A and -B gene expression in alveolar macrophages of individuals with idiopathic pulmonary fibrosis. J Clin Invest 1990; 85:2023–2027.

91. Bauman MD, Jetten AM, Bonner JC, Kumar RK, Bennett RA, Brody AR. Secretion of a platelet-derived growth factor homologue by rat alveolar macrophages exposed to particulates in vitro. Eur J Cell Biol 1990; 51:327–334.

92. Bonner JC, Brody AR. Asbestos-induced alveolar injury. Evidence for macrophage-derived PDGF as a mediator of the fibrogenic response. Chest 1991; 99:54S–55S.

93. Schapira RM, Osornio-Vargas AR, Brody AR. Inorganic particles induce secretion of a macrophage homologue of platelet-derived growth factor in a density-and-time-dependent manner in vitro. Exp Lung Res 1991; 17:1011–1024.

94. Mossman BT, Bignon J, Corn M, Seaton A, Gee JB. Asbestos: scientific developments and implications for public policy. Science 1990; 247:294–301.

95. Cote RJ, Jhanwar SC, Novick S, Pellicer A. Genetic alterations of the *p53* gene are a feature of malignant mesotheliomas. Cancer Res 1991; 51:5410–5416.

96. Metcalf RA, Welsh JA, Bennett WP, Seddon MB, Lehman TA, Pelin K, Linnainmaa K, Tammilehto L, Mattson K, Gerwin BI, Harris CC. *p53* and Kirsten-*ras* mutations in human mesothelioma cell lines. Cancer Res 1992; 52:2610–2615.

97. Van der Meeren A, Kispert J, Seddon MB, Linnainmaa K, Mattson K, Gerwin BI. Retinoblastoma gene expression in human mesothelioma cell lines. Eur Respir Rev 1993 (in press).

98. Almoguera C, Forrester K, Winter E, Lama C, Perucho M. Activated *ras* genes in pulmonary carcinoma. Lung Cancer 1988; 4:168–170.

99. Rodenhuis S, Slebos RJ, Boot AJ, Evers SG, Mooi WJ, Wagenaar SS, van

Bodegom PC, Bos JL. Incidence and possible clinical significance of K-*ras* oncogene activation in adenocarcinoma of the human lung. Cancer Res 1988; 48:5738–5741.

100. Bos JL. *ras* oncogenes in human cancer: a review. Cancer Res 1989; 49:4682–4689.

101. Kobayashi T, Tsuda H, Noguchi M, Hirohashi S, Shimosato Y, Goya T, Hayata Y. Association of point mutation in c-Ki-*ras* oncogene in lung adenocarcinoma with particular reference to cytologic subtypes. Cancer 1990; 66: 289–294.

102. Doolittle RF, Hunkapiller MW, Hood LE, Devare SG, Robbins KC, Aaronson SA, Antoniades HN. Simian sarcoma virus *onc* gene, v-*sis*, is derived from the gene (or genes) encoding a platelet-derived growth factor. Science 1983; 221:275–277.

103. Downward J, Yarden Y, Mayes E, Scrace G, Totty N, Stockwell P, Ullrich A, Schlessinger J, Waterfield MD. Close similarity of epidermal growth factor receptor and v-*erb*-B oncogene protein sequences. Nature 1984; 307:521–527.

104. Sherr CJ, Rettenmier CW, Sacca R, Roussel MF, Look AT, Stanley ER. The c-*fms* proto-oncogene product is related to the receptor for the mononuclear phagocyte growth factor, CSF-1. Cell 1985; 41:665–676.

105. Masuda A, Kizaka-Kondoh S, Miwatani H, Terada Y, Nojima H, Okayama H. Signal transduction cascade shared by epidermal growth factor and platelet-derived growth factor is a major pathway for oncogenic transformation in NRK cells. New Biol 1992; 4:489–503.

106. Gronwald RG, Seifert RA, Bowen-Pope DF. Differential regulation of expression of two platelet-derived growth factor receptor subunits by transforming growth factor-beta. J Biol Chem 1989; 264:8120–8125.

107. Mercola M, Wang CY, Kelly J, Brownlee C, Jackson-Grusby L, Stiles C, Bowen-Pope D. Selective expression of PDGF A and its receptor during early mouse embryogenesis. Dev Biol 1990; 138:114–122.

108. Siegbahn A, Hammacher A, Westermark B, Heldin CH. Differential effects of the various isoforms of platelet-derived growth factor on chemotaxis of fibroblasts, monocytes, and granulocytes. J Clin Invest 1990; 85:916–920.

109. Olashaw NE, Kusmik W, Daniel TO, Pledger WJ. Biochemical and functional discrimination of platelet-derived growth factor alpha and beta receptors in BALB/c-3T3 cells. J Biol Chem 1991; 266:10234–10240.

110. Eriksson A, Rorsman C, Ernlund A, Claesson-Welsh L, Heldin CH. Ligand-induced homo- and hetero-dimerization of platelet-derived growth factor alpha- and beta-receptors in intact cells. Growth Factors 1992; 6:1–14.

111. Eriksson A, Siegbahn A, Westermark B, Heldin CH, Claesson-Welsh L. PDGF alpha- and beta-receptors activate unique and common signal transduction pathways. EMBO J 1992; 11:543–550.

112. Pierce GF, Mustoe TA, Lingelbach J, Masakowski VR, Gramates P, Deuel TF. Transforming growth factor beta reverses the glucocorticoid induced wound-healing deficit in rats: possible regulation in macrophages by platelet-derived growth factor. Proc Natl Acad Sci USA 1989; 86:2229–2233.

# 13

## Chromosomal Abnormalities in Human Malignant Mesothelioma

**SAKARI KNUUTILA**

University of Helsinki
Helsinki, Finland

**K. MATTSON**

Helsinki University Central Hospital
Helsinki, Finland

**L. TAMMILEHTO**

The Finnish Institute of Occupational
 Health
Helsinki, Finland

## I. Introduction

After the introduction of chromosome-banding techniques some 20 years ago, the possibility arose of using chromosomal study to facilitate diagnosis and prognosis and to help understanding the biology of neoplasms. Today, there is no doubt about the benefits of chromosomal study in assessing leukemias and lymphomas, as well as several solid tumors (1). We present findings that illustrate the clinical and biological significance of chromosomal study in mesothelioma.

## II. Description of Chromosomal Abnormalities in Human Malignant Mesothelioma

### A. All Patients with Mesothelioma Have Chromosomal Abnormalities

A large proportion of patients whose cases have been described in the literature (2–12) have had clonal chromosomal abnormalities (Table 1). In fact, we are inclined to believe that all of these patients would have had a

**Table 1** Karyotypes of Patients with Mesothelioma. Compilation from the Literature

| No. of patients | Source of specimen | No. of patients with clonal abnormality | bp −1 | bp 1p11-12 | bp 3p− | −4 | +5 | −6 | +7 | −9 | 9p− | +11 | +12 | −14 | −15 | −18 | −19 | +20 | −22 | Ref. |
|---|---|---|---|---|---|---|---|---|---|---|---|---|---|---|---|---|---|---|---|---|
| 38 | T/PF | 25 | + |  | + | + | + | + | + | + | + | + | + | + | + |  |  |  | + | 2,3 |
| 40 | PF/T | 30 | + | + | + | + | + | + | + | + | + | + | + | + |  |  |  | + | + | 4 |
| 5 | T | 4 | + | + | + |  |  |  |  |  |  |  |  |  |  | + | + |  | + | 5 |
| 9 | PF/T/CL | 7 | + | + | + |  |  | + | + |  |  |  |  |  |  |  |  |  |  | 6 |
| 1 | PF | 1 |  |  |  |  |  |  | + |  |  |  |  |  |  |  |  |  |  | 7 |
| 2 | PF | 2 |  |  |  |  |  |  |  |  |  |  |  | + |  |  |  |  | + | 8 |
| 14 | PF/T | 9 | +? |  |  |  |  |  |  |  | + |  |  |  |  |  |  |  | + | 9 |
| 2 | PF | 2 |  |  |  |  |  |  |  |  |  |  |  | + |  |  |  |  | + | 10 |
| 5 | CL[b] | 5 | + | + |  |  | + | + | + | + | + | + | + |  |  |  |  |  | + | 11 |
| 1 | PF | 1 |  |  |  |  |  | + |  |  |  |  |  |  |  |  |  |  |  | 12 |

[a]On the basis of results by Tiainen and co-workers and Hagemeijer et al. these abnormalities were chosen as recurrent abnormalities. Additional recurrent abnormalities have been reported by other researchers.

[b]The cell lines were set up from specimens obtained from patients on whom the karyotype analysis was primarily performed by Tiainen and co-workers.

bp, break point; CL, cell line; PF, pleural fluid; T, tumor.

chromosomal abnormality in their neoplastic cells. The chromosomal study of mesothelioma is usually performed on cultured cells and, even in short-term cultures, there is a tendency for normal cells to overgrow the neoplastic cells. Recently, we performed an interphase cytogenetic study, using in situ hybridization with a biotinylated chromosome 7-specific probe, on uncultured tumor cells from two patients for whom no abnormality had been revealed by standard G-banding analysis of cultured tumor cells. Interphase cytogenetic analysis revealed cells with three hybridization signals, (i.e., trisomy 7, in these patients). The normal results obtained by G-banding analysis appear to have been due to overgrowth by normal cells in the cultures.

### B. None of the Chromosomal Abnormalities Are Specific to Mesothelioma

The abnormalities are usually extremely complex, even chaotic, involving both the chromosomal structure and number (2–4,13). Although the chromosomal number is most often aneuploid, great variation is seen among the cells of a single specimen. Polyploid forms of the near-diploid clone are frequent. Diplochromosomes (originating from endoreduplication) are also found, which suggests that polyploidy in mesothelioma is at least partly due to endoreduplication (2). We have also come across a combination clone, evidently produced by cell fusion (2). Polyploidy in which some, but not all, chromosomes are multiplied several times over is most probably the result of a nondisjunction type of event.

Structural chromosomal abnormalities in mesothelioma are also highly variable (see Table 1), consisting of translocations, deletions, insertions, and inversions. Double minutes and homogeneously staining regions, representing cytological manifestations of gene amplification, may occasionally be seen (2).

The most common chromosomal abnormalities reported in the mesothelioma literature are presented in Table 1. The most common numerical abnormalities are trisomies or polysomies of chromosomes 5, 7, 11, 12, and 20 and monosomies or partial monosomies of chromosomes 1, 3, 4, 6, 9, 14, 15, 18, 19, and 22. Structural abnormalities are most frequent in the short arms of chromosomes 1 and 3.

The presence of several related subclones indicates the occurrence of a process known as clonal evolution. Together with the complexity of the abnormalities, this is evidence that the malignant process has reached an advanced stage.

None of the abnormalities are specific to malignant mesothelioma (2–4,13), and the complexity of the karyotypes makes the deduction of primary chromosomal changes difficult.

### C.  Polysomy 7 and Hyperdiploid Chromosomal Number Correlates with Shorter Survival

Of the recurrent abnormalities, only polysomy 7 has prognostic significance. The number of copies of the short arm of chromosome 7 was negatively correlated with survival ($p = 0.02$) (2–4,13). The median survival of patients with hyperdiploid (>46) mean chromosomal number and diploid karyotype was 31 months ($p = 0.0007$) (14).

### D.  Coexisting Groups of Chromosomal Abnormalities

Two coexisting groups of chromosomal abnormalities could be separated in our study (3): a group of chromosomal gains accompanying polysomy 7, and a group of chromosomal losses associated with chromosome 3 or break point 1 p11-22. These correlations suggest cooperation between different oncogenes or growth factor genes, and the loss of suppressor gene activity.

## III.  Asbestos and Chromosomal Abnormalities

Structural aberrations in the short arm of chromosome 1, and loss of material in chromosomes 1 and 4, were associated with a high asbestos lung burden in our patients (3).

Various types of asbestos fibers cause numerical and structural chromosomal abnormalities in many different kinds of cultured cells (15). Asbestos appears to induce polyploidy and aneuploidy, as well as stable and unstable structural chromosomal aberrations. Of the human cell types, pleural mesothelial cells are the most sensitive (16). Compared with most other mutagenic agents, the aberrations caused by asbestos are highly variable. In addition to causing straightforward structural changes, asbestos fibers also interfere with mitotic cell division. The exact mechanisms by which asbestos fibers bring about endoreduplication, cell fusion, and nondisjunction, causing polyploidization in mesothelioma, are largely unknown. There are indications that the fibers have direct effects on cell membranes, the mitotic apparatus, chromatin, and DNA (17). The indirect influences may be mediated, at least partly, by free oxygen radicals, because asbestos fibers induce the formation of hydroxy radicals in vitro (17,18) and free radicals are known to cause chromosomal aberrations (19).

Despite their complexity, the chromosomal abnormalities in mesothelioma are not random. This leads one to ask whether the abnormalities in cell cultures exposed to asbestos are also nonrandom and, if so, whether the nonrandom abnormalities found in cell cultures and mesothelioma might not be the same. According to Olofsson and Mark (20), chromosomes 2, 4, 7, 15, 17, 19, 21, 22, and X were overpresented and add numerical abnormalities in human pleural cell cultures exposed to asbestos. Even though no distinct hot spot was seen in any chromosomal band, chromosome 1 seemed to be involved more often than the other chromosomes (20). Interestingly, a break point at 1 p11-22 is a recurring abnormality in mesothelioma and is also associated with a high asbestos fiber burden, as mentioned earlier (3). Another chromosomal segment with recurring break points in mesothelioma is the short arm of chromosome 3. This segment was not, however, affected in the Olofsson and Mark experiment (20). In studies on immortal Syrian hamster cell lines transformed by asbestos (21), six of eight cell lines studied had an extra chromosome 11, and other recurrent abnormalities were also seen. In these cells, mechanical induction of aneuploidy by asbestos may contribute to their transformation, with trisomy 11 playing an essential role in the neoplastic process.

## IV. Role of Chromosomal Abnormalities in Tumorigenesis of Mesothelioma

It is difficult to pinpoint the phase of the malignant process in mesothelioma at which the recurrent chromosomal abnormalities are produced. It is conceivable that the abnormalities caused by asbestos are preponderantly random, and that the abnormalities required for malignant transformation are selected from this pool (Fig. 1). Both the complex clonal evolution of the karyotype abnormalities, and the long latent period between asbestos exposure and the appearance of clinical mesothelioma, support the importance of chromosomal selection in mesothelioma.

It is believed that carcinogenesis requires the presence of both cellular oncogenes and suppressor genes. Thus, the large variety of chromosomal changes caused by asbestos exposure would seem to provide an excellent basis for neoplastic transformation (see Fig. 1). Figure 1 indicates which chromosomal abnormalities may be important at each step in the tumorigenesis.

## V. Importance of Early Diagnosis

In mesothelioma, diagnosis often takes place very late in the malignant process, when effective treatment is no longer possible. For improved prognosis, it is important to identify the disease at the premalignant stage (i.e., several decades earlier than it is now). Identification of specific chromo-

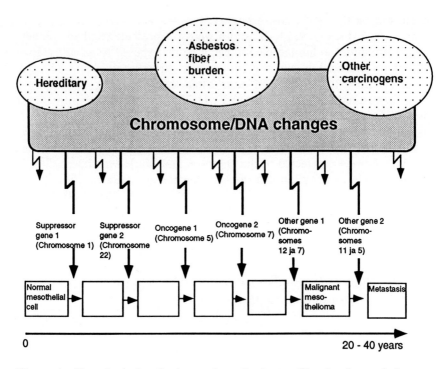

**Figure 1**  Hypothesis for the interaction of asbestos fiber burden and chromosomal abnormalities in the multistep tumorigenesis of mesothelioma. (Modified according to Ref. 22.)

somal aberrations seems to offer the possibility of early diagnosis of mesothelioma and the prediction of the development of cancer in asbestos-exposed individuals.

Standard cytogenetic methods appear to be inadequate for detecting clonal chromosomal abnormalities in asbestos-exposed persons and for predicting the development of mesothelioma. An improvement in mesothelioma diagnosis is offered by interphase cytogenetics using in situ hybridization (23–25), which allows the study of numerical and even some structural chromosomal abnormalities in nondividing cells. Interphase cytogenetic methods are faster than conventional karyotype analysis and do not require such high numbers of cells. Furthermore, many different kinds of preparations can be used, including paraffin-embedded sections (14), cytospin preparations, smears, and sputum specimens. Interphase cytogenetics can also be carried out on histologically, morphologically, and immunologically characterized cells (25).

## VI. Summary

With some exceptions, the chromosomal abnormalities associated with malignant mesothelioma are very complex, involving both structural and numerical changes. The chromosome number is usually hypodiploid, but this varies greatly within a given specimen, and polyploid forms of the hypodiploid clone are common. The structural chromosome abnormalities are also highly variable. The most common numerical abnormalities are trisomies or polysomies of chromosomes 5, 7, 11, 12, and 20, and monosomies or partial monosomies of chromosomes 1, 3, 4, 9, 14, 15, 18, 19, and 22. Structural abnormalities are most frequent on the short arms of chromosomes 1 and 3. Clonal evolution, as demonstrated by the presence of several related subclones, and the complexity of the abnormalities, indicates that the malignant process is at an advanced stage. None of the abnormalities are specific to malignant mesothelioma, only polysomy 7 has been found to have prognostic significance. In our studies the number of copies of the short arm of chromosome 7 was negatively correlated with survival ($p = 0.02$). Also hyperdiploid mean chromosomal number correlated with shorter survival ($p = 0.0007$). Structural aberrations in the short arm of chromosome 1, and loss of material in chromosomes 1 and 4, were associated with a high asbestos burden.

## References

1. Heim S, Mitelman F. Cancer cytogenetics. New York: Alan R Liss, 1987.
2. Tiainen M, Tammilehto L, Mattson K, Knuutila S. Cancer Genet Cytogenet 1988; 33:251.
3. Tiainen M, Tammilehto L, Rautonen J, Tuomi T, Mattson K, Knuutila S. Br J Cancer 1989; 60:618.
4. Hagemeijer A, Versnel MA, Van Drunen E, Moret M, Bouts MJ, van der Kwast TH, Hoogsteden HC. Cancer Genet Cytogenet 1990; 47:1.
5. Flejter WL, Li FP, Antman KH, Testa JR. Genes Chromosomes Cancer 1989; 48:148.
6. Popescu NC, Chahinian AP, DiPaolo JA. Cancer Res 1988; 48:142.
7. Bello MJ, Rey JA, Aviles MJ, Arevalo M, Benitez J. Cancer Genet Cytogenet 1987; 29:75.
8. Stenman G, Olofsson K, Mansson T, Hagmar B, Mark J. Hereditas 1986; 105:233.
9. Gibas Z, Li FP, Antman KH, Bernal S, Stahel R, Sandberg AA. Cancer Genet Cytogenet 1986; 20:191.
10. Mark J. Acta Cytol 1978; 22:398.
11. Pelin-Enlund K, Husgavel-Pursiainen K, Tammilehto L, Klockars M, Jantunen K, Gerwin BI, Harris CC, Tuomi T, Vanhala E, Mattson K, Linnainmaa K. Carcinogenesis 1990; 11:673.

12. Meloni AM, Stephenson CF, Li FP, Sandberg AA. Cancer Genet Cytogenet 1992; 59:57.
13. Tiainen M, Tammilehto L, Rautonen J, Tuomi T, Mattson K, Knuutila S. In: Brinkley B, Lechner J, Harris C, eds. Cellular and molecular fiber carcinogenesis. current communications in molecular biology. Cold Spring Harbor, NY: Cold Spring Harbor Laboratory Press, 1992:41.
14. Tiainen M, Rautonen J, Pyrhonen S, Tammilehto L, Mattson K, Knuutila S. Chromosome number correlates with survival in patients with malignant pleural mesothelioma. Cancer Genet Cytogenet 1992; 62:21–24.
15. Knuutila S. Chromosomal changes associated with asbestos exposure. In: Sluyser M, ed. Asbestos related cancer. London: Ellis Horwood, 1991:124–132.
16. Lechner JF, Tokiwa T, La Veck M, Benedict WF, BanksSchlegel S, Yeager H, Danerjee A, Harris CC. Asbestos-associated chromosomal changes in human mesothelial cells. Proc Natl Acad Sci USA 1985; 82:3884–3888.
17. Jaurand MC. Particulate-state carcinogenesis: a survey of recent studies on the mechanisms of action of fibers. IARC Sci Publ 1989; 90:54–73.
18. Zalma R, Bonneau L, Jaurand MC, Guignard J, Pezerat H. Formations of oxy-radicals by oxygen reduction arising from the surface activity of asbestos. Can J Chem 1987; 65:2338–2341.
19. Knuutila S. Role of free radicals in genetic damage (mutation). Med Biol 1984; 62:110–114.
20. Olofsson K, Mark J. Specificity of asbestos-induced chromosomal aberrations in short-term cultured human mesothelial cells. Cancer Genet Cytogenet 1989; 41:33–39.
21. Oshimura M, Hesterberg TW, Barret JC. An early nonrandom karyotypic change in immortal Syrian hamster cell lines transformed by asbestos: trisomy of chromosome 11. Cancer Genet Cytogenet 1986; 22:225–237.
22. Knuutila S, Tiainen M, Tammilehto L, Rautonen J, Pyrhonen S, Mattson K. Cytogenetics of human malignant mesothelioma. Eur Respir Rev 1993; 3:25–28.
23. Cremer T, Landegent J, Brueckner A, Scholl HP, Schardin M, Hager HD, Devilee P, Pearson P, van der Ploeg M. Detection of chromosome aberrations in the human interphase nucleus by visualization of specific target DNAs with radioactive and non-radioactive in situ hybridization techniques: diagnosis of trisomy 18 with probe L1.84. Hum Genet 1986; 74:346–352.
24. Hopman AHN, Ramaekers FCS, Raap AK, Beck JLM, Devilee P, van der Ploeg M, Voojis GP. In situ hybridization as a tool to study numerical chromosome aberrations in solid bladder tumors. Histochemistry 1988; 89:307–316.
25. Wessman M, Knuutila S. A method for the determination of cell morphology, immunologic phenotype and numerical chromosomal abnormalities on the same mitotic or interphase cancer cell. Genet (Life Sci Ad) 1988; 7:127–130.

# 14

## Immunobiology and Immunotherapy of Malignant Mesothelioma

BRUCE W. S. ROBINSON

University of Western Australia and
Sir Charles Gairdner Hospital
Perth, Western Australia, Australia

## I. Introduction

Malignant mesothelioma is an unusual tumor, arising from serosal surfaces. Until the middle of this century it was rare, occurring with a frequency of less than 1 case per million population; consequently, the number of cases presenting with mesothelioma to a single institution was small and little was known about the biology of the disease. With the widespread utilization of asbestos in industry, there has been a marked increase in the incidence of this disease. The worldwide rates are now thought to be 10,000–20,000 cases per annum, with relatively large numbers focused in particular institutions that service areas of high risk (e.g., industrial and ship-building areas, asbestos mining and manufacturing areas). This increase in incidence of the disease, together with the abject failure of standard forms of therapy (surgery, radiotherapy, and chemotherapy) to impinge on survival statistics in this disease (1,2), is the stimulus for our recent efforts to try to understand the biology of this disease, with a view to developing improved therapeutic approaches. In this chapter I will describe the immunobiology of malignant mesothelioma and our efforts to use this information to develop improved immunotherapeutic approaches to this

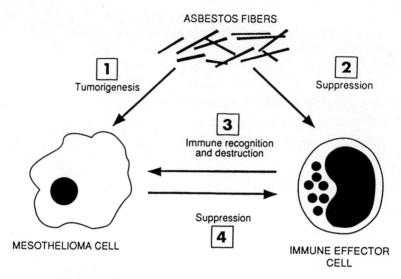

ASBESTOS FIBERS

**1**
Tumorigenesis

**2**
Suppression

**3**
Immune recognition
and destruction

Suppression
**4**

MESOTHELIOMA CELL

IMMUNE EFFECTOR
CELL

**Figure 1** Relation between asbestos fibers, antitumor immune effector cells, and mesothelioma cells. Whereas most studies have evaluated the carcinogenic or transformational relation between asbestos fibers and mesothelial–mesothelioma cells (1), there is evidence that involvement of immune anticancer systems represent and important component of this relation. Asbestos fibers profoundly suppress the activity of immune anticancer systems (2), immune effector cells are able to recognize and destroy mesothelioma cells under certain circumstances (3), and mesothelioma cells release molecules that exert suppressive effects on immune anticancer effector cells (4).

disease. The relation between asbestos fibers, mesothelial cells, and the immune systems is schematized in Figure 1.

## II.  Asbestos Fibers and the Immune System

There have been a substantial number of published studies describing immune abnormalities in individuals exposed to asbestos. Although these studies are complicated by the indirect effects of the presence of asbestosis (i.e., the effects of a progressive fibrotic lung disease, rather than asbestos per se) and the effects of cigarette smoking, there is evidence suggesting that the inhalation of asbestos can cause immune dysregulation. One consistent finding has been the elevation of serum immunoglobulins, and there have been suggestions of reduced circulating T-cell numbers and, in some studies, reduced blood lymphocyte mitogen responsiveness (3–19). In terms of systemic and anticancer defenses, natural killer (NK) activity is probably unaffected in asbestos-exposed persons (20); however, Manning et al. have demonstrated that lymphokine-activated killer (LAK) cell generation is reduced in asbestos-exposed subjects, compared with non–asbestos-exposed controls, with 29% of patients demonstrating levels of lysis of mesothelioma targets that were greater than 2 standard deviations (SD) below the control mean (21). Whether these persons are at greater risk of developing malignancy is yet to be determined.

In vitro studies of the effects of asbestos on immune function have been numerous. Alveolar macrophages exposed to asbestos become activated to release several inflammatory and immune mediators (22–25). Importantly, in terms of anticancer defenses, all forms of asbestos profoundly suppress NK-cell activity in a dose-dependent fashion. Interestingly, this suppression is contact-dependent and is not related to toxicity of the NK cells, and NK cells can recover their activity when removed from the asbestos fibers. Furthermore, interleukin-2 (IL-2) is able to partially reverse this depression of activity (20). Similarly, asbestos fibers inhibit the generation of human LAK cells as well as suppressing their activity (21). Thus, it appears that asbestos fibers can alter the cellular milieu to create conditions favorable for the development of malignancy partly by suppressing immune surveillance mechanisms that may be responsible for destroying transformed cells.

## III.  Asbestos Fibers and Mesothelial Cells

Asbestos fibers alter the biology of mesothelial cells in defined ways (see Chap. 11; 26–29). From an immunobiological point of view, the effects of asbestos fibers on mesothelial cells in terms of cell transformation involve genetic changes that may have important implications for immune recognition. The induction of oxidant-mediated damage, with the generation of karyotypic abnormalities plus other ill-defined mechanisms, likely leads to a number of mutations that will produce altered peptides which may be recognized as foreign by the immune system (see later). Although few mutations have yet been studied, it is clear that a significant proportion of mesothelioma cells have mutations in the *p53* tumor suppressor gene (30,31).

## IV.  Mesothelioma and Immune Function

Patients with mesothelioma, similar to other patients with advanced malignancy, have depressed immune function. Although most patients maintain normal white cell counts, total serum proteins, and immunoglobulin levels

(32), mitogen responsiveness is reduced (19) and, importantly, LAK cell activity against mesothelioma tumor targets is significantly depressed to about 60% of the value seen in normal persons (33). Interestingly, this depression of LAK cell activity could be restored by the addition of indomethacin during the LAK cell generation, whereby LAK cell suppression occurs in these patients (Fig. 2). This suggests that at least some of the systemic immunosuppressive processes present in patients with this disease may be reversed pharmacologically.

Recent studies of mesothelioma tumor cells demonstrate that these cells undergo autocrine growth stimulation by several growth factors, including platelet-derived growth factor (PDGF) (34) and, importantly, transforming growth factor-beta (TGF-$\beta$) (in preparation). A powerful immuno-

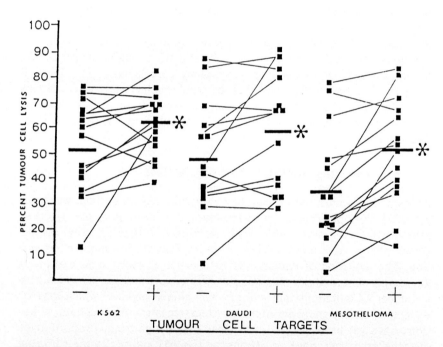

**Figure 2** Reversal of depressed LAK cell activity in patients with mesothelioma by indomethacin. Blood from 14 patients was cultured for 3–7 days in medium plus IL-2 in the absence (−) or the presence (+) of 10 μg/ml indomethacin, following which LAK cell activity was measured against K562 targets (a standard NK target), Daudi cells (a standard LAK target), and six cultured human mesothelioma cell lines (Manning et al., results pooled) assessed using a standard $^{51}$Cr-release assay. *$p > 0.05$ (paired Student's $t$ test) comparing LAK cell activity generated in the absence or presence of indomethacin.

suppressant, TGF-$\beta$ is capable of generating both immune deviation and down-regulation of human T cells. As the TGF-$\beta$ produced by mesothelioma cells is released into the surrounding milieu, rather than acting as a private autocrine growth factor, we believe that this factor likely suppresses the activity of T cells entering mesotheliomas. In this context, Bielefeldt-Ohmann et al. have shown that T cells within murine mesotheliomas demonstrate features of down-regulated activity, with low surface expression of CD3 (35). This local production of TGF-$\beta$ is likely to be important in protecting the tumor from immune destruction. It is particularly important to understand this, as many of the other criteria for an appropriate immune response [e.g., expression of major histocompatibility (MHC) molecules and systemic immune recognition] appear to be present in mesothelioma, raising the prospect that if local immunosuppression within tumors can be blocked, along with blockaded systemic immunosuppression, then an effective antitumor response may be generated.

### V. Mesothelioma Cells as Targets of Immune Effector Cells

Immune anticancer effector cell activity can occur by either non–MHC-restricted processes (NK, LAK, and $\gamma$–$\delta$ T-cell recognition) or by MHC-restricted processes ($\alpha$–$\beta$ T-cell mechanisms).

To evaluate the capacity of human mesothelioma cells to act as targets for immune effector cells, we first generated a number of human mesothelioma lines from the pleural fluids of patients with established malignant mesothelioma. Approximately 15 of these lines have been established with 5 of them used as long-term mesothelioma cultures and fully characterized in terms of cytology, immunocytochemistry, and ultrastructure (36).

When evaluated as targets for NK cell activity, these mesothelioma cells proved to be resistant to NK cell lysis. In contrast, both cultured and fresh mesothelioma cells were susceptible to lysis by LAK cells (37). Furthermore, this lysis could be augmented by tumor necrosis factor (TNF) (38). Lysis of mesothelioma targets by $\gamma$–$\delta$ T cells was evaluated by Mavaddat et al., who used cloned $\gamma$–$\delta$ T cells (39). This study demonstrated that individual $\gamma$–$\delta$ T-cell clones demonstrated unique cytotoxic profiles that, in contrast with the lysis of standard LAK (Daudi) or NK (K562) targets, did not parallel with T-cell receptor V$\gamma$ or V$\delta$ gene utilization. In addition there was no correlation between $\gamma$–$\delta$ lysis of mesothelioma targets and the production of interferon $\gamma$ (IFN-$\gamma$), TNF, IL-2, or IL-4, nor with the expression of the MHC-class I-binding molecule CD8 (39). Thus, despite having a common tissue of origin, these mesothelioma targets did not exhibit a common γ-δ recognition structure, such as the superantigen described for Daudi cells.

Recognition and lysis of tumor targets by antigen-specific T cells require the presentation of antigen-derived peptides on the surface of the target by MHC class I or class II molecules. Christmas et al. have evaluated the expression of histocompatibility locus antigen (HLA) molecules on human mesothelioma cells (40). They demonstrated that class I MHC molecules are expressed constitutively at a high level on all mesothelioma cell lines, as determined by indirect immunofluorescence and fluorescence-activated cell-sorter analysis (Fig. 3), and Northern blot analysis, using class I locus-specific probes, has demonstrated constitutive transcription of *HLA-A, -B,* and *-C* genes in each of the cell lines. None of the cell lines constitutively expressed HLA class II (DR or DQ) antigens. Treatment with IFN-α and IFN-γ increased class I mRNA in most cell lines; however, surface expression was not augmented, likely because of the already high expression. IFN-γ-induced membrane HLA-DR expression in three of the cell lines but not of HLA-DQ expression (40). These studies did not support the contention that mesothelioma is able to grow because of loss of surface expression of the class I molecules responsible for presenting mutant peptides to the immune system. To evaluate the possible presence of mutant or new peptides, we have evaluated murine mesothelioma cells for their immunogenicity in standard vaccination–challenge experiments and demon-

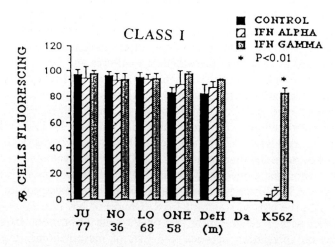

**Figure 3** Class I MHC surface antigen expression in mesothelioma cell lines in the presence or absence of interferons compared with control cell lines (Daudie, Da) and K562.

strated that few of the mesothelioma lines are able to afford protection against subsequent challenge (41). Interestingly, this failure of protection occurs despite the generation of some form of immune response in the animals by the challenged mesothelioma cells, suggesting that the vaccination procedures do induce an immune response, but that this is insufficient to overcome the resistance of the tumor cells to destruction, no doubt partly owing to the release of immunosuppressive factors, as described earlier.

One other method of evaluating the susceptibility of mesothelioma cells to immune destruction is to evaluate their susceptibility to immune cell-derived cytokines. Bowman et al. (42) have used five human mesothelioma cell lines in vitro, in a tetrazolium bromide assay system (MTT), to evaluate the susceptibility of mesothelioma cells to IFN-$\alpha$, IFN-$\gamma$, TNF, and combinations of these cytokines. They demonstrated that all of the mesothelioma lines were resistant to TNF, but displayed varying degrees of sensitivity to the interferons, with IFN-$\alpha$ inhibiting the growth of one of the lines and IFN-$\gamma$ inhibiting the growth of two of the lines. No significant interactions between the cytokines were seen when used in combination. With the same technique, they screened the sensitivity of these cells to eight commonly used neoplastic drugs and demonstrated that these cell lines were as resistant, if not more so, than lung and colon carcinoma cell lines. This lack of sensitivity of mesothelioma cell lines to the direct growth-inhibitory effects of the interferons, in conjunction with similar observations in the animal model of mesothelioma, suggest that the in vivo efficacy of IFN-$\alpha$ in this disease is mediated by immunological, rather than direct growth-inhibitory, mechanisms.

## VI. Immunotherapy of Mesothelioma: Animal Studies

Human mesothelioma cells can be transplanted into immune-deficient nude mice for screening of the direct effects of immune cell cytokines on mesothelioma growth. Chahinian et al. have demonstrated that IFN-$\alpha$ in this xenograft model augments the antitumor effects of the drug combination mitomycin and cisplatin (43). Griffin et al. have used this model to evaluate the efficacy of site-directed toxins administered locally (44). By using the ricin toxin linked to a monoclonal antibody specific for human transferrin receptor, they demonstrated reduction in tumor growth following intraperitoneal injection of human mesothelioma cells, with survival extended from 150 to 400% of controls. Similarly, the intraperitoneal injection of diphtheria toxin using this model produced tumor regression and prolonged disease-free survival (45). Although these results are interesting, they have been demonstrated only in this animal model, which is complicated by the innate resistance of mouse cells to the detrimental effects of diphtheria toxin and that heterotransplanted cell lines are clonal and lack the partial heterogeneity of primary human tumors.

Bowman et al. have evaluated the capacity of TNF administered systematically with doctinomycin (actinomycin D); (46), a combination with marked in vitro efficacy, in human mesothelioma heterotransplanted into nude mice. The combination produced marked wasting of the animals, with little reduction in tumor growth, suggesting synergism in terms of side effects with little antitumor effect in this model.

Because the nude mouse is immunodeficient, only the direct effects of immune cytokines can be evaluated. Consequently, we established a murine model of mesothelioma. BALB/c and CBA mice were injected intraperitoneally with crocidolite asbestos and, from the primary tumors produced, 12 continuously growing cell lines (5 BALB/c, 7 CBA) have been fully characterized by cytological and ultrastructural analyses. All cell lines produced tumors when injected into syngeneic mice, and this murine model appears to replicate the human disease in terms of histology, ultrastructure, morphology, MHC expression, PDGF autocrine growth features, TGF-$\beta$ production, and *p53* tumor suppressor gene abnormalities (47). Thus, this model appears to represent a faithful model of the human tumor (Table 1) and, because of the presence of an intact immune system, provides the opportunity to study the immunobiology of this tumor in vivo. We are currently using this model to evaluate the efficacy of several immunothera-

**Table 1**  Comparison of Human and Murine Mesothelioma

| Feature | Human MM | Murine MM |
|---|---|---|
| Asbestos induction | Yes | Yes |
| Associated effusion | Yes | Yes |
| Epithelial histology | Yes | Yes |
| Sarcomatous histology | Yes | Yes |
| Mixed histology | Yes | Yes |
| Ultrastructural microvilli | Yes | Yes |
| Ultrastructural glycogen granules | Yes | Yes |
| Ultrastructural type junctions | Yes | Yes |
| Variable morphology in culture | Yes | Yes |
| MHC class I expression | Yes | Yes |
| MHC class II expression | No | No |
| PDGF autocrine growth | Yes | Yes |
| TGF-$\beta$ autocrine growth | Yes | Yes |
| p53 abnormalities | Unusual | Unusual |

peutic strategies. Interferon-$\alpha$ produces reduction in tumor growth, despite absence of in vitro sensitivity of this tumor to interferon, suggesting that interferon acts by an immunomodulatory mechanism (35).

One additional type of animal study of immunotherapy has been undertaken. As malignant pleural mesothelioma remains localized to the pleural cavity for a large part of its natural history, a clinical trial using intrapleural IL-2 administration was planned. To evaluate the capacity of intrapleural IL-2 to boost local and systemic LAK cell activity, Flexman et al. administered intrapleural IL-2 in escalating doses to rats and evaluated systemic, pleural, and pulmonary NK and LAK cell activity (48). Intrapleural IL-2 administration boosted systemic and pulmonary NK activity. Pleural LAK cell was markedly enhanced by the intrapleural IL-2 administration, which also boosted systemic NK and, to a lesser extent, LAK cell activity. This route of administration was well tolerated by the animals.

## VII.  Immunotherapy of Mesothelioma: Human Studies

Following the success of our preclinical studies using IL-2 and LAK cells in animals and the published clinical success in a number of patients with advanced malignancy using systematically administered IL-2 and LAK cells (49), we enrolled five patients in a phase I/II clinical trial using recombinant human IL-2 (Cetus), in doses escalating from $4 \times 10^6$ to $16 \times 10^6$ units/ $m^2$ per day intrapleurally, with a single intrapleural administration of autologous LAK cells ($0.85 \times 10^9$–$2.75 \times 10^9$ cells) that had been harvested by leukophoresis and cultured for 4 days in recombinant human IL-2 to generate LAK cells. All of the patients experienced systemic symptoms (fever, rigors, nausea), and all had weight gain and transient hypotension and, in all but one patient, therapy was ceased because of severe additional side effects, including liver and renal dysfunction, encephalopathy, pulmonary edema, and local pleural problems (loculation, empyema) (50,51). This approach was, therefore, ceased. Stoter et al. (52) have also used IL-2 intrapleurally without LAK cells and have demonstrated partial responses in early mesothelioma (i.e., patients with localized, nodular disease).

From our foregoing observations with IFN-$\alpha$ in animals with mesothelioma, we have conducted several clinical trials with this agent. When used alone in 25 patients with malignant mesothelioma [$3 \times 10^6$–$18 \times 10^6$ units of interferon alpha 2a (Roferon-A) daily for 12 weeks] 4 responses were seen (16%), which included 1 complete response, 2 partial responses ($> 50\%$ reduction in tumor area on thoracic CT scan, Fig. 4), and 1 patient had a delayed partial response (complete disappearance of a large, rapidly growing subcutaneous lesion over 18 months following cessation of ther-

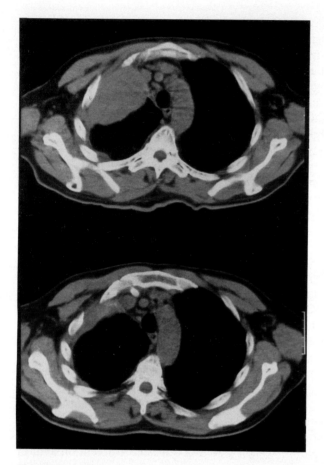

**Figure 4**   Interferon alfa 2A (Roferon A) and mesothelioma: A thoracic CT scan is shown for a patient with established mesothelioma (above) and a repeat CT scan following 12 weeks of therapy with IFN-α (below).

apy). Although all patients experienced the usual interferon-related side effects of flulike symptoms, lethargy, and weight loss, the therapy was reasonably well tolerated (53).

Because doxorubicin (Adriamycin) has some antimesothelioma activity in approximately 15–20% of patients, we combined this therapy with recombinant human IFN-α2a in a further 25 patients. Four patients exhibited partial responses; however, side effects were substantial, with virtually all patients experiencing nausea and vomiting, severe lethargy and weight loss, and leukopenia (54). On this basis it was felt that the doxorubicin did not add substantially to the effects of IFN-α alone.

## VIII. Conclusions and Future Studies

It is clear from the foregoing studies that immunological approaches to the therapy of mesothelioma are worth further study, as they offer the potential to produce tumor reduction by entirely different mechanisms from standard chemotherapeutic and radiotherapeutic approaches. Our preliminary immunobiological studies have demonstrated that mesothelioma cells can be rendered susceptible to immune destruction in vitro and in vivo. Although it is encouraging that mesothelioma cells can constitutively express the class I MHC molecules responsible for presentation of antigenic tumor peptides, it is not yet known whether or not costimulatory molecules (e.g., B7, ICAM-1, and such) are expressed. We are currently employing gene-transfer studies to evaluate this issue. Additional studies will be required to determine whether or not T-cell epitopes are being presented by these mesothelioma cells, as has been recently described in melanoma (55). Several obstacles exist, however, the most important of these being the immunosuppressive milieu of the tumor. Mesothelioma cells produce large quantities of TGF-$\beta$, a powerful T-cell immunosuppressant, and any immunotherapeutic strategy that augments specific immune responses to mesothelioma will inevitably be thwarted because this antitumor response will be suppressed as soon as it enters the tumor milieu. It has recently been demonstrated that agents such as IFN-$\alpha$ can suppress the production of TGF-$\beta$ (56), and we are currently undertaking other studies using inducible TGF-$\beta$ antisense transfectants to evaluate the role of this molecule in subverting tumor-specific antitumor responses.

Although there is no guarantee that immunotherapy will ultimately offer patients with malignant mesothelioma any tumor regression or prolongation of life, the preliminary studies just described are encouraging and suggest that further laboratory and clinical studies employing modern immunotherapeutic approaches offer the prospect of enhancing the outlook for this otherwise uniformly fatal, aggressive, and treatment-resistant disease.

### Acknowledgments

This work was funded by the National Health and Medical Research Council of Australia, the Sir Charles Gairdner Hospital, the Cancer Foundations of Western Australia, and a Jarnes Hardie Industries Medical Research Fellowship.

The secretarial assistance of Mrs. Trudy Turner is gratefully acknowledged.

## References

1. Musk AW, Bowman R, Christmas T, Robinson BWS. Management of malignant mesothelioma. In: Henderson DW, Shilkin K, Langlois S, Whitaker D, eds. Malignant mesothelioma. New York: Hemisphere Publishing, 1992:292–304.

2. Robinson BWS. Development of new therapeutic strategies for mesothelioma. Lung Cancer 1993; 9:413–418.

3. Morris DL, Greenberg SD, Lawrence EC. Immune responses in asbestos-exposed individuals. Chest 1985; 87:278–280.

4. deShazo RD, Hendrick JH, Diem JE, et al. Immunological aberrations in asbestos cement workers: dissociation from asbestosis. J Allergy Clin Immunol 1983; 72:454–461.

5. Pernis B, Vigliani EC, Selikoff LT. Rheumatoid factor in serum of individuals exposed to asbestos. Ann NY Acad Sci 1965; 132:112–120.

6. Turner-Warwick M, Parkes WR. Circulating rheumatoid and antinuclear factors in asbestos workers. Br Med J 1970; 3:492–495.

7. deShazo RD, Daul CB, Morgan JE, et al. Immunologic investigation in asbestos-exposed workers. Chest 1986; 89:162S–165S.

8. Wagner MMF, Campbell MF, Edwards RF. Sequential immunological studies on an asbestos exposed population. I. Factors affecting peripheral blood leukocytes and T-lymphocytes. Clin Exp Immunol 1979; 38:323–331.

9. Kagan E, Solomon A, Cochrane JC, et al. Immunological studies of patients with asbestosis. II. Studies of circulating lymphoid cell numbers and humoral immunity. Clin Exp Immunol 1977; 28:268–275.

10. Gaumer HR, Doll NH, Kaimal J, et al. Diminished suppressor cell function in patients with asbestosis. Clin Exp Immunol 1981; 44:108–116.

11. Miller LG, Sparrow D, Ginns LC. Asbestos exposure correlates with alterations in circulating T cell subsets. Clin Exp Immunol 1983; 51:110–116.

12. Tsang PH, Chu FN, Fischbein A, Bekesi JG. Impairments in functional subsets of T-suppressor (CD8) lymphocytes, monocytes and natural killer cells among asbestos-exposed workers. Clin Immunol Immunopathol 1988; 47:323–332.

13. Campbell MJ, Wagner MMF, Scott MP, Brown DG. Sequential immunological studies in an asbestos-exposed population. II. Factors affecting lymphocyte function. Clin Exp Immunol 1980; 39:176–183.

14. Kagan E, Solomon A, Cochrane JC, et al. Immunological studies of patients with asbestosis. I. Studies of cell mediated immunity. Clin Exp Immunol 1977; 28:261–267.

15. Kubota M, Kagamimori S, Yokoyama K, Okada A. Reduced killer cell activity of lymphocytes from patients with asbestosis. Br J Ind Med 1985; 42:276–280.

16. Ginns LC, Ryu JH, Rogol PR, et al. Natural killer cell activity in cigarette smokers and asbestos workers. Am Rev Respir Dis 1985; 131:831–834.

17. deShazo RD, Morgan J, Bozelka B, Chapman Y. Natural killer cell activity in asbestos workers. Interactive effects of smoking and asbestos exposure. Chest 1988; 94:482–485.

18. Kagamimori S, Watanabe M, Kubota M, et al. Serum interferon levels and natural killer cell activity in patients with asbestosis. Thorax 1984; 39:65–66.

19. Haslam PL, Lukoszek A, Merchant JA, Turner-Warwick M. Lymphocyte responses to phytohemagglutinin in patients with asbestosis and pleural mesothelioma. Clin Exp Immunol 1978; 31:178–188.

20. Robinson BWS. Asbestos and cancer: human natural killer cell activity is suppressed by asbestos fibres but can be restored by recombinant interleukin 2. Am Rev Respir Dis 1989; 139:897–902.

21. Manning L, Davis M, Robinson BWS. Asbestos fibres inhibit the in vitro activity of lymphokines activated killer (LAK) cells from healthy individuals and patients with malignant mesothelioma. Clin Exp Immunol 1991; 83: 85–91.

22. Hayes A, Mullan B, Lovegrove FT, Robinson BWS, Musk AW. Gallium lung scanning and bronchoalveolar lavage in crocidolite-exposed workers. Chest 1989; 96:22–26.

23. Hayes AA, Venaille TJ, Rose AH, et al. Asbestos-induced release of a human alveolar macrophage-derived neutrophil chemotactic factor. Exp Lung Res 1990; 16:121–130.

24. Case BW, Ip MPC, Padilla M, Kleinerman J. Asbestos effects on superoxide production. An in vitro study of hamster alveolar macrophages. Environ Res 1986; 39:299–306.

25. DuBois CM, Bissonnette E, Rola-Pleszczynski M. Asbestos fibers and silica particles stimulate rat alveolar macrophages to release tumour necrosis factor. Autoregulatory role of leukotriene $B_4$. Am Rev Respir Dis 1989; 139:1257–1264.

26. Whitaker DW, Manning LS, Robinson BWS, Shilkin K. The pathobiology of the mesothelium. In: Henderson DW, Shilkin K, Langlois S, Whitaker D, eds. Malignant mesothelioma. New York: Hemisphere Publishing, 1992:25–68.

27. Mossman B, Light W, Wei E. Asbestos: mechanisms of toxicity and carcinogenicity in the respiratory tract. Annu Rev Pharmacol Toxicol 1983; 23:595–615.

28. Jaurand MC, Pinchon MC, Bignon J. Mesothelial cells in vitro. Pleura Health Dis 1985; 30:43–67.

29. Barrett JC, Lamb PW, Wiseman RW. Multiple mechanisms for the carcinogenic effects of asbestos and other mineral fibers. Env Health Perspect 1989; 81:81–89.

30. Metcalf RA, Welsh JA, Bennett WP, Seddon MB, Lehman TA, Pelin K, Linnainmaa K, Tammilehto L, Mattson K, Gerwin BI, Harris CC. *p53* and Kirsten-*ras* mutations in human mesothelioma cell lines. Cancer Res 1992; 52: 2610–2615.

31. Cote RJ, Jhanvar SC, Novick S, Pellicer A. Cancer Res 1991; 51:5410.

32. Garlepp MJ, Fitzpatrick D, Mutsaers S, Bielefeldt-Ohmann H, David M, Robinson BWS. Mesothelioma: recent studies of growth regulation. In: Peters G, ed. Sourcebook on asbestos diseases, vol. 5. Asbestos medical research. New York: Garland Publishing, 1992: (in press).

33. Manning LS, Bowman RV, Davis MR, Musk A, Robinson BWS. Clin Immunol Immunopathol 1989; 53:68.

34.  Garlepp MJ, Christmas TI, Manning LS, Mutsaers S, Dench J, Leong C, Robinson BWS. The role of platelet derived growth factor in the growth of human malignant mesothelioma. Eur Respir Rev 1993; 3:189–191.
35.  Bielefeldt et al. Manuscript in preparation.
36.  Manning LS, Murch A, Garlepp MJ, Davis MR, Musk A, Robinson BWS. Int J Cancer 1990; 47:285.
37.  Manning LS, Bowman RV, Darby SB, Robinson BWS. Am Rev Respir Dis 1989; 139:1369.
38.  Bowman R, Manning LS, Davis M, Robinson BWS. Capacity of tumour necrosis factor to augment lysis of tumour targets by cytotoxic lymphocytes. Clin Immunol Immunopath 1991; 58:80–91.
39.  Mavaddat N, Robinson BWS, Rose AH, Manning LS, Garlepp MJ. An analysis of the relationship between $\gamma\delta$ T-cell receptor V gene usage and nonMHC restricted cytotoxicity. Immunol Cell Biol 1993; 71:27–37.
40.  Christmas TI, Manning LS, Davis MR, Robinson BWS, Garlepp M. HLA antigen expression and malignant mesothelioma. Am J Respir Cell Mol Biol 1991; 5:213–220.
41.  Manning LS, Davis MR, Bielefeldt-Ohmann H, Marzo AL, Garlepp MJ, Whitaker D, Robinson BWS. Evaluation of immunogenicity of murine mesothelioma cells by immunization. Eur Respir Rev 1993; 3:234–237.
42.  Bowman R, Whitaker D, Manning LS, Davis MR, Robinson BWS. Interaction between dactinomycin and tumor necrosis factor in mesothelioma cachexia without oncolysis. Cancer 1991; 67:2495–2500.
43.  Chahinian AP, Norton L, Holland JF, et al. Experimental and clinical activity of mitomycin C and cis-diamminedichloroplatinum in malignant mesothelioma. Cancer Res 1984; 44:1688–1692.
44.  Griggin TW, Richardson C, Houston L, et al. Antitumor activity of intraperitoneal immunotoxins in a nude mouse model of human malignant mesothelioma. Cancer Res 1987; 47:4266–4270.
45.  Raso V, McGrath J. Cure of experimental human malignant mesothelioma in athymic mice by diphtheria toxin. JNCI 1989; 81:622–627.
46.  Bowman R, Manning LS, Davis MR, Robinson BWS. Chemosensitivity and cytokine sensitivity of malignant mesothelioma. Cancer Chemother Pharmacol 1991; 28:420–426.
47.  Davis MR, Manning LS, Whitaker D, Robinson BWS. Tumorigenic mouse malignant mesothelioma cell lines – a representative model for the human disease. Int J Cancer 1992; 52:881–886.
48.  Flexman J, Manning L, Robinson BWS. In vivo boosting of lung natural killer (NK) and lymphokine-activated killer (LAK) cell activity by interleukin-2 (IL-2): comparison of systemic, intrapleural and inhalation routes. Clin Immunol Immunopathol 1990; 82:151–156.
49.  Rosenberg SA, Lotze MT, Muul LM, Chang AE, Avis FP, Leitman S, Linehan WM, Robertson GN, Lee RE, Rubin JT, Seipp CA, Simpson CG, White DE. A progress report on the treatment of 157 patients with advanced cancer using lymphokine-activated killer cells and interleukin-2 or high-dose interleukin-2 alone. N Engl J Med 1987; 316:889–897.

50. Robinson BWS, Bowman R, Christmas T, Musk AW, Manning LS. Immunotherapy for malignant mesothelioma: use of interleukin-2 and interferon alpha. Interferons Cytokines 1991; 18:5-7.

51. Robinson BWS, Bowman RV, Manning LS, Musk AW, Van Hazel GA. Interleukin-2 and lymphokine-activated killer cells in malignant mesothelioma. Eur Respir Rev 1993; 3:220-222.

52. Stoter G, Goey SH, Slingerland R, et al. Intrapleural interleukin-2 (IL-2) in malignant pleural mesothelioma: a phase I-II study [abstr 1630]. Proc Am Assoc Cancer Res 1990; 31:275.

53. Christmas TI, Manning LS, Garlepp MJ, Musk AW, Robinson BWS. Effect of interferon alpha-2a on malignant mesothelioma. J Interferon Res 1992; 13: 912.

54. Upham J, Musk AW, Robinson BWS. Interferon alpha and doxorubicin in mesothelioma. Aust NZ J Med (in press).

55. van der Bruggen P, Traversari C, Chomez P, Lurquin C, De Plaen E, van den Eynde B, Knuth A, Boon T. A gene encoding an antigen recognized by cytolytic T lymphocytes on a human melanoma. Science 1991; 254:1643-1647.

56. Dhanani S, Huang M, Dubinett S. Interferon-alpha inhibits murine macrophage transforming growth factor-beta production. Am Rev Respir Dis 1993; 147:A758.

# 15

## Chemotherapy of Malignant Mesothelioma

**PIERRE RUFFIÉ**

Institut Gustave-Roussy
Villejuif, France

## I. Introduction

There is no uniform agreement on the most appropriate therapeutic modalities to manage this tumor. Local treatment, such as surgery and/or radiation therapy, are technically difficult, in view of the extent of the disease (1). If the tumor tends to spread locally, the frequency of metastases is often underestimated, as shown at postmortem examination (2,3).

The results remain poor and, in retrospective studies, there are no drastic differences in survival among groups of patients treated with different therapeutic procedures (4,5) and others did not find any differences between treated and untreated patients (6).

The median survival from the time of diagnosis is less than 1 year, and confirms the poor outcome of diffuse malignant mesothelioma (DMM). The cure of mesothelioma is exceptional, with 5-years survival estimated to be less than 5%. But some individual untreated cases with an unpredictable long outcome have been described (6); thus, in treated patients this may be falsely attributed to the effects of treatment.

Although cure of mesothelioma is exceptional, the identification of prognostic factors may help us understand the results of future therapeutic

**Table 1**  Prognostic Factors[a]

| Authors (Ref.) | Chahinian (7) | Antman (8) | Alberts (4) | Ruffié (5) |
|---|---|---|---|---|
| No. of cases | 69 | 136 | 262 | 118 |
| Prognostic factors | Platelet count | PS[b] | PS | Stage |
|  | Histological type | Histological type | Ethnic | Platelet count |
|  | Age | Chest pain | Duration of symptoms | Asbestos exposure |
|  |  | Duration of symptoms | Stage |  |

[a]Multivariate analysis.
[b]PS, performance status.

endeavors. The factors reported to have a favorable influence on survival (4,5,7,8) include epithelial cell type, age younger than 50 years, female sex, dyspnea as initial symptom, delay of diagnosis longer than 6 months, stage of disease, platelet count fewer than 400,000, absence of weight loss, good performance status (PS), absence of exposure to asbestos, and resection of the tumor.

The results obtained with multivariate analysis are shown in Table 1; they may be useful in determining stratification variables for future therapeutic trials.

## II. Methodology: Assessment of Response to Chemotherapy

The role of chemotherapy in the management of these tumors is currently unclear (9–11). One of the greatest problems in the interpretation of the efficacy of cytostatic agent is the way of evaluating an objective response (OR). For evaluable disease, a *complete response* (CR) was defined as the total disappearance of all measurable disease. A *partial response* (PR) was defined as a reduction of 50% in the product of two perpendicular diameters of reproducible measurable lesions for at least 4 weeks. The criteria for *stable disease* was either an increase of $<25\%$ or a decrease of $<50\%$ in tumor size. So it is easy to imagine the difficulty of the assessment of response with evaluating measurable target in DMM, sometimes based only on subjective criteria or the notion of stable disease, which is very frequent in DMM, that are considered as a genuine antitumor responses. That explains some optimistic or overestimated results with objective response (addition of PR and CR) more than 40% (12).

Pleural effusion is not considered as a measurable target, since, as the disease progresses, the pleural space is obliterated and recurrent pleural effusion ceases to be a problem, and most mesotheliomas are not measurable on chest x-ray films by classic criteria. The introduction of new technologies such as computed tomography (CT) scan may have partially solved the problem of measurable disease and appears to be accurate in documenting progression.

In another way, a TNM-staging system appears to be useful. The first classification for pleural mesothelioma was proposed by Butchart (13), in 1976, and was modified by Chahinian, in 1983 (7). More recently, the International Union Against Cancer TNM-staging system has been adopted officially (Table 2). The TNM classification defines the extent of the disease in terms of three components: the primary tumor, designated by letter T; the regional lymph nodes, designated by the letter N; and the distant metastases, designated by the letter M. However, no totally satisfactory-staging system exists for peritoneal mesothelioma.

The role played by chemotherapy is difficult to assess when it is associated with multiple combined modalities. The tumor is uncommon, the number of patients too few, anecdotal reports often emphasize responders (14), nonresponders may not be reported, and this results in a tendency toward overestimation of pooled activity. For that matter, the preliminary results are not confirmed by a larger number of patients in cooperative group trials. That is a common finding in chemotherapy practice. To rule out this bias, only prospective studies with a sufficient number of patients ( > 14) are analyzed in this review.

## III. Review of Chemotherapy Trials

### A. Single-Agent Chemotherapy

A list of 13 agents tested with a sufficient number of patients ( > 14) can be considered as probably inactive, so that investigation with these drugs is not warranted (Table 3) (15–28).

The group of anthracyclines (Table 4) appears to be the most interesting. In the past, doxorubicin was considered the most active compound, with an OR estimated at more than 40% (9). But the results were not confirmed by others with a larger number of patients: 0–14% of OR in, respectively, 0 of 21 and 7 out of 51 patients (18,29). When the number of evaluable cases was pooled (11) a total of 197 patients have been treated, 35 of whom achieved an OR (18%).

**Table 2**  TNM-Staging System in Diffuse Malignant Mesothelioma Proposed by the UICC

| | |
|---|---|
| T: primary tumor and extent | |
| TX | Primary tumor cannot be assessed |
| T0 | No evidence of primary tumor |
| T1 | Primary tumor limited to ipsilateral parietal/or visceral pleura |
| T2 | Tumor invades any of the following: ipsilateral lung, endothoracic fascia, diaphragm, pericardium |
| T3 | Tumor invades any of the following: ipsilateral chest wall muscle, ribs, mediastinal organs or tissues |
| T4 | Tumor extends to any of the following: contralateral pleura of lung direct extension, peritoneum of intra-abdominal organs by direct extension, cervical tissues |
| N: lymph nodes | |
| NX | Regional lymph nodes cannot be assessed |
| N0 | No regional lymph node metastases |
| N1 | Metastases in ipsilateral bronchopulmonary or hilar lymph nodes |
| N2 | Metastases in mediastinal lymph nodes |
| N3 | Metastases in contralateral mediastinal, internal mammary, supraclavicular, or scalene lymph nodes |
| M: metastases | |
| MX | Presence of distant mestastases cannot be assessed |
| M0 | No (known) distant mestastases |
| M1 | Distant mestastases present |

Stage I = T1,N0,M0 T2,N0,M0
Stage II = T1,N1,M0 T2,N1,M0
Stage III = T3, any N,M0 Any T,N2,M0
Stage IV = Any T,N3,M0 T4, any N,M0 Any T, any N M1


Detorubicin has been used in only one clinical trial, with an OR of 43% (in 9 out of 21 patients) (12). This study needs confirmation; here, the criteria of response were mostly subjective.

Other analogues of doxorubicin, such as 4-epidoxorubicin (Epirubicin) (30,31) or tetrahydropyran (THP)-doxorubicin (Pirarubicin) (32,34) were tested, with quite similar results: respectively, 8 OR in 69 evaluable patients (11%) and 6 OR in 58 evaluable patients (10%) (see Table 4).

The dose may be a very important issue, as shown by the clear dose-response relation shown in a randomized trial in breast cancer between high-dose (100 mg/m$^2$) and low-dose (50 mg/m$^2$) of Epiburicin (35). For mesothelioma, Mattson et al. (30) found 7 OR in 48 evaluable patients treated with high-dose (110–130 mg/m$^2$) compared with 1 OR in 21 assessable patients treated by lower doses (75 mg/m$^2$) in another trial (31). For

**Table 3**  Single Agents (Probably Inactive or Inactive)

| Association agent | Response OR/no. patients | Ref. |
|---|---|---|
| Acivicin | 0/21 | 15 |
| Aclarubicin (Aclacinomycine A) | 1/17 | 16 |
| Bleomycin | 2/19 | 17 |
| Cyclophosphamide | 0/21 | 18 |
| Diaziquone | 0/21 | 19 |
| Diazonorleucine | 0/15 | 16 |
| 5-Fluorouracil | 1/20 | 20 |
| Amsacrine (m-AMSA) | 1/17 | 21 |
| Mitoxantrone | 2/28 | 22 |
| Mitoxantrone | 1/34 | 23 |
| N-Propargyldieazafolic | 1/18 | 24 |
| Vinblastine | 0/20 | 25 |
| Vincristine | 0/23 | 26 |
| Vindesine | 1/17 | 27 |
| Vindesine | 0/21 | 28 |

THP-doxorubicin, we had no responders in 15 evaluable patients, as opposed to the previous promising results from Sridhar (34).

When pooling, all evaluable cases for the anthracycline trials (except detorubicin), the final result is an OR of 15% (in 342 patients). So anthracyclines have to be considered as only marginally active.

Five other drugs can also be considered as being marginally active (Table 5):

**Table 4**  Single Agents: Anthracyclines (Marginally Active)

| Agent | Response | (CR) | Ref. |
|---|---|---|---|
| Doxorubicin | 7/51 | (2) | 29 |
| Doxorubicin | 0/21 | | 18 |
| Detorubicin | 9/21 | (2) | 12 |
| 4-Epidoxorubicin (75 mg/m$^2$) | 1/21 | | 30 |
| 4-Epidoxorubicin (120 mg/m$^2$) | 7/48 | | 31 |
| THP-Adriamycin | 3/35 | | 32 |
| THP-Adriamycin | 0/15 | | 33 |
| THP-Adriamycin | 3/8 | (1) | 34 |

**Table 5**  Single Agent: Marginally Active

| Agent | Response | Ref. |
|---|---|---|
| Mitomycin | 4/19 | 36 |
| Dihydro-5-azacytidine | 6/41 | 37 |
| Dihydro-5-azacytidine | 0/14 | 38 |
| Ifosfamide | 4/17 | 39 |
| Ifosfamide | 2/26 | 40 |
| Ifosfamide | 1/39 | 41 |

1. Mitomycin, tested by Bajorin (36), with 4 PR in 19 evaluable patients, but with some significant pulmonary toxicity.
2. Dihydro-5-azacytidine, a water-soluble analogue of azacitidine (5-azacytidine) is a well known old drug previously tested with promising result 15 years ago (7). Recently, the Cancer and Leukemia Group B (CALGB) has tested this new drug (37), with interesting results (1 CR and 6 PR in 41 evaluable patients), but not confirmed by another group from the M. D. Anderson Cancer Research Group (no OR out of 14 patients) (38).
3. Ifosfamide, an analogue of cyclophosphamide, was tested by two groups (39,40), with an overall OR of 13%, with 6 OR in 43 evaluable patients. A further clinical trial has been conducted by the Eastern Cooperative Oncology Group (41), with a larger number of patients. Of the 39 cases evaluable for response, only 1 patient had a partial response lasting 6.3 months. The severe toxicity (at least one episode of severe or life-threatening toxicity) documented in more than half of the patients precludes any further dose escalation in patients with DMM. It is uncertain whether the results are superior to cyclophosphamide (11–18).
4. Cisplatin (CDDP) has been widely tested (Table 6) (42–46), showing an activity comparable with doxorubicin when the number of

**Table 6**  Single Agent: Cisplatin (Marginally Active)

| Dose (course) | Response | Ref. |
|---|---|---|
| 100 mg/m$^2$ | 1/9 | 42 |
| 100 mg/m$^2$ (3 S) | 5/35 | 43 |
| 120 mg/m$^2$ (4 S) | 3/24 | 44 |
| 80 mg/m$^2$ (6 S) | 4/9 | 45 |
| 200 mg/m$^2$ (3 S) | 3/8 | 46 |

**Table 7** Single Agent: Carboplatin (Marginally Active)

| Dose/course (mg/m$^2$) | No. of patients | Response[a] | | | Ref. |
|---|---|---|---|---|---|
| | | CR | PR | OR | |
| 300–400 | 17 | 1 | 1 | 2 | 47 |
| 400 | 9 | 0 | 2 | 2 | 48 |
| 400 | 37 | 0 | 2 | 2 | 49 |
| 450 | 31 | 1 | 4 | 5 | 50 |
| 800–1200–1600 | 4 | 0 | 0 | 0 | 51 |

[a]CR, complete response; OR, objective response; PR, partial response.

evaluable cases (131) was pooled (11), with an OR of 18% (42–44). The use of very high doses gave some promising results, as demonstrated by Planting et al. in Rotterdam (45). With a dosage of 80 mg/m$^2$ weekly for 6 courses a significant activity with four PR in nine evaluable patients was observed, without great toxicity. These results are very close to those of Rebattu et al. (46) using 200 mg/m$^2$ of cisplatin every 3 weeks with three OR out of eight evaluable patients.

5. Carboplatin, an analogue of cisplatin, did not provide better results, (47–50), even when used at very high doses (51). The cumulative data give an OR of 12% in 98 evaluable patients (Table 7).

In conclusion, only a small number of drugs have a marginal activity (Table 8): OR is constantly lower than 15%, CR is an exception, the dura-

**Table 8** Single Agent: Pooled Data

| Agent | No. of trials | No. of cases | No. of responses[a] | | OR (%) |
|---|---|---|---|---|---|
| | | | CR | PR | |
| Doxorubicin | 15 | 197 | 7 | 2 | 18 |
| 4-Epidoxorubicin | 2 | 69 | 0 | 8 | 10 |
| THP-Doxorubicin | 3 | 58 | 2 | 4 | 10 |
| Dihydro-5-azacytidine | 2 | 55 | 1 | 5 | 11 |
| Ifosfamide | 3 | 82 | 0 | 7 | 9 |
| Cisplatin | 8 | 131 | 8 | 16 | 18 |
| Carboplatin | 5 | 98 | 2 | 9 | 12 |

[a]CR, complete response; PR, partial response; OR, objective response.

**Table 9**  High-Dose Methotrexate

| Combination | Response | Ref. |
|---|---|---|
| MTX + CF (1.5 mg/m$^2$) | 4/9 | 52 |
| MTX + CF + VCR | 6/9 | 53 |
| MTX + CF + Cisplatin | 4/6 | 52 |

tion of the response being short, and the median survival being only a little better in the responders.

### B.  Combination Chemotherapy

High dose of methotrexate (MTX) combined with leucovorin (CF) alone (52) or with either vincristine (53) or cisplatin (52) showed some activity, with 14 OR out of the 24 patients tested in these three trials awaiting confirmation (Table 9).

Since doxorubicin was the first well-studied agent with some reported activity, most of the standard combination regimens contained doxorubicin (54–56) (Table 10). However, the results with combination chemotherapy using doxorubicin are comparable with those of doxorubicin alone in terms of response, duration of response, and median survival (9–11).

More interesting is the association of doxorubicin and cisplatin (57–59) (Table 11). With the two apparent best drugs as a single agent, this combination is well-known to be synergistic, and the preliminary results were promising with four responses (1 CR) in six patients (57). When the number of evaluable cases was pooled (89 patients), the overall OR was 31%, with a few CR (7%) (11) (Table 12). The association etoposide

**Table 10**  Combined Cytostatic Agents (with Doxorubicin)

| Combination | Response | (CR) | Ref. |
|---|---|---|---|
| 5-Azacytidine + DOX | 8/36 | 3 | 7 |
| CPM + DTIC + DOX | 2/40 | 1 | 54 |
| versus | | | |
| CPM + DOX | 9/36 | 3 | 54 |
| IFO + DOX | 2/16 | | 55 |
| IFO + EPI | 1/17 | | 56 |

DOX, doxorubicin; CR, complete response; CPM, cyclophosphamide; IFO, ifosfamide; EPI, epirubicine; DTIC, deticene.

**Table 11** Combined Cytostatic Agents (with Cisplatin)

| Combination | Response | (CR) | Ref. |
|---|---|---|---|
| DOX + CISPLAT | 4/6 | (1) | 57 |
| DOX + CISPLAT | 8/19 | (2) | 58 |
| DOX + CISPLAT | 6/24 | | 59 |
| VP16 + CISPLAT | 3/26 | | 60 |
| MITO + CISPLAT | 4/12 | (1) | 61 |

VP16, etoposide (Vepeside); CR, complete response; CISPLAT, cisplatin; MITO, mitomycin; DOX, doxorubicin.

(VP16)-cisplatin seems to be less interesting with only 3 OR out of 26 patients in a National Cancer Institute (NCI) Canada trial (60).

On the basis of an in vivo screening of multiple single agents in nude mice transplanted with two human malignant mesotheliomas, Chahinian (61) developed his combination of mitomycin and cisplatin. The preliminary results gave 4 OR (I CR) in 12 evaluable patients. These data then served as the basis for a randomized trial of mitomycin plus cisplatin versus doxorubicin plus cisplatin, the reference combination. The CALGB should be credited for conducting this only available randomized trial. The results showed a little better OR with the combination of mitomycin plus cisplatin (26% vs 14%), but there was no difference in median survival (62).

In conclusion, the presenting therapeutic combination reference is the mitomycine–cisplatin, rather than doxorubicin–cisplatin. But in their modest activity, this represents the least questionable available combina-

**Table 12** Combination Chemotherapy: Pooled Data

| Combination | No. of trials | No. of cases | No. of responses | | OR (%) |
|---|---|---|---|---|---|
| | | | CR | PR | |
| 5-Azacytidine + DOX | 3 | 45 | 5 | 6 | 24 |
| CPM + DTIC + DOX | 5 | 77 | 3 | 14 | 22 |
| CPM + DOX | 5 | 54 | 1 | 8 | 17 |
| CDDP + MITOMYCIN | 2 | 37 | 3 | 3 | 16 |
| CDDP + DOX | 7 | 89 | 6 | 22 | 31 |

CDDP, cisplatin; CPM, cyclophosphamide; CR, complete response; DOX, doxorubicin; DTIC, deticene; OR, objective response; PR, partial response.

tion, rather than the best. Indeed, the results of the combination are not particularly superior to those obtained with a single agent, the response being generally short (6–8 months), with no real change in median survival.

From a pessimistic point of view, the available data do not justify the routine use of chemotherapy as a standard therapy. Actually, DMM remains a chemoresistant tumor. However, we must recall that this was the situation for chemotherapy of non–small-cell lung cancer 10 years ago. Since then things have changed and are still changing.

### C. Intracavitary Chemotherapy

Another way to give a cytotoxic drug is the intracavitary route. What the potential advantages of this approach? First, treating the underlying malignancy as well as controlling the effusion; second, modeling studies have suggested a major pharmacokinetic advantage for the intracavitary route, compared with the systemic delivery: peak intracavitary concentrations of cisplatin are 20–240 times higher than peak plasma concentrations when cisplatin is administered into the pleural or peritoneal cavities (63,64). Third, this benefit has already been demonstrated in studies using local administration of drugs in ovarian carcinoma.

Cisplatin was the most frequent drug used by the intracavitary route. Cumulated data for 58 patients (65) indicate that the best results are obtained with peritoneal mesothelioma, with 63% OR (22 out of 35 evaluable patients), whereas only 17% OR (4 out of 23 evaluable patients) was obtained in pleural mesothelioma. The addition of mitomycin to cisplatin does not appear to have improved the efficacy of such therapy, but it increases local toxicity (66).

The conclusions and the limitations of this approach are the following: chemotherapeutic agents act mainly by sclerosis, rather than cytotoxicity, so they have a symptomatic palliative effect in effusion, as opposed to an antitumoral activity. The results are more interesting in peritoneal mesothelioma than in pleural mesothelioma, for which they are rather disappointing. Intracavitary chemotherapy has several limitations. It requires good dispersion throughout the serosal cavity to be effective; the drugs penetrate the tumor to a distance of only a few millimeters. So patients having either a bulky DMM tumor or intrapleural adhesions, cannot benefit from this therapeutic modality. In the model of ovarian carcinoma, the intraperitoneal chemotherapy was effective only in patients whose disease was minimal residual (<5 mm). Therefore, this approach can be effective only in the early stage I of pleural mesothelioma which is rather rare or in combination with other treatment modalities (67), with a curative approach associating intraperitoneal induction chemotherapy, followed by cytoreductive surgery and early postoperative intraperitoneal chemotherapy in peritoneal mesothelioma (68).

## IV. Conclusions

The cure of mesothelioma seems exceptional. The diagnosis of mesothelioma is too late, with a bulky tumoral disease incurable by local treatments. An early detection of high-risk patients is necessary.

The cytostatic drugs are not without effect, but the results are still poor. Further investigation is required with phase II trials, which may identify new drugs with better activity.

The selection of active agents can be made by using experimental models, either human, such as mesothelioma cell lines (HMCL) (69), or the Chahinian's nude mice model (61). There has been substantial experimental evidence suggesting an increase of activity of cytotoxic drugs by cytokines (70). It seems promising to associate these synergistic modalities for the treatment of mesothelioma either by local treatment or systemic treatment. There are some ongoing phase I/II clinical trials based on these hypotheses.

As this tumor is uncommon and several different prognostic categories exist, a cooperative effort will be necessary for carefully planned future therapeutic trials, comparing a treatment modality versus a best supportive care arm to demonstrate the value of any new therapeutic approach.

## References

1. Rush VW. Diagnosis and treatment of pleural mesothelioma. Semin Surg Oncol 1990; 6:279–285.
2. Roberts GH. Distant visceral metastases in pleural mesothelioma. Br J Dis Chest 1976; 70:246–250.
3. Huncharek M, Muscat J. Metastases in diffuse pleural mesothelioma: influence of histological type. Thorax 1987; 42:897–898.
4. Alberts AS, Falkson G, Goedhals L, Vorobiof DA, Van der Merwe LA. Malignant pleural mesothelioma. A disease unaffected by current therapeutic maneuvers. J Clin Oncol 1988; 6:527–535.
5. Ruffié P, Feld R, Minkin S, Cormier Y, Boutan-Laroze A, Ginsberg R, Ayoub J, Shepherd FA, Evans WK, Figueredo A, Pater JL, Pringle JF, Kreisman H. Diffuse malignant mesothelioma of the pleura in Ontario and Quebec: a retrospective study of 332 patients. J Clin Oncol 1989; 7:1157–1168.
6. Law MR, Gregor A, Hodson ME, Bloom HJG. Malignant mesothelioma of the pleura: a study of 52 treated and 64 untreated patients. Thorax 1984; 39: 255–259.
7. Chahinian AP, Pajak TF, Holland JF, Norton L, Ambinder RM, Mandel

EM. Diffuse malignant mesothelioma: prospective evaluation of 69 patients. Ann Intern Med 1982; 96:746–755.

8. Antman KH, Shemin R, Ryan L, Klegar KL, Osteen RT, Herman T, Lederman G, Corson JM. Malignant mesothelioma, prognostic variables in a registry of 180 patients, the Dana–Farber Cancer Institute and Brigham and Women's Hospital experience over 2 decades, 1965–1985. J Clin Oncol 1988; 6:147–153.

9. Aisner J, Wiernik PH. Chemotherapy in the treatment of malignant mesothelioma. Semin Oncol 1981; 8:335–343.

10. Falkson G, Alberts AS, Falkson HC. Malignant pleural mesothelioma treatment, the current state of art. Cancer Treat Rev 1988; 15:231–242.

11. Krarup-Hansen A, Hansen HH. Chemotherapy in malignant mesothelioma: a review. Cancer Chemother Pharmacol 1991; 28:319–330.

12. Colbert N, Izrael V, Vannetzel JM, Schlienger M, Milleron B, Blanchon F, Herman D, Akoun G, Roland J, Chatelet F, Laugier A. A prospective study of detorubicin in malignant mesothelioma. Cancer 1985; 56:2170–2174.

13. Butchart EG, Ashcroft T, Barnsley WA, Holden MP. Pleuropneumonectomy in the management of diffuse malignant mesothelioma of the pleura. Thorax 1976; 31:15–24.

14. Usawasdi T, Dhingra HM, Charnsangavej C, Luna MA. A case report of malignant pleural mesothelioma with long term disease control after chemotherapy. Cancer 1991; 67:48–54.

15. Falkson G, Vorobiof DA, Simon IW, Borden E. Phase II trial of acivicin in malignant mesothelioma. Cancer Treat 1987; 7:545–546.

16. Earhart RH, Amato DJ, Chang A, Borden EC, Shiraki M, Dowd ME, Comis RL, Davis TE, Smith TJ. Phase II trial of 6-diazo-5-oxo-L-norleucine versus aclacinomycin-A in advanced sarcomas and mesotheliomas. Invest New Drugs 1990; 8:113–119.

17. Amato DA, Borden EC, Shiraki M, Enterline HT, Rosenbaum C, Davis HL, Paul AR, Stevens CM, Lerner HJ. Evaluation of bleomycin, chlorozotocin, MGGB and bruceantin in patients with advanced soft tissue sarcoma, bone sarcoma or mesothelioma. Invest New Drugs 1985; 3:397–401.

18. Sorensen PG, Bach F, Bork E, Hansen HH. Randomized trial of doxorubicin versus cyclophosphamide in diffuse malignant mesothelioma. Cancer Treat Rep 1985; 69:1431–1432.

19. Eagan RT, Frytak S, Richardson RL, Creagan ET, Nichols WC. Phase II trial of diaziquone in malignant mesothelioma. Cancer Treat Rep 1986; 70:429.

20. Harvey VJ, Slevin ML, Ponder BAJ, Blackshaw AJ, Wrigle PFM. Chemotherapy of diffuse malignant mesothelioma. Cancer 1984; 54:961–964.

21. Falkson G, Vorobiof DA, Lerner HJ. A phase II study of m-AMSA in patients with malignant mesothelioma. Cancer Chemother Pharmacol 1983; 11:94–97.

22. Eisenhauer EA, Evans WK, Raghaven D, Desmeules MJ, Murray NR, Stuart-Harris R, Wilson KS. Phase II study of mitoxantrone in patients with mesothelioma. A National Cancer Institute of Canada clinical trials group study. Cancer Treat Rep 1986; 70:1029–1030.

23. Van Breukelen FJM, Mattson K, Giaccone G, Van Zandwijk N, Planteydt

HT, Kirkpatrick A, Dalesio O. Mitoxantrone in malignant pleural mesothelioma: a study by the EORTC lung cancer cooperative group. Eur J Cancer 1991; 27:1627–1629.

24. Cantwell BMJ, Earnshaw M, Harris AL. Phase II study of a novel antifolate, N-10-propargyl-5, 8-dideazafolic, in malignant mesothelioma. Cancer Treat Rep 1986; 70:1335–1336.

25. Cowan JD, Green S, Lucas J, Weick JK, Balcerzak SP, Rivkin SE, Coltman CA, Baker LH. Phase II trial of five day intravenous infusion vinblastine sulfate in patients with diffuse malignant mesothelioma: a Southwest Oncology Group Study. Invest New Drugs 1988; 6:247–248.

26. Martensson G, Sorenson S. A phase II study of vincristine in malignant mesothelioma – a negative report. Cancer Chemother Pharmacol 1989; 24:133–134.

27. Kelsen D, Gralla R, Cheng E, Martin N. Vindesine in the treatment of malignant mesothelioma, a phase II study. Cancer Treat Rep 1983; 67:821–822.

28. Boutin C, Irisson M, Guerin JC, Roegel E, Paramelle B, Brambilla C, Jeannin L, Dabouis G, Le Caer H, Viallat JR. Phase II trial of vindesine in malignant pleural mesothelioma. Cancer Treat Rep 1987; 71:205–206.

29. Lerner HJ, Schoenfeld DA, Martin A, Falkson G, Borden E. Malignant mesothelioma; the Eastern Cooperative Oncology Group experience. Cancer 1983; 52:1981–1985.

30. Magri MD, Veronesi A, Foladore S, De Giovanni D, Serra C, Crismancich F, Tuveri G, Nicotra M, Tommasi M, Morassut S, Larbone A, Grandi G, Mon Fardini S, Bianchi C. Epirubicin in the treatment of malignant mesothelioma: a phase II cooperative study. Tumori 1991; 77:49–51.

31. Mattson K, Giaccone G, Kirkpatrick A, Evrard D, Tammilehto L, Van Breukelen FJM, Planteydt HT, Van Zandwijk N. Epirubicin in malignant mesothelioma: a phase II study for the European Organization for Research and Treatment of Cancer Lung Cancer Cooperative Group. J Clin Oncol 1992; 10:824–828.

32. Kaukel E, Koschel G, Gatzemeyer U, Salewski E. A phase II study of pirarubicin in malignant pleural mesothelioma. Cancer 1990; 66:651–654.

33. Ruffié P. Unpublished data.

34. Sridhar KS, Hussein AM, Feun LG, Zubrod C. Activity of pirarubicin in malignant mesothelioma. Cancer 1989; 63:1084–1091.

35. Habeshaw T, Paul J, Jones R, Stallard S, Stewart M, Kaye SB, Soukop M, Symonos RP, Reed NS, Rankin EM. Epirubicin at two-dose levels with prednisolone as treatment for advanced breast cancer: the results of a randomized trial. J Clin Oncol 1991; 9:295–304.

36. Bajorin D, Kelsen D, Mintzer DM. Phase II trial of mitomycin in malignant mesothelioma. Cancer Treat Rep 1987; 71:857–858.

37. Harmon D, Vogelzang N, Roboz J, Goutsou M, Antman K, Coughlin K, Green MR. Dihydro-5-azacytidine in malignant mesothelioma using serum hyaluronic acid as a tumor marker. A phase II trial of the CALG B [abstr]. Proc ASCO 1991; 10:351.

38. Dhingra HM, Murphy WK, Winn RJ, Raber MN, Hong WK. Phase II trial

of 5,6-dihydro-5-azacytidine in pleural malignant mesothelioma. Invest New Drugs 1991; 9:69–72.

39. Alberts AS, Falkson G, Van-Zyl L. Malignant pleural mesothelioma: phase II pilot study of ifosfamide and mesna. JNCI 1988; 80:698–700.

40. Zidar B, Metch B, Ballerzak S, Pierche H, Militello L, Keppen M, Berenberg J. A phase II evaluation of ifosfamide and mesna in unresectable diffuse malignant mesothelioma: a Southwest Oncology Group Study. Cancer 1992; 70:2547–2551.

41. Falkson G, Hunt M, Borden EC, Hayes JA, Falkson CI, Smith TJ. An extended phase II trial of ifosfamide plus mesna in malignant mesothelioma. Invest New Drugs 1992; 10:337–343.

42. Dabouis G, Le Mevel B, Coroller J. Treatment of diffuse malignant mesothelioma by cis-dichlorodiammine platinum in nine patients. Cancer Chemother Pharmacol 1981; 5:209–210.

43. Zidar B, Green S, Pierce H, Roach R, Balcerzak S, Militello L, Keppen M, Berenberg J. A phase II evaluation of cisplatin in unresectable diffuse malignant mesothelioma. A Southwest Oncology Group study. Invest New Drugs 1988; 6:223–226.

44. Mintzer DM, Kelsen D, Frimmer D, Heelan R, Gralla R. Phase II trial of high dose cisplatin in patients with malignant mesothelioma. Cancer Treat Rep 1985; 69:711–712.

45. Planting A, Goey H, Verweij J. Phase II study of six weekly courses of high dose cisplatinum in mesothelioma [abstr]. Proc AACR 1991; 32:194.

46. Rebattu, Personal communication.

47. M Bidde EK, Harland SJ, Calvert AH, Smith IE. Phase II trial of carboplatin in treatment of patients with malignant mesothelioma. Cancer Chemother Pharmacol 1986; 18:284–285.

48. Cantwell BMJ, Franks CR, Harris AL. Phase II study of the platinum analogues JM8 and JM9 in malignant pleural mesothelioma. Cancer Chemother Pharmacol 1986; 18:286–288.

49. Vogelzang NJ, Goutsou M, Corson JM, Suzuki Y, Graziano S, Aisner J, Cooper MR, Coughlin KM, Green MR. Carboplatin in malignant mesothelioma: a phase II study of the Cancer and Leukemia Group B. Cancer Chemother Pharmacol 1990; 27:239–242.

50. Raghavan D, Gianoutsos P, Bishop J, Lee J, Young I, Corte P, Bye P, McLaughan B. Phase II trial of carboplatin in the management of malignant mesothelioma. J Clin Oncol 1990; 8:151–154.

51. Gore ME, Calvert AH, Smith IE. High dose carboplatin in the treatment of lung cancer and mesothelioma: a phase I dose escalation study. Eur J Cancer Clin Oncol 1987; 23:1391–1397.

52. Djerassi I, Kim JS, Kasserov L, Reggev A. Response of mesothelioma to large doses of methotrexate with CF rescue used alone or with cisplatinum [abstr]. Proc ASCO 1985; 4:191.

53. Dimitrov N, Egner J, Balcueva E, Suhrland LG. High-dose methotrexate with citrovocum factor and vincristine in the treatment of malignant mesothelioma. Cancer 1982; 50:1245–1247.

54. Samson MK, Wasser LP, Borden E, Wanebo HJ, Creech RH, Philips M, Baker LH. Randomized comparison of cyclophosphamide, imidazole carboxamide, and Adriamycin versus cyclophosphamide and Adriamycin in patients with advanced stage malignant mesothelioma: a Sarcoma Intergroup Study. J Clin Oncol 1987; 5:86–91.

55. Carmichael J, Cantwell BMJ, Harris AL. A phase II trial of ifosfamide–mesna with doxorubicin for malignant mesothelioma. Eur J Cancer Clin Oncol 1989; 25:911–912.

56. Magri MP, Foladores S, Veronesi A, Serra C, Nicotra M, Tommasi M, Grandi G, Monfardini S, Bianchi C. Treatment of malignant mesothelioma with epirubicin and ifosfamide: a phase II cooperative study. Ann Oncol 1992; 3:237–238.

57. Zidar BL, Pugh RP, Schiffer LM, Raju RN, Vaidya KA, Bloom RL, Horne D, Baker LH. Treatment of six cases of mesothelioma with doxorubicin and cisplatin. Cancer 1983; 52:1788–1791.

58. Henss H, Fiebig H, Schildge J, Arnold H, Hasse J. Phase II study with the combination of cisplatin and doxorubicin in advanced malignant mesothelioma of the pleura. Onkologie 1988; 1:118–120.

59. Ardizzoni A, Rosso R, Salvati F, Fusco V, Cinquegrana A, De Palma M, Serrano J, Pennucci MC, Soresi E, Crippa M, Gulisano M, Castagneto B, Scagliotti G, Rinaldi M, Santi L. Activity of doxorubicin and cisplatin combination chemotherapy in patients with diffuse malignant pleural mesothelioma. An Italian Lung Cancer Task Force (FONICAP) phase II study. Cancer 1991; 6:2984–2987.

60. Eisenhauer EA, Evans WK, Murray NR, Kocha W, Wierzbicki R, Wilson KS. Phase II of VP16 and cisplatin in patients with unresectable malignant mesothelioma. Invest New Drugs 1988; 6:327–329.

61. Chahinian AP, Norton L, Holland JF, Szrajer L, Hart RD. Experimental and clinical activity of mitomycin C and cisplatin in malignant mesothelioma. Cancer Res 1984; 44:1688–1692.

62. Chahinian AP, Antman KH, Goutson M, Corson JM, Suzuki Y, Modeas C, Herdon JE, Aisner J, Ellison RR, Leone L, Vogelzang NJ, Green MR. Randomized phase II trial of cisplatin with mitomycin or doxorubicin for malignant mesothelioma. J Clin Oncol 1993; 11:1559–1565.

63. Markman M, Cleary S, Pfeifle C, Howell SB. Cisplatin administered by the intracavitary route as treatment for malignant mesothelioma. Cancer 1986; 58: 18–21.

64. Rusch VW, Niedzwiecki D, Tao Y, Menendez-Botet C, Cnistrian A, Kelsen D, Saltz L, Markman M. Intrapleural cisplatin and mitomycin for malignant mesothelioma following pleurectomy: pharmacokinetic studies. J Clin Oncol 1992; 10:1001–1006.

65. Vlasveld LT, Gallee MPW, Rodenhuis S, Taal BG. Intraperitoneal chemotherapy for malignant peritoneal mesothelioma. Eur J Cancer 1991; 27:732–734.

66. Markman M, Kelsen D. Intraperitoneal cisplatin and mitomycin as treatment for malignant peritoneal mesothelioma. Regul Cancer Treat 1989; 2:49–53.

67. Antman KH, Osteen RT, Klegar KL, Amato DA, Pomfret EA, Larson DA,

Corson JM. Early peritoneal mesothelioma: a treatable malignancy. Lancet 1985; 3:977–981.

68. Vidal Jove J, Sweatman TW, Israel M, Graves T, Litwin FP, Davidson ED, Sugarbaker PH. A curative approach to malignant peritoneal mesothelioma: case report and review of the literature. Reg Cancer Treat 1991; 3:269–274.

69. Bowman RV, Manning LS, Davis R, Robinson BWS. Chemosensitivity and cytokine sensitivity of malignant mesothelioma. Cancer Chemother Pharmacol 1991; 28:420–426.

70. Sklarin NT, Chahinian AP, Fever EJ, Lahman LA, Szrajer L, Holland JF. Augmentation of activity of cisplatin and mitomycin C by interferon in human malignant mesothelioma xenograft in nude mice. Cancer Res 1988; 48:64–67.

# 16

## Therapeutic Studies of Malignant Mesothelioma in Nude Mice

**A. PHILIPPE CHAHINIAN**

Mount Sinai School of Medicine
New York, New York

## I.  Introduction

Malignant mesothelioma is a type of tumor that is ideally suited for experimental therapeutic studies in nude mice. Although its incidence is increasing, mesothelioma remains a rare tumor (1). Clinical data on the efficacy of chemotherapy are scarce. Prospective clinical trials can evaluate only a very limited number of regimens, mostly as phase II-type trials of existing or new single agents. To conduct large-scale studies of combination chemotherapy or randomized phase III trials of different regimens comparing single agents or different combinations would take many years, even for cooperative groups. Finally, mesothelioma is a tumor refractory to most agents, and selection of treatments by experimental studies before clinical trials is highly desirable. Correlation between the nude mouse model and corresponding clinical therapeutic results in various types of cancers, including mesothelioma, has been remarkably good (2,3). Finally, the nude mouse model allows keeping the tumor lines for as long as necessary to conduct as many experiments as required.

## II.  Historical Aspects

The discovery of the nude (hairless) mouse by Flanagan (4) marked an important event in cancer research. After it was shown that such mice, homozygous for the autosomal recessive gene *nu*, lack a normal thymus (5), it became evident that these animals are deficient in functional mature T cells, thus permitting heterotransplantation of tumors in these animals. Indeed, the first human tumor, an adenocarcinoma of the colon, was successfully transplanted in nude mice by Rygaard and Povlsen (6). The possibility of serial growth of such tumors by successive transfer to other nude mice was reported later by the same authors (7).

Since then, many different human tumors have been transplanted into nude mice. The original histological characteristics of the parent tumor as well as the production of tumor markers and ectopic hormones usually remain preserved in xenografts (8–10).

The predictive value of this laboratory model has been evaluated. Many experiments in tumors, other than mesothelioma, have shown that the results of chemotherapy in nude mice xenografts have correlated well with clinical experience for each tumor type (8–11). In the most compelling cases for which a direct comparison between the results of chemotherapy in patients and their corresponding xenografts was possible, there was a close and remarkable agreement, thereby further validating this system (11,12).

Our experiments at the Mount Sinai Medical Center in New York began in 1978, when we successfully transplanted mesothelioma in nude mice from two patients (13). These two lines, one epithelial, and the other mixed type, but preponderantly epithelial, have been maintained by serial transplantation in nude mice up to the present time. Their human nature and close resemblance to the original tumors have been confirmed by karyotypic, histological, and ultrastructural studies (13,14). At about the same time, Arnold et al. (15), from the Central Institute for Cancer research in Berlin, Germany, reported a successful transplantation of a human mesothelioma into nude mice. The histological type of mesothelioma, however, was not mentioned, except that it was obtained from a female patient with peritoneal carcinomatosis.

## III.  Chemotherapy Studies in Nude Mice

Our initial chemotherapy experiments at Mount Sinai included testing of many single agents and confirmed the clinical experience that malignant mesothelioma is rather refractory to most agents (2,3,16). We observed that doxorubicin azacitidine, (5-azacytidine), fluorouracil (5-fluorouracil), methotrexate, vincristine, and vindesine were ineffective against both of our initial mesothelioma lines. It is of note that the patient from whom onc line was derived was treated with a combination of doxorubicin and azacitidine without clinical response. The active single agents for the first line (by decreasing order of activity) were mitomycin, dacarbazine, carmustine (BCNU), bleomycin, and cyclophosphamide. The second line was more resistant, but cisplatin and bleomycin showed activity.

As a result of these experiments, we then elected to test a combination of the most active single agent in one line (mitomycin) with the most active one for the other (cisplatin). The combination of mitomycin and cisplatin proved to be the most effective regimen for both lines, and addition of the inactive agent increased the antitumor effect of the active one in each respective cell line (16). Figure 1 shows the antitumor effect of a combination of mitomycin and cisplatin compared with either drug alone in four distinct lines of human mesothelioma xenografts in our laboratory.

Given these studies, we then conducted a pilot clinical trial at Mount Sinai with a combination of these two agents. Objective tumor response was seen in 4 of 12 patients (33%) with malignant mesothelioma, including one complete response (16). A direct patient–xenograft correlation was also

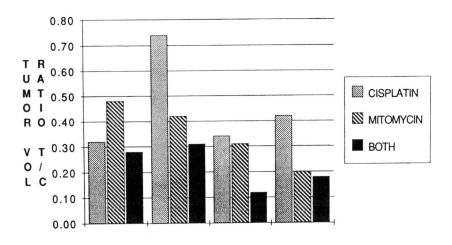

**MESOTHELIOMA LINE**

**Figure 1**   Effect of cisplatin or mitomycin alone and in combination against four lines of human malignant mesothelioma xenografts in nude mice. The tumor volume ratio T/C represents the mean tumor volume of animals treated with chemotherapy (T) over controls treated with normal saline (C).

obtained at Mount Sinai in a patient who underwent surgery (pleuropneumonectomy) for malignant mesothelioma and who relapsed 3 months later. The corresponding xenografts showed complete response to mitomycin and cisplatin, and so did the patient when treated with that drug combination (17). That patient unfortunately experienced mitomycin-induced pulmonary toxicity after two cycles, which led to the discontinuation of that agent. He also developed brain metastases. Nevertheless, duration of response was 15 months and survival from onset of chemotherapy was 18 months.

On the basis of these results, a cooperative trial by the Cancer and Leukemia Group B (CALGB) in the United States performed a randomized phase II clinical study of doxorubicin and cisplatin versus mitomycin and cisplatin in 70 patients with malignant mesothelioma (18). Final results showed a response rate of 26% (including two complete responses) for 35 patients treated with mitomycin and cisplatin, versus 14% (with no complete response) for 35 patients treated with doxorubicin and cisplatin. Survival, however, was similar for the two groups, with a median of 7.7 and 8.8 months, respectively. Intracavitary administration of mitomycin and cisplatin has been evaluated at Memorial Sloan–Kettering Cancer Center in New York in 11 patients with peritoneal mesothelioma (19). Reduction of ascites was seen in 6 of them, and 2 patients remained without evidence of recurrent disease for 32+ and 41+ months, respectively. The use of this combination, given intrapleurally after surgery for pleural mesothelioma, is currently being evaluated in that institution as well (20). Hence, wide clinical applications resulted from the discovery of this regimen in the nude mouse model.

Testing of other agents, such as anthracycline derivatives and analogs of cisplatin, has also been conducted in the nude mouse system. We have compared the activity of carboplatin (CBDCA) and iproplatin (CHIP) with cisplatin in our first two mesothelioma lines (21). In the line resistant to cisplatin, carboplatin was inactive, but iproplatin showed borderline activity. In the line sensitive to cisplatin, iproplatin was ineffective, but carboplatin showed mild activity. These three platinum analogs, therefore, showed different levels of activity in these tumors. Daunorubicin, as a single agent given intravenously, was evaluated in nude mice by Arnold et al. (15). A 79% increase in life span of nude mice with an ascitic form of mesothelioma was observed. Additional experiments by the same group of investigators on this mesothelioma line revealed sensitivity (measured by percentage inhibition of tritiated thymidine or uridine incorporation in tumor cells) to 4-hydroperoxy-cyclophosphamide, vinblastine and, to a lesser extent, fluorouracil, whereas methotrexate was ineffective (22).

## IV.  Studies of Tumor Markers in Nude Mice

Buhl et al. (23), in Denmark, transplanted a human mesothelioma (type not specified) into nude mice and studied the effect of a combination of vincristine, cyclophosphamide, doxorubicin, and prednisolone. This treatment resulted in no measurable regression of the tumors, but only in their stabilization. There was, however, a concomitant decrease in urinary excretion of pseudouridine and hypoxanthine in these animals. This work was based on the observation of increased urinary levels of pseudouridine in asbestos workers with mesothelioma (24).

A more specific tumor marker for mesothelioma, hyaluronic acid (HA), has been studied in nude mice with human mesothelioma xenografts by Roboz et al. (25). By using a new high-performance liquid chromatography (HPLC) technique for the quantification of intact HA, serum levels of HA were measured before and after transplantation of human mesothelioma in nude mice. The HA concentration rose to 8–16 $\mu$g/ml as early as the fourth to fifth day after subcutaneous tumor transplantation, before the tumors became clinically palpable. Experimental and clinical studies of serum levels of HA are currently being evaluated, not only for the diagnosis of mesothelioma, but also to monitor the effect of treatment on the tumor.

## V.  Biological and Immunological Agents in Nude Mice

The role of interferon (IFN) was examined in our laboratory for its antitumor effects against mesothelioma xenografts in nude mice (26). Whereas human recombinant IFN-$\alpha$ 2a alone, given at a dose of $2 \times 10^5$ IU subcutaneously 5 days per week for 5 weeks showed very little antitumor effect, the addition of IFN to an effective agent (mitomycin in one line and cisplatin in the other) increased tumor response when compared with chemotherapy alone (Table 1). The role of various IFNs has been evaluated in small series of patients with mesothelioma (1). Interferon-alpha, given intrapleurally produced two partial responses among 13 cases of mesothelioma (27). Intrapleural IFN-$\gamma$ seemed effective for very early-staged mesothelioma (nodules smaller than 5 mm), with four complete response and one partial response out of nine patients. At a more advanced stage, it produced only one partial response in ten patients (28). Interferon-$\beta$ showed no appreciable activity in a trial including 14 patients with mesothelioma (29). Clinical trials combining interferon with chemotherapy are currently being evaluated. Preliminary results seem encouraging. A combination of cisplatin and IFN-$\alpha$ given systematically to 19 evaluable patients with advanced pleural

**Table 1**  Activity of Human Recombinant Interferon-alfa With or
Without Chemotherapy in Two Lines of Human Malignant Mesothelioma
Xenografts in Nude Mice

| Mesothelioma cell line | Treatment arms compared with controls | Mean tumor volume ratio[a] |
|---|---|---|
| Line 1 | Interferon/control | 0.70 |
| | Cisplatin/control | 0.29 |
| | Cisplatin + interferon/control | 0.05 |
| | Cisplatin + interferon/cisplatin | 0.16 |
| Line 2 | Interferon/control | 0.54 |
| | Mitomycin/control | 0.33 |
| | Mitomycin + interferon/control | 0.13 |
| | Mitomycin + interferon/mitomycin | 0.40 |

[a]Mean tumor volume ratio denotes mean tumor volume of treated animals over control animals.
Source: Ref. 26.

mesothelioma resulted in 7 partial responses (37%) (30). Another trial of cisplatin and IFN-$\alpha$, together with tamoxifen, resulted in three partial responses and one minor response in nine patients with pleural mesothelioma (31). The mechanisms by which interferons may potentiate the activity of chemotherapy are complex and are being evaluated experimentally and clinically in several tumors, such as colon cancer and melanoma (32). Complex, and as yet poorly understood, interactions may take place, involving various mechanisms, such as direct antiproliferative effects of IFNs, host protective effects of IFNs, immunomodulatory effects, as well as effects on drug-metabolizing enzymes and drug pharmacokinetics.

The effect of immunotoxins directed against human transferrin receptor has been evaluated in another nude mouse model of human mesothelioma using the H-MESO-1 cell line (33). In these experiments, monoclonal murine IgG antibodies against that receptor, coupled to ricin A, were potent in vitro cytotoxins against H-MESO-1 cells. When such immunotoxins were given intraperitoneally 24 h after intraperitoneal administration of 6 $\times$ $10^6$–9 $\times$ $10^6$ H-MESO-1 cells in nude mice, survival of tumor-bearing mice was extended by 149–404%. Specificity of this response was confirmed by the ineffectiveness of irrelevant control immunotoxin as well as blockade of specific antitransferrin immunotoxin action by excess free antibody. The carboxylic ionophore monensin potentiated the cytotoxicity of these immunotoxins.

Spectacular results and even "cure" of human mesothelioma (H-

MESO-line) in nude mice was reported by investigators at the Dana–Farber Cancer Institute in Boston with the use of diphtheria toxin (34). A single intravenous or intraperitoneal dose of 1–3 μg of diphtheria toxin apparently eradicated malignant ascites and tumor masses in such treated animals, whereas lower doses were not as effective. It was estimated that as little as 10,000 molecules of diphtheria toxin per target cell was sufficient to kill H-MESO cells. A rapid and complete direct cytotoxic effect on tumor cells was demonstrated by measuring protein synthesis by incorporation of [³H]leucine, both by the intravenous and intraperitoneal routes of administration of diphtheria toxin. This treatment did not appear to produce toxic symptoms in mice, and the low susceptibility of murine cells to diphtheria toxin allowed a selective elimination of sensitive human tumor cells. Formalin-attenuated diphtheria toxoid or diphtheria toxin plus neutralizing sheep antidiphtheria toxin were ineffective.

## VI.  Physical Agents: Photodynamic Therapy in Nude Mice

Photodynamic therapy (PDT) is a novel and elegant treatment modality that is being investigated experimentally and clinically in several tumors. Its use for the treatment of mesothelioma is logical, since this peculiar tumor involves serosal surfaces diffusely and, at least initially, superficially over a large area. Surgical resection is often difficult and incomplete. Use of PDT has been evaluated in a nude mouse model of mesothelioma, using the H-MESO-1 cell line transplanted subcutaneously. A porphyrin-type photosensitizing agent (porfimer; Photofrin II) given intraperitoneally was present at higher concentrations in tumor tissues than in normal lung and heart (35). Twenty-four hours after intraperitoneal administration of Photofrin II at doses of 2 or 5 mg/kg in nude mice, subcutaneous human mesothelioma transplants were exposed for 30 min to laser light at 630 nm, 200 mW/cm² (360 J/cm²) using an ion-pumped dye laser. Tumors were exposed transcutaneously with the laser fiber positioned 1.5 cm from the surface, producing a 1-cm-diameter spot size. There was a significant decrease in tumor volume up to 18 days after treatment for both doses of Photofrin II when compared with controls, with a greater effect in the higher-dose group.

The cytotoxic effects of PDT were also evaluated in vitro against the same H-MESO-1 line, demonstrating rapid uptake of Photofrin II by the mesothelioma cells, with a 50% uptake within 2 h and a plateau reached at 8 h (36). Gold vapor laser light alone and Photofrin II alone produced little cytotoxicity, as measured by a tritiated thymidine assay, whereas the combination of both was cytotoxic in vitro at all doses, with an increasing effect for higher doses of light or drug.

Clinical applications of this technique have already begun. At the National Cancer Institute in the United States, a phase I trial of intraoperative photodynamic therapy of malignant pleural mesothelioma is being conducted (37). The photosensitizing agent (dihematoporphyrin ether) is administrated to the patient 2 days before surgery. After thoracotomy and debulking of the tumor to a thickness less than 5 mm, the ipsilateral chest cavity is filled with an intralipid solution for better light-scattering and then exposed to a 630-nm light, using an argon pump-dye laser during about 30 min. Results of this phase I trial are pending (38). So far, this approach seems to be well tolerated. Reported side effect included a transient rise in serum creatinine, with no evidence of myoglobinuria. A similar approach was reported in Europe using a chlorin derivative as a photosensitizing agent (39). Four patients with malignant mesothelioma received intraoperative PDT with that agent. Its tissue concentration was up to 14 times higher in the tumor than in normal tissues. Postoperative side effects included anorexia, fluid retention, hypoproteinemia, and severe chest pain. One patient died of aspiration pneumonia on the sixth postoperative day. Autopsy revealed tumor necrosis of mesothelioma throughout the chest cavity and the lung surface. The depth of necrosis ranged from 0.5 to 1 cm at the diaphragmatic area and from 0.3 to 0.5 cm at the lung surface. These results indicate that the doses and side effects of PDT should be carefully investigated before large-scale clinical trials.

An alternative approach is to deliver the light through a thoracoscope rather than thoracotomy. This technique has been described in Sweden (40). One patient received Photofrin II and underwent thoracoscopy 48 h later. The pleural surface was exposed to light from a gold vapor laser. The procedure lasted 6 h under epidural anesthesia. Following this procedure, the patient was "very tired" and in poor general condition for 2 days. Serum creatinine rose temporarily. A CT scan of the chest 2 weeks posttreatment showed "striking reduction in pleural tumors." To reduce the risk of tumor seeding along the puncture channels, that patient also received superficial electron radiotherapy to the ipsilateral thorax. Follow-up 10 months after treatment revealed no sign of tumor progression.

## VII. Conclusions

In summary, the nude mouse model has been of great value for the study of new effective therapies for this rare disease, which has a reputation of being untreatable. Novel approaches have been investigated in this experimental model. The antitumor activity of original regimens in the nude mouse using chemotherapy, biological or immunological agents, as well as physical agents has already been applied to the clinic, with some success and good prospects for future clinical trials. Considerable time has been saved by selecting only the most effective experimental therapies for clinical research.

### Acknowledgments

Supported in part by Public Health Service Grant CA36283 awarded by the National Cancer Institute, Department of Health and Human Services, Bethesda, Maryland, and by the T. J. Martell Foundation for Leukemia, Cancer, and AIDS Research.

### References

1. Chahinian AP. Malignant mesothelioma. In: Holland JF, Frei E III, Bast RC Jr, Kufe DW, Morton DL, Weichselbaum RR, eds. Cancer medicine, 3rd ed. Philadelphia: Lea & Febiger, 1993:1337–1355.
2. Chahinian AP. Laboratory models for the treatment of mesothelioma. In: Antman K, Aisner J, eds. Asbestos-related malignancy. Orlando: Grune & Stratton, 1987:375–383.
3. Chahinian AP. The nude mouse model in mesothelioma research and therapy. Eur Respir Rev 1993; 3:204–207.
4. Flanagan SP. Nude, a new hairless gene with pleiotropic effects in the mouse. Genet Res 1966; 8:295–309.
5. Pantelouris EM. Absence of thymus in a mouse mutant. Nature 1968; 217: 370–371.
6. Rygaard J, Povlsen CO. Heterotransplantation of a human malignant tumor to "nude" mice. Acta Pathol Microbiol Scand 1969; 77:758–760.
7. Povlsen CO, Rygaard J. Heterotransplantation of human adenocarcinomas of the colon and rectum to the mouse mutant nude. A study of nine consecutive transplantations. Acta Pathol Microbiol Scand 1971; 79:159–169.
8. Giovanella BC, Stehlin JS Jr, William LJ, Lee SS, Shepard RC. Heterotransplantation of human cancers into nude mice. A model system for human cancer chemotherapy. Cancer 1978; 42:2269–2281.
9. Ovejera AA, Houchens DP, Barker AD. Chemotherapy of human tumor xenografts in genetically athymic mice. Ann Clin Lab Sci 1978; 8:50–56.
10. Povlsen CO. Status of chemotherapy, radiotherapy, endocrine therapy and immunotherapy studies of human cancer in the nude mouse. In: Fogh J, Giovanella BC, eds. The nude mouse in experimental and clinical research. New York: Academic Press, 1978:437–456.
11. Steel GG, Courtenay VD, Peckham MJ. The response to chemotherapy of a variety of human tumor xenografts. Br J Cancer 1983; 47:1–13.

12. Shorthouse AJ, Peckham MJ, Smyth JF, Steel GG. The therapeutic response of bronchial carcinoma xenografts. A direct patient–xenografts comparison. Br J Cancer 1980; 41(suppl 4):142–145.
13. Chahinian AP, Beranek JT, Suzuki Y, Bekesi JG, Wisniewski L, Selikoff IJ, Holland JF. Transplantation of human malignant mesothelioma into nude mice. Cancer Res 1980; 40:181–185.
14. Suzuki Y, Chahinian AP, Ohnuma T. Comparative studies of human malignant mesothelioma in vivo, in xenografts in nude mice and in vitro. Cancer 1987; 60:334–344.
15. Arnold W, Naundorf H, Wilder GP, Nissen E, Tanneberger S. Biological characterization of mesothelioma line in nude mice. I. Transplantation of in vitro cultivated cells of a human ascitic tumor effusion. Arch Geschwulst-forsch 1979; 49:495–507.
16. Chahinian AP, Norton L, Holland JF, Szrajer L, Hart RD. Experimental and clinical activity of mitomycin C and *cis*-diamminedichloroplatinum in malignant mesothelioma. Cancer Res 1984; 44:1688–1692.
17. Chahinian AP, Kirschner PA, Gordon RE, Szrajer L, Holland JF. Usefulness of the nude mouse model in mesothelioma based on a direct patient–xenograft comparison. Cancer 1991; 68:558–560.
18. Chahinian AP, Antman K, Goutsou M, Corson JM, Suzuki Y, Modeas C, Herndon JE, Aisner J, Ellison RR, Leone L, Vogelzang NJ, Green MR. Randomized phase II trial of cisplatin with mitomycin or doxorubicin for malignant mesothelioma by the Cancer and Leukemia Group B. J Clin Oncol 1993 (in press).
19. Markman M, Kelsen D. Intraperitoneal cisplatin and mitomycin as treatment for malignant peritoneal mesothelioma. Regul Cancer Treat 1989; 2:49–53.
20. Rush V, Kelsen D, Saltz L, Ginsberg R, McCormack P, Burt M, Markman M. A phase II trial of intrapleural and systemic chemotherapy for malignant pleural mesothelioma [abstr]. Proc Am Soc Clin Oncol 1992; 11:352.
21. Chahinian AP, Szrajer L, Malamud S, Schwartz PH, Holland JF. Comparative activity of three platinum analogs against human malignant mesothelioma xenografts in nude mice [abstr]. Proc Am Assoc Cancer Res 1985; 26:261.
22. Nissen E, Arnold W, Weis H, Naundorf H, Tanneberger S. Biological characterization of a mesothelioma line in the nude mice. II. Some characteristics of cells cultivated in vitro prior to and after transplantation in nude mice. Arch Geschwulstforsch 1979; 49:544–550.
23. Buhl L, Dragsholt C, Svendsen P, Hage E, Buhl MR. Urinary hypoxanthine and pseudouridine as indicators of tumor development in mesothelioma-transplanted nude mice. Cancer Res 1985; 45:1159–1162.
24. Borek E, Sharma OK, Waalkes TP. New applications of urinary nucleoside markers. Recent Results Cancer Res 1983; 84:301–316.
25. Roboz J, Chahinian AP, Holland JF, Silides D, Szrajer L. Early diagnosis and monitoring of transplanted human malignant mesothelioma by serum hyaluronic acid. JNCI 1989; 81:924–928.
26. Sklarin NT, Chahinian AP, Feuer EJ, Lahman LA, Szrajer L, Holland JF. Augmentation of activity of *cis*-diamminedichloroplatinum (II) and mitomy-

cin C by interferon in human malignant mesothelioma xenografts in nude mice. Cancer Res 1988; 48:64–67.

27. Christmas TI, Musk AW, Robinson BWS. Phase II trial of recombinant human alpha interferon therapy in malignant pleural mesothelioma [abstr]. Proc Am Assoc Cancer Res 1990; 31:283.

28. Boutin C, Viallat JR, Van Zandwijk N, Douillard JT, Paillard JC, Guerin JC, Mignot P, Migueres J, Varlet F, Jehan A, Delepoulle E, Brandely M. Activity of intrapleural recombinant gamma-interferon in malignant mesothelioma. Cancer 1991; 67:2033–2037.

29. Von Hoff DD, Metch B, Lucas JG, Balcarzak SP, Grunberg SM, Rivkin SE. Phase II evaluation of recombinant interferon-beta (IFN-Beta Ser) in patients with diffuse mesothelioma. A Southwest Oncology Group study. J Interferon Res 1990; 10:531–534.

30. Soulié P, Ruffié P, Trandafir L, Monnet A, Tardivon A, Cvitkovic E, Le Chevalier T, Bignon J, Armand JP. Combined systemic CDDP–interferon alpha in advanced pleural malignant mesothelioma [abstr]. Proc Am Soc Clin Oncol 1993; 12:400.

31. Pogrebniak H, Kranda K, Steinberg S, Temeck B, Feuerstein I, Pass H. Cisplatin, interferon alpha, and tamoxifen (CIT) for malignant pleural mesothelioma [abstr]. Proc Am Soc Clin Oncol 1993; 12:398.

32. Hoffman MA, Wadler S. Mechanisms by which interferon potentiates chemotherapy. Cancer Invest 1993; 11:310–313.

33. Griffin TW, Richardson C, Houston LL, LePage D, Bogden A, Raso V. Antitumor activity of intraperitoneal immunotoxins in a nude mouse model of mesothelioma. Cancer Res 1987; 47:4266–4270.

34. Raso V, McGrath J. Cure of experimental human malignant mesothelioma in athymic mice by diphtheria toxin. JNCI 1989; 81:622–627.

35. Feins RH, Hilf R, Ross H, Gibson SL. Photodynamic therapy for human malignant mesothelioma in the nude mouse. J Surg Res 1990; 4:311–314.

36. Keller SM, Taylor DD, Weese JL. In vitro killing of human malignant mesothelioma by photodynamic therapy. J Surg Res 1990; 48:337–340.

37. Pass HI, Tochner Z, DeLaney T, Smith P, Friauf W, Glatstein E, Travis W. Intraoperative photodynamic therapy for malignant mesothelioma [letter]. Ann Thorac Surg 1990; 50:687–688.

38. Pass HI. Photodynamic therapy in oncology. Mechanisms and clinical use. JNCI 1993; 85:443–456.

39. Ris HB, Altermatt HG, Inderbitzi R, Hess R, Nachbur B, Stewart JCM, Wang Q, Lim CK, Bonnett R, Berenbaum MC, Althaus U. Photodynamic therapy with chlorins for diffuse malignant mesothelioma. Initial clinical results. Br J Cancer 1991; 64:1116–1120.

40. Lofgren L, Larsson M, Thaning L, Hallgren S. Transthoracic endoscopic photodynamic treatment of malignant mesothelioma [letter]. Lancet 1991; 337:359.

# 17

## New Therapeutic Approaches in Mesothelioma

**JEAN BIGNON**

University of Paris Val de Marne and
Institut National de la Santé et de
la Recherche Médicale
Créteil, France

**ISABELLE MONNET**

Centre Hospitalier Intercommunal de
Créteil
Créteil, France

**PIERRE RUFFIÉ and
HEDDI HADDADA**

Institut Gustave Roussy
Villejuif, France

**MARIE-CLAUDE JAURAND**

Institut National de la Santé et de
la Recherche Médicale
Créteil, France

## I. Introduction

Malignant mesothelioma (MM) is a tumor of the pleura and peritoneum that has a poor prognosis; the classic treatments, such as surgery, chemotherapy, and radiotherapy, are considered to have little or no effect (1–3). To improve survival of this incurable malignancy, fundamental and clinical studies are being carried out to develop new therapeutic strategies, based on immunotherapy and gene therapy.

## II. Rationale for Immunotherapy of Mesothelioma

There is now substantial convergent scientific data suggesting that human malignant mesothelioma could respond to different immunotherapeutic approaches.

### A. Immune Cell Imbalances Associated with Asbestos Exposure in Human Pleural Mesothelioma

A solid link has been demonstrated between asbestos exposure and subsequent development of several types of malignancies, mainly lung carcinoma and MM (4). Although the pathogenesis of MM is not totally understood, impairment of the host immune system by inhalation of asbestos fibers is now thought to be a major concern. Indeed, several studies suggest that depression of cellular immune defenses represents a marked increased risk for developing asbestos-related respiratory malignancies, either lung cancer or mesothelioma.

There are data obtained in a certain number of asbestos workers showing that the most usual immunological imbalance associated with asbestos exposure was a decrease of CD8 cells in the blood associated with a redistribution of T-helper/inducer CD4 cells from the blood to the lung resulting in enhanced CD4/CD8 ratio in bronchoalveolar lavage (BAL). These results suggested an immune imbalance favoring the T-helper-inducer function, as opposed to the T-cytotoxic–suppressor activity, in subjects with asbestos exposure, with or without asbestosis as well as pleural plaques.

The suppressive effect of asbestos fibers on natural killer (NK) cells' activity has been demonstrated in vivo as well as in vitro. Several studies have shown inconsistent alterations in NK-cell numbers, proportions, and activities in the peripheral blood of asbestos-exposed persons (5,9–15). In most of these studies, NK cells were identified by the CD16 (Leu-11a) antibody. However, the human NK cells possess another antigen, CD57 (Leu-7), defining a subset of NK cells. Recently, Al Jarad et al. (15), studying these two antigens, have shown a reduction of the absolute number and proportion of the circulating CD16-positive lymphocytes in subjects exposed to asbestos compared with a control group, whereas the CD57 did not differ between either group. This result is consistent with the hypothesis that asbestos fibers suppress NK-cell activity.

The suppressive effect of asbestos on NK-cells' activity has been confirmed in vitro, suggesting that the down-regulation was dependent on a direct contact of NK cells with fibers (16,17).

For mesothelioma, a few clues indicate that there are immune changes in such patients, possibly related to a reduction of the anticancer defenses. As in most solid tumors in humans, a biopsy of MM tumor usually shows an infiltration of the stroma, with a variable number of mononuclear immune cells (particularly monocytes and lymphocytes). However, we do not know if a more favorable prognosis of some malignant mesotheliomas might be related to the magnitude of infiltrating cells in the tumor [either tumor-infiltrating lymphocytes (TIL) or monocytes–macrophages]. On the other hand, it is questioned whether this local immune surveillance might explain why metastasis at a distance from the thorax happens rather rarely and late in this malignancy.

Immune cells in malignant pleural effusions are of great interest because they may contain a biologically significant antitumor effector cell population of particular immunological interest. Lymphocytosis is a usual cytological characteristic in pleural MM, corresponding mainly to T lymphocytes with a preponderant intrapleural influx of CD4 (Leu-3 +), resulting in a high CD4/CD8 ratio compared with blood (18–20). However, Hoogsteden et al. (20), when evaluating the leukocytes in pleural fluid of 20 patients with pleural MM, found no correlation between the CD4/CD8 ratio and survival time. Moreover, the average percentage of monocytes-macrophages are increased (about 30% for the mean) in pleural exudate, suggesting an influx of monocytic cells (18). These modifications are not specific for primary MM, as they are observed in other malignant exudative pleurisies. However, the relative increase of monocytes–macrophages in malignant pleural effusions may play an important immune role, contributing to antigen presentation to T lymphocytes and producing interleukin-2 (IL-2) capable of up-regulating the induction of lymphokine-activated killer (LAK) cells (21). The percentages of B lymphocytes in pleural fluid were rather small (0–26%) (18,20), suggesting that the local production of antitumor antibodies should be limited in MM.

More information concerning intraserosal cytokines is needed. In a study now in progress in collaboration with Dr. Emilie, we found a dramatic increase of interleukin-6 (IL-6) levels in pleural effusion associated with MM. This has also been observed by Yokoyama et al. (21) in nonmalignant pleural exudates, as well as in metastatic malignant effusions, with a significant correlation with peripheral blood platelet counts. It will be of great interest to determine the significance of such an increase of IL-6 in MM and to explore the cellular and humoral immunological changes that occur during intrapleural therapeutic trials using various recombinant human cytokines [IL-2, interferons (IFNs), tumor necrosis factor (TNF); see further].

In pleural effusions, it has been shown that lysis of malignant cells is mediated mainly by NK cells and by LAK cells. Thus, high LAK activity can be generated in cells of pleural effusions in vitro as well as in vivo, and pleural macrophages in the pleural effusion up-regulate the induction of LAK activity by IL-2 (22,23).

### B. Arguments in Favor of Immunotherapy in Cancer

Various immune effectors have been identified with a potential to kill tumor cells or inhibit their growth. This can be mediated by different cells, such as cytotoxic T cells (CTL) (24), NK cells (25,26), LAK cells (27), and macrophages. The other option is the intervention of cytokines that work either by interaction with immune cells (such as IL-2-activated LAK) or directly, such as TNF-$\alpha$ and IFN-$\gamma$ (28).

The sensitivity of mesothelioma cells of individual patients to various biotherapies has been tested on human mesothelioma cell lines (HMCL) developed in several laboratories (30,31). The HMCL represent a useful tool for assessing the direct toxic effects of cytokines, allowing one to correlate the in vitro responses to drugs with cell phenotypes (cell morphology, immunocytochemistry, electron microscopy). About a third of HMCL are prone to lysis by recombinant human (rHu)-IFN-γ (32,33). They are also sensitive to rHu-IFN-α, but to a smaller degree (32,34). In contrast, they did not respond to rHu-TNF-α, but this cytokine potentiated the cytotoxic effect of IFNs (32,34). The HMCL express the IFN-γ receptor, but without any correlation with their in vitro response to rHu-IFN-γ (35). Thus, from the same patient it is possible to obtain several cell lines, which may have different in vitro responses to different recombinant cytokines, given alone or in association. These data might explain why some patients are resistant to treatment, even when their cell lines appear sensitive in vitro to rHu-IFN-γ (35).

On the other hand, fresh and cultured human malignant mesothelioma cells have been insensitive in vitro to NK cells, whereas they were susceptible to LAK cells (36). Moreover, the HMCL are very useful for studying the intracellular penetrability of any gene vectors that might be used for gene transfer (see Sec. IV).

### C. Advantages of Local Immunotherapy in Intracavitary Tumors

Immunotherapy by intrapleural or intraperitoneal inoculation of recombinant cytokines (rHu-IFNs, rHu-IL-2) has several advantages. First, it allows higher local concentrations of the drug in direct contact with the tumor cells, as well as with the local immune effector cells [cytotoxic T lymphocytes (CTL) and macrophages]. Second, it generates less systemic diffusion of the recombinant cytokines, thereby decreasing the risk of general adverse effects and avoiding the disadvantage of activating large numbers of irrelevant T cells, NK cells, monocytes, and macrophages. The benefit of the direct intracavitary inoculation of recombinant cytokines has been demonstrated in pleural mesothelioma for rHu-IFN-γ (37,38) as well as for the highly toxic rHu-IL-2 (39). The same advantage has been previously reported in the context of local immunotherapy with rHu-IL-2 for ovarian cancer disseminated to the peritoneum (40) and, more recently, by using rHu-IFN-γ (41). The same route might be used, on one hand, for immune gene therapy by inoculating intraserosally LAK/TIL cells or monocytes–macrophages, carrying cytokine gene vectors or, on the other hand, a viral vector prone to directly infect the intraserosal tumor cells themselves, with local expression of the transferred cytokine gene. This approach is more attractive because it suppresses the systemic toxicity of recombinant cytokines, as will be discussed later on (see Sec. IV).

## III. Clinical Trials Using Immunotherapy in Pleural Malignant Mesothelioma

### A. Protocols Using Recombinant Human Cytokines

Because of the disappointing results obtained with classic treatments, several clinical groups, taking into account the aforementioned clues in favor of immunotherapy, have recently performed phase I and II trials in pleural MM by using recombinant human cytokines. The recombinant cytokines were administered either by the systemic or intraserosal routes.

Recombinant interferons have been tested in several phase I and II trials. Preliminary clinical reports suggest that systemic interferon alpha produced antitumoral activity, with an average objective response (OR) of about 15% (32,42,43).

Interferon gamma has been used in three phase II trials for malignant mesothelioma. The trials involve European and multicenter studies, with the objective of testing the efficacy and tolerance to local injections of human recombinant interferon gamma (rHu-IFN-$\gamma$) in mesothelioma. The protocol was as follows: the pretherapeutic staging consisted of a thoracic computed tomography (CT) scan and a thoracoscopic examination with biopsies; a pleural catheter was then implanted. The treatment consisted of endocavity injections of rHu-IFN$\gamma$ twice a week during 8 weeks. Fifteen days after the last injection, a thoracic CT scan was again performed; in the absence of progression, a new thoracoscopy with biopsies was carried out. Patients with proved stage I–III mesothelioma, according to Butchard's modified classification (37), were included. Two phase II studies were performed at a dosage of 40 million units of rHu-IFN-$\gamma$ per injection twice a week during 2 months. The first study was a pilot study (37), the second was an extended trial with 17 participating centers in Europe (38). The data of these two trials were pooled, and the results for the 96 eligible patients are reported. Sixty percent of the patients had a stage IIa disease and 20% stage I disease. The histological type was epithelial in 80% of the patients, corresponding to tumor localized only to parietal or to visceral pleura (IA), or with a double localization to both parietal and visceral pleura (IIB). A more rare response was observed in patients with extension to the mediastinal pleura (stage IIA). The global objective response (OR) rate was 19.3%, with 8% a complete response (CR), which means normal pleura at the second thoracoscopic examination and no tumor cells in the biopsy samples. Patients with stage IA had a response rate of 58% and a median survival of 36 months, whereas the median survival of the entire population was 11 months. Fever occurred in 83% of patients, but grade 3–4 adverse events were observed in only 23% of the cases (fever in 17 patients and infection in 6 patients). Biologically severe adverse events were neutropenia (4%) and an increase in hepatic enzymes (6%).

Thus, we can conclude that IFN-γ showed a clear efficacy in malignant mesothelioma, with a global response rate of about 20%, which compares favorably with the best drug tested. It was noticeable that complete responses were observed and that the response rate was particularly encouraging in stage IA patients.

A more recent study (Feb. 1991–Nov. 1992), tested IFN-γ at a dose of 60 million units per injection. Inclusion and exclusion criteria were the same as previously detailed, and 51 patients were eligible. Preliminary results indicate that this higher dosage had no advantage in terms of efficacy and toxicity.

### B.  Protocols Combining Immunotherapy with Chemotherapy

Although MM is considered a chemoresistant tumor, unresponsive to most single cytotoxic agents, cisplatin has shown marginal activity (less than 15% of response rate) (44); weekly high-dose cisplatin (CDDP) may increase the response rate with four OR in nine patients treated by six weekly courses of 80 mg/m$^2$ of cisplatin (45).

There is substantial experimental evidence (in human malignant mesothelioma cell lines or nude mice xenografts) suggesting a synergy between cytotoxic drugs and IFN-α (34,46). On the other hand, clinical trials in other tumors have shown a potentiation of cisplatin by interferon alfa (47,48). These data encouraged three of us to undertake a clinical trial combining rHu-IFN-α and cisplatin. Weekly CDDP delivery provides a basis for optimal dose intensity and durable interaction in a combined CDDP–IFN-α program. Therefore, we began a phase I–II study, designed to assess the clinical and biological tolerance for this combination, as well as its antitumoral activity (49). Twenty-three previously untreated patients with an evolving disease were treated with this combination. The weekly schedule of administration was 60 mg/m$^2$ of CDDP systemically combined with $3 \times 10^6$ units of rHu-IFN-α subcutaneously administered at day 0, 1, 2, and 3 ($12 \times 10^6$ units/week). One cycle was 5 weeks, followed by a rest period of 4 weeks. The treatment was planned for five cycles with two 5-weekly courses, one 4-weekly course, and two 3-weekly courses, for a maximum of 20 weeks of treatment and an optimal dose of 1200 mg/m$^2$ of CDDP. According to clinical tolerance, the initial schedule was shortened after the first ten patients (two 4-week courses and two 3-week courses). Twenty-one patients are now evaluable for toxicity evaluation (41 cycles), the median cumulative dose of CDDP was 480 mg/m$^2$ (240–1200) and the median dose intensity was 31 mg/m$^2$ per week. The major secondary effect with the initial dose was a progressive deterioration of the general status, with a median weight loss of 7.5%. The shortening of our initial program provided better acceptance and tolerance. Renal, neurological, and hematological toxicities were rare and cumulative. The responses were eight OR, three stable disease, and ten progressive disease. The duration of response was short. This 37% rate of OR is encouraging, supporting the concept of an interaction between both drugs. This needs additional trials with a higher dosage of IFN-α2a to confirm these preliminary data.

### C. Protocols Using Interleukin-2 Lymphokine-Activated Killer Cells

Biotherapy consisting of the reinjection of autologous peripheral blood T lymphocytes, stimulated in vitro by IL-2 to become lymphokine-activated killer (LAK) cells, was the first tentative trial for a more physiological approach to immunotherapy (50,51). Clinical trials based on this concept allowed Rosenberg et al. (52,53) and West et al. (54) to obtain significant clinical effects by the reinjection of these LAK cells into patients with either renal cancer or melanoma. For mesothelioma, Yanagawa et al. (55) have adapted this strategy in two cases of mesothelioma, injecting LAK cells into the pleural cavity, combined with daily systemic injection of IL-2. Although these two cases are isolated, the authors concluded from this treatment that local adoptive immunotherapy, which resulted in reduction of pleural effusion and a decline of hyaluronic acid in the effusions of one patient, could be useful for malignant effusion caused by mesothelioma. On the other hand, Ottow et al. (56), in a murine model of intraperitoneal cancer, observed that LAK cells plus exogenous rHu-IL-2 resulted in a greater reduction in tumor burden than the systemic administration.

Recent studies in several laboratories have investigated the antitumor efficiency of reinjecting patients with their own tumor infiltrating lymphocytes (TIL) after in vitro activation by rHu-IL-2 (57–60). From these studies, it appeared that there was a better antitumor efficiency of rIL-2-expanded TIL in comparison with LAK-IL-2 in different types of human malignancies (61,62). These results suggest that IL-2 should be more efficient and have less toxicity if its effect is mediated by local immune cells.

When studying cells of pleural or ascitic fluids obtained from 13 patients with ovarian or metastatic breast cancer, Blanchard et al. (63) have shown that the effusion-associated lymphocytes (EAL) were readily activated by rHu-IL-2 in medium containing autologous effusion fluid, suggesting that in situ increase of tumoricidal activity can occur by locally injecting rHu-IL-2 or other immune cell-activating cytokines, such as interferons. Human mesothelioma tumors usually contain a large proportion of infiltrating lymphocytes that are amenable to local stimulation by IL-2 or by other cytokines. Such a protocol, employing autologous LAK cells plus intrapleural rHu-IL-2, combined with indomethacin, has been carried out in patients with mesothelioma; but the trial had to be stopped because of major local and systemic side effects (64). These results somewhat contradict those reported by Astoul et al. (39) after intrapleural injections of rHu-IL-2 alone.

## IV. Gene Therapy in Mesothelioma

Severe systemic toxicities associated with the use of high doses of rHu-IL-2 alone, or with LAK or TIL cells plus rHu-IL-2 or other cytokines (rHu-TNF-α) are responsible for difficult general conditions that limit reaching effective doses at the tumor site for treatment of various cancers in humans. The ideal would be a continuous delivery of an adequate cytokine(s) dose, in close contact with malignant cells, with a minimal release to other tissues and cells through the general circulation, thereby avoiding systemic toxicity. These limitations have stimulated several laboratories to explore other hypotheses and to develop more advanced biological and molecular manipulations. Gene therapy of cancer has become a reality, and several modalities of this alternative approach can now be envisioned (65–67). We will focus mainly on those modalities that can be applied to mesothelioma.

### A. Candidate Genes for Gene Therapy in Cancer

There are so many genes that can be candidates for gene therapy for cancer that the choice now appears difficult.

An efficient approach could be to transfer into cancer cells genes encoding enzymes able to convert a nontoxic prodrug into an active tumoricidal drug. This has been done experimentally for the treatment of brain tumors, by Culver et al. (68), who introduced the thymidine kinase gene from a herpes virus into brain tumor cells to render them more sensitive to the herpes virus drug, ganciclovir. The other possibilities are to introduce into cancer cells drug-resistance genes or genes able to modify the antigenic recognition of human tumor cells by the cytotoxic T lymphocytes (CTL).

Nowadays, we have acquired a better understanding of the mechanisms involved in the recognition of cell surface antigens by CTL. The specific T-cell receptor of CTL binds to a complex that comprises a class I major histocompatibility molecule (MHC class I) plus a small tumor-specific antigen peptide. Thus, this observation implies the presence of MHC class I molecules at the surface of the target tumor cells. In mesothelioma, most HMCL express histocompatibility locus antigen (HLA) class I and II molecules (69,70).

Besides the direct contact of the killer T-cell receptors with the MHC class I–antigenic peptide, a costimulation occurs through the B7 receptor that is present only at the surface of the "professional" antigen-presenting cells (APC), such as macrophages and dendritic cells (71). This B7 receptor interacts as a second signal with the CD28 molecule of CTL. As tumor cells do not usually carry the B7 antigen on their surface, they escape destruction by immune cells. Given this concept, a new strategy, which consists of introducing the *B7* gene into cancer cells in a mouse model of melanoma, has been recently published. Chen et al. (72) have shown that all of the mice with melanoma that were treated by transduction of *B7* gene, along with a gene of a viral antigen, into the tumor lived longer than untreated controls: 40% survived the experiment and were tumor-free. Townsend and Allison (73) obtained the same regression of tumor cells injected into animals by transfecting the *B7* gene into melanoma cell lines, but without cotransfection of a viral gene. These results indicate that transfecting only the *B7* gene is sufficient to provide antitumor activity. They also demonstrated that a first injection into mice of B7-positive melanoma cells worked like a kind of vaccine, which protected 89% of the mice for more than 3 months. From these experiments, it can be deduced that an autocrine production of IL-2 was induced by the contact of the two surface antigens of tumor cells (MHC classes I and B7) with the two receptors of CD8 cells, thereby stimulating CTL to multiply. Thus, this model of gene therapy in experimentally induced mice tumors demonstrates that a bifocal stimulation of CD8 T cells is capable of bypassing the exogenous help of CD4 + cell-derived lymphokines usually necessary to initiate the multiplication of activated killer cells. This stimulating new strategy for cancer treatment, favorably commented on in *Science* by J. Travis (74), seems to be promising. However, we must be cautious because we do not know if this costimulatory strategy will be effective for treating naturally occurring cancers in humans.

Other candidate tumor genes could be those encoding specific peptidic antigens, such as the new family of *MAGE* genes, recently identified in a melanoma cell line as well as in other cancer cell lines (75). However, the usual great heterogeneity of human tumors from one patient to another and from one tumor cell clone to another (as clearly demonstrated in mesothelioma for the in vitro response to IFN-γ) precludes transfer of specific tumor antigen genes, even if they are effective in vitro on cell lines. This is also true for tumor suppressor genes. Indeed, the cancer cells that do not have the specific tumor gene should escape destruction, thereby facilitating a clonal selection of cells responsible for the worst tumor progression.

Another approach to genetic immunomodulation is vaccine development. Thus, the potential immunogenicity of mesothelioma has been recently investigated by Manning et al. (76) by immunization of BALB/c mice with irradiated cells from two MM cell lines of the same strain. Immunization of mice with one of the cell lines significantly reduced the rate of tumor development when challenged with a tumorigenic dose of these cell lines. By contrast, there was no protection in another strain of syngeneic CBA mice. However, in humans, genetic vaccination is not easily feasible, because of the polyclonality of antigens and because we do not know the candidate gene(s) for the development of such vaccines.

### B. Transgenic Immunotherapy Based on the Transfer of Cytokine Genes

Many of the current prospects for gene therapy involve the use of gene vectors encoding cytokines, for a specific, direct in vivo transfection to tumor tissues or cells. It is thought that this approach will be efficient because of the promising responses obtained after the intrapleural injection of rHu-IFN-$\gamma$ or rHu-IL-2 in human MM. Thus, the genes of different recombinant cytokines, such as rHu-IL-2, rHu-IFN-$\gamma$, rHu-TNF-$\alpha$, as well as rHu-IL-4 (77,78), can be candidates for gene therapy. The expressed cytokines work either by a direct cytotoxic effect on tumor cells, as demonstrated in vitro on cell lines of human mesothelioma (79), or indirectly by enhancing the local antitumor immune responses (80). This method of cytokine delivery would be more physiological than the systemic or intraserosal route. Indeed, the cells transfected with a gene are capable of expressing the corresponding cytokine in the microenvironment of the tumor. Such a procedure would probably limit the side effects that are usually attendant with the systemic excess of the most toxic human recombinant cytokines, such as IL-2 or TNF-$\alpha$.

Such a project first requires identification of the human recombinant cytokine(s)' cDNA, which is necessary for transfer, to promote an efficient immunotherapy of mesothelioma.

The cytokine rHu-TNF-$\alpha$, which has a potent cytolytic and immunomodulatory action in carcinoma, might be a good candidate for gene therapy. Actually, Hand et al. (34) did not show any significant direct in vitro cytotoxic effect of rHu-TNF-$\alpha$ on HMCL. Moreover, the toxicity of TNF-$\alpha$ should make one extremely cautious in using this gene for gene therapy of MM in humans.

### C. What Vectors and What Cell Manipulations Can Be Used for Transgenic Immunotherapy?

There are several systems that have been explored for gene transfection of cytokine(s). So far, by comparison with liposomes or derived systems, it seems that virus vectors (retrovirus, adenoassociated virus, bovine papillomavirus, adenovirus) are the most efficient for gene transduction because of their potential to easily infect tumor cells and possibly also any associated immune cells (CTL or monocytes–macrophages) (65–67).

Several authors are using retrovirus for transfecting foreign genes (80,81). Rosenberg's group at the National Cancer Institute have been allowed to start a protocol of immune gene therapy in patients with advanced melanoma by reinjecting the patients with their own TIL that have been previously modified in vitro by transduction of the TNF-$\alpha$ gene with a retrovirus vector (81). Apparently, the retrovirus, although having integrated the gene in its genome, does not produce a sufficient amount of rHu-TNF-$\alpha$, as stressed in the criticisms of the NCI's Division of Cancer Treatment Board of scientific advisers (82). Elsewhere, doubt was expressed concerning the homing of the TILs back into the tumor tissue, as TIL are capable of ending up in the liver, where TNF-$\alpha$ might create severe cellular toxicity. Moreover, there is the inherent risk of the retrovirus activating other genes, with potential carcinogenesis. Adenoassociated virus, which is a parvovirus, has also been proposed as a vector. As it also integrates the genome of target cells, it has the same disadvantages as the retrovirus.

Currently, an adenovirus seems the most efficient viral vector. In France, a replication-deficient recombinant adenovirus-5 (Ad-5) has been developed, by Perricaudet et al. (83,84), which appeared to be an efficient vector for in vivo expression of various genes (85–87).

We are presently developing a project of gene therapy for mesothelioma that is based on the intrapleural or intraperitoneal inoculation of this viral vector expressing rHu-cytokine gene, namely IFN-$\gamma$. When used in vivo, the recombinant Ad-5 bearing the cDNA of IFN-$\gamma$ will be able to induce the expression of the foreign gene locally in the serosal cavity into the infected cells, either the tumor cells or the monocyte–macrophage-associated cells. Thus, the cytokine will work in a more physiological way, avoiding the systemic deleterious effects of toxic rHu-cytokines, such as IL-2. Preliminary experiments carried out in our laboratories in vitro on HMCL as well as in vivo on nude mice and monkeys have given promising results, indicating a feasibility in humans (in preparation).

## V. Conclusion

Nowadays, the treatment of cancer is mainly based on killing a maximum number of cancer cells. During the last decade, new strategies of immunotherapy (LAK or TIL cells plus IL-2 or different recombinant cytokines, such as IL-2, IFN-$\gamma$, or -$\alpha$, TNF, or others) have been developed to improve the survival from cancers, particularly those resistant to chemotherapy. In mesothelioma, some OR have been recently observed with three recombinant human cytokines: namely, rHu-INF-γ, rHu-IFN-α, and rHu-IL-2, administered either intrapleurally or by the systemic route, sometimes in association with chemotherapy. But as yet the design of such protocols is decided more as a lottery than on the basis of solid background scientific justification. Actually, we need to better understand how these drugs work at the cellular and molecular levels. Transgenic immunotherapy seems to be a rational way to acquire this knowledge and possibly to develop new therapeutic protocols for humans, with the hope of improving the prognosis of diffuse malignant mesothelioma and probably also of metastatic tumors of the pleura and peritoneum. Theoretically, the ideal aim of gene therapy would be an attempt to achieve a normal, or at least an inoffensive, phenotype for cancer cells. The transfer of cytokine genes proceeds by two mechanisms to obtain direct cell toxicity and to achieve the recovery of normal immune control against foreign antigens such as those of cancer cells. However, it will probably require some time before these different approaches will be successful.

## References

1. Schemin RJ. In: Antman K, Aisner J, eds. Asbestos-related malignancy. New York: Grune & Stratton, 1987:332.
2. Alberts A, Falkson G, Goedhals L, Vorobiof DA. J Clin Oncol 1988; 6:527.
3. Ruffié P, Feld R, Minkin S, Cormier Y, Boutan-Loroze A, Ginsberg R, Ayoub J, Shepherb FA, Evans WK, Figueredo A, Pater JL, Pringle JF, Kreisman H. J Clin Oncol 1989; 7:1157.
4. Bignon J, Brochard P, De Cremoux H, Nebut M, Jaurand MC. In: Deslauriers J, Lacquet LK, eds. International trends in general thoracic surgery. Delarue NC, Eschapasse. Thoracic surgery: surgical management of pleural diseases. Toronto: CV Mosby, 1990:327.
5. Tsang PH, Chu FN, Fischbein A, Bekesi JG. Clin Immunol Immunopathol 1988; 47:323.
6. Gellert AR, Langford JA, Winter RJD, Untayakumar S, Sinha G, Rudd RM. Thorax 1985; 40:508.
7. Wallace JM, Oishi JS, Barbers RG, Batra P, Aberle DR. Am Rev Respir Dis 1989; 139:33.
8. Sprince NL, Oliver LC, McLoud TC, Eisen EA, Christiani DC, Ginns LC. Am Rev Respir Dis 1991; 143:822.
9. Kubota M, Kagaminmari S, Yokoyama K, Okada A. Br J Ind Med 1985; 42:276.
10. Ginns LC, Ryu JH, Rogol PR, Prine NL, Oliver LC, Larsson CD. Am Rev Respir Dis 1985; 131:831.

11. Lew F, Tsang P, Holland JF, Warner N, Selikoff IJ, Bekesi JG. J Clin Immunol 1986; 6:225.
12. Yoneda T, Kitamura H, Nikami R, Yokoyama K. Eur J Respir Dis 1986; 68: 64.
13. De Shazo RD, Morgan J, Bozelka B, Chapman Y. Chest 1988; 94:482.
14. Robinson BWS. Am Rev Respir Dis 1989; 139:897.
15. Al Jarad N, Macey M, Uthayakumar S, Newland AC, Rudd RM. Br J Ind Med 1992; 49:811.
16. Manning LS, Bowman RV, Davis MR, Musk A, Robinson BWS. Clin Immunol Immunother 1989; 53:68.
17. Manning LS, Davis MR, Robinson BWS. Clin Exp Immunol 1991; 83:85.
18. Guzman J, Bross KJ, Würtemberger G, Costabel P. Chest 1989; 93:590.
19. Kabbani-Lazreq A, Poron F, Defouilloy C, Vojtek AM, Bignon J, Fleury-Feith J. Eur Respir Rev 1993; 3:216.
20. Hoogsteden HC, Versnel MA, Hop W, Van der Kwast THH, Hilvering C. Eur Respir Rev 1993; 3:30.
21. Yokohama A, Maruyama M, Ito M, Khono N, Hiwada K, Yano S. Chest 1992; 102:155.
22. Yanakawa H, Sone S, Nii A, Fukuta K, Nakanishi M, Maeda K, Honda M, Ogura T. Jpn J Cancer Res 1989; 80:1220.
23. Okubo Y, Nakata M, Kuroiwa Y, Wada S, Kusama S. Chest 1987; 92:500.
24. Khavari P. J Biol Med 1987; 60:409.
25. Oldham RK. Cancer Metastasis Rev 1983; 2:323.
26. Herberman RB. Concepts Immunopathol 1985; 1:96.
27. Rosenbergs A. Immunol Today 1988; 9:58.
28. Old LJ. Cancer Res 1981; 41:361.
29. Gerwin BI, Lechner JF, Redder RR. Cancer Res 1987; 47:6180.
30. Manning LS, Whitaker D, Murch AR, Garlepp MJ, Davis MR, Musk AW, Robinson BWS. Int J Cancer 1990; 47:285.
31. Jaurand MC, Buard A, Zeng L. Eur Respir Rev 1993; 3:126.
32. Bowman RV, Manning LS, Davis MR, Robinson BWS. Cancer Chemother Pharmacol 1991; 28:420.
33. Zeng L, Monnet I, Brochard P, Bignon J, Jaurand MC. J Interferon Res 1991; 11:5111.
34. Hand AM, Husgafvel-Pursiainen K, Tammilehto L, Mattson K, Linnainmaa K. Cancer Lett 1991; 58:205.
35. Jaurand MC, et al. (in preparation).
36. Manning LS, Bowman RV, Darby SB, Robinson BWS. Am Rev Respir Dis 1989; 139:1369.
37. Boutin C, Viallat JR, Van Zandwijk N, Douillard JT. Cancer 1991; 67:2033.
38. Boutin C, Bignon J, Coetmer D, Douillard Y. Am Rev Respir Dis 1992; 145: A511.
39. Astoul P, Viallat JR, Laurent JC, Brandely M, Boutin C. Chest 1993; 103: 209.
40. Lotze M, Custer M, Rosenberg SA. Arch Surg 1986; 121:1373.

41. Pujade-Lauraine E, Guastella JP, Colombo N, François E. Bull Cancer 1993; 80:163.
42. Robinson BWS, Bowman RV, Christmans TT. Lung Cancer 1991; 7:172.
43. Ardizzoni A, Rosso R, Salvati F. Lung Cancer 1991; 7:171 [abstr].
44. Zidar BL, Green S, Pierce HI. Invest New Drugs 1988; 6:223.
45. Plating A, Goey H, Verweij J. Proc AACR 1991; 32 [abstr].
46. Sklarin NT, Chahinian AP, Flever L. Cancer Res 1988; 48:64.
47. Wadler S, Schwartz EL. Cancer Res 1990; 50:3473.
48. Margolin KA, Diroshow JH, Akman SA. J Clin Oncol 1992; 10:1574.
49. Soulié P, Ruffié P, Transdafir L. Ann Oncol 1992; 3(suppl 5):[abstr].
50. Taniguchi T, Matsui H, Fujita T, Takaoka C, Kashima N, Yoshimoto R, Hamuro J. Nature 1983; 302:305.
51. Ottow RT, Steller EP, Sugarbaker PH, Wesley RA, Rosenberg SA. Cell Immunol 1987; 104:366.
52. Rosenberg SA, Lotze MT, Muul LM. N Engl J Med 1985; 313:1485.
53. Rosenberg SA, Lotze MT, Muul LM. N Engl J Med 1987; 316:889.
54. West WH, Tauer KW, Yanelli JR, Marshall GD, Orr DW, Thurman GB, Oldham RK. N Engl J Med 1987; 316:898.
55. Yanagawa H, Sone S, Fukuta K. Jpn J Clin Oncol 1991; 21:377.
56. Ottow RT, Steller EP, Sugarbaker PH. Cell Immunol 1987; 104:
57. Itoh K, Tilden AB, Balch CM. Cancer Res 1986; 46:3011.
58. Kradin RL, Boyle LA, Preffer FI. Cancer Immunol Immunother 1987; 24:76.
59. Muul LM, Spiess P, Director E. J Immunol 1987; 138:989.
60. Belldegrun A, Muul LM, Rosenberg SA. Cancer Res 1988; 48:206.
61. Itoh K, Platsoucas CD, Balch CM. J Exp Med 1988; 168:1419.
62. Rosenberg SA, Packard BS, Aebersold PM. N Engl J Med 1988; 319:1676.
63. Blanchard DK, Kavanach JJ, Sinkovics JG. Cancer Res 1988; 48:6321.
64. Manning LS, Davis MR, Robinson BWS. Clin Immunol Immunopathol 1989; 53:68.
65. Rosenberg SA. Cancer Res 1991; 51:5074s.
66. Gutierrez AA, Lemoine NR, Sikora K. Lancet 1992; 339:715.
67. Russell SJ. Cancer J 1993; 6:21.
68. Culver KW, Ram Z, Ishii H, Olfield EH, Blaise RM. Science 1992; 256:1550.
69. Christmas TI, Manning LS, Davis MR, Robinson BWS, Garlepp MJ. Am J Respir Cell Mol Biol 1991; 5:213.
70. Jaurand MC et al. (in preparation).
71. Holt PG. Eur Respir J 1993; 6:120.
72. Chen L, Ashe S, Brady WA. Cell 1992; 71:1093.
73. Townsend SE, Allison JP. Science 1993; 259:368.
74. Travis J. Science 1993; 259:310.
75. van der Bruggen P, Traversari C, Chomez P, Lurquin C, De Plaen E, van den Eynde B, Knuth A, Boon T. Science 1991; 254:1643.
76. Manning LS, Davis MR, Bielefeldt-Ohmann H. Eur Respir Rev 1993; 3:234.
77. Tepper R, Pattengale PK, Leder P. Cell 1989; 57:503.
78. Golumbek PT, Lazenby AJ, Levitsky HI. Science 1991 (1 Nov).

79. Zeng L, Buard A, Monnet I. (in press).
80. Gansbacher B, Bannerji R, Daniels B, Zier K, Cronin K, Gilboa E. Cancer Res 1990; 50:7820.
81. Rosenberg SA, Aebersold P, Cornetta K. N Engl J Med 1990; 323:570.
82. Anderson C. Science 1993; 259:1391.
83. Gilardi P, Courtney M, Pavirani A, Perricaudet M. FEBS Lett 1990; 267:60.
84. Stratford-Perricaudet LD, Levrero M, Chasse JF, Perricaudet M, Briand P. Hum Gene Ther 1990; 1:241.
85. Rosenfeld MA, Siegfried W, Yoshimura K, Yoneyama K, Fukayama M, Stier LE, Paakko PK, Gilardi P, Stratford-Perricaudet LD, Perricaudet M. Science 1991; 252:431.
86. Rosenfeld MA, Yoshimura K, Trapnell BC, Yoneyama K, Rosenthal ER, Dalemans W, Fukayama M, Bargon J, Stier LE, Stratford-Perricaudet L, Perricaudet M. Cell 1992; 68:143.
87. Le Gal La Salle G, Robert JJ, Berrard S, Ridoux V, Stratford-Perricaudet LD, Perricaudet M, Mallet J. Science 1993; 259:988.

# AUTHOR INDEX

*Italic numbers give the page on which the complete reference is listed.*

# SUBJECT INDEX

## A

Asbestos bodies, 3, 4, 82
Asbestos fibers,
  animal exposure, 14, 194, 199, 232
  building exposure, 20, 21
  cellular effects,
    active oxygen species, 81, 85, 215,
      216, 233, 235
    chromosome damage, 215, 224,
      248
    cytokine production, 87, 228, 233,
      234, 255
    DNA damage, 86, 216
    fiber dimensions and, 81, 224,
      231
    growth factor production, 233,
      234
    mutations, 86
    phagocytosis, 81, 85, 87
    radical production (*see* active
      oxygen species)
  exposure-response relationship, 22
  exposure levels, 23, 24
  immune system, 254
Asbestosis, 2, 10, 20

## C

Computed tomography, 2, 72, 271,
  301
Cytochrome P450, 49, 216

## F

Fiber burden,
  fiber size, 7, 43, 53
  fiber type, 8, 43
  lung, 6, 7
  pleura, 6, 7, 9
Fiber durability, 201

## L

Lung cancer, 4, 62
  smoking, 3, 4, 48

## M

Mesothelial cell,
  cellular interactions, 231, 233
  cytokine production, 226, 227
  established cell lines,
    culture, 173
    cytogenetics, 86, 178
    cytokine production, 181, 213, 229,
      260
    cytokine susceptibility, 259, 300
    growth factor production, 90, 181,
      212, 228, 256, 260
    as immune effector cells, 257
    immunostaining, 177
    molecular changes, 86, 211
    morphology, 174

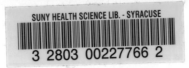
X